Instructor's Manual and Test Bank to accompany

POTTER • PERRY

CANADIAN FUNDAMENTALS OF NURSING

Second Edition

Patricia A. Castaldi, BSN, MSN
Associate Dean
Trinitas School of Nursing
Elizabeth, New Jersey
A Cooperative Program
  with Union County College
Cranford, New Jersey

CANADIAN EDITORS

Janet C. Ross-Kerr, RN, BScN, MS, PhD
Professor
Faculty of Nursing, University of Alberta
Edmonton, Alberta

Marilynn J. Wood, RN, BSN, MSN, DrPH
Professor
Faculty of Nursing, University of Alberta
Edmonton, Alberta

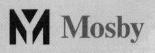

Mosby

A Harcourt Canada Health Sciences Company

Toronto Montreal Fort Worth New York Orlando
St. Louis Philadelphia London Sydney

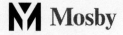 Mosby

Copyright © 2001 Harcourt Canada Ltd.

ISBN 0-9205-1342-5

Acquisitions Editor: Ann Millar
Developmental Editor: Liz Radojkovic
Production Editor: Laurie Thomas
Production Coordinator: Jon Pressick
Copy Editor: Susan Harrison
Permissions Editor: Cindy Howard
Cover Design: Kathi Gosche
Interior Design: Kathi Gosche
Typesetting and Assembly: Jansom
Printing and Binding: Maracle Press Limited

Harcourt Canada Ltd.
55 Horner Avenue, Toronto, ON, Canada M8Z 4X6
Customer Service
Toll-Free Tel.: 1-800-387-7278
Toll-Free Fax: 1-800-665-7307

Printed in Canada
1 2 3 4 5 05 04 03 02 01

INTRODUCTION

This Instructor's Manual and Test Bank to accompany the second edition of *Canadian Fundamentals of Nursing* has been developed to assist in the preparation of classroom, laboratory, and clinical educational activities for fundamentals of nursing courses. Although there are differences in curricula and teaching styles, this manual will assist in class preparation by highlighting chapter information, thus saving valuable time and effort.

This manual includes two sections. In Section I, suggestions for classroom discussions, interactive exercises, clinical skills, and client care experiences (clinical activities) are provided for each chapter in the text. Resources for student activities are available to reproduce and assign to students for use individually or in a group. Teaching strategies in the manual correspond with the emphasis of the content in the text. In addition, the critical thinking exercises from the text and respective answers are provided.

Section II of the manual is a revised test bank that includes over 700 questions and answers. The questions are keyed to the page in the text where the content is covered.

The primary intent of this Instructor's Manual and Test Bank is to be a quick reference and resource for you, the instructor, to use with your students. Your suggestions for future editions are welcomed.

CANADIAN CONTRIBUTORS

Debbie Fraser Askin, RNC, MN
Assistant Professor
Faculty of Nursing, University of Manitoba
Winnipeg, Manitoba

Barbara J. Astle, RN, BScN, MN
Nurse Educator, Faculty of Nursing
University of Calgary
Calgary, Alberta
Doctoral Student, Faculty of Nursing
University of Alberta
Edmonton, Alberta

Andrea Baumann, RN, BScN, MScN, PhD
Associate Dean Health Science (Nursing)
Professor and Director, School of Nursing
Faculty of Health Science, McMaster
    University
Hamilton, Ontario

L. Dawn Kapler, RN
Instructor
Health Careers, NorQuest College
Edmonton, Alberta

Kaysi Eastlick Kushner, RN, MN
Doctoral Candidate and Lecturer
Faculty of Nursing, University of Alberta
Edmonton, Alberta

Jeanne M. Molnar, RN, BN, MEd
Professor/Coordinator
Health and Life Sciences Sector
Algonquin College of Applied Arts and
    Technology
Nepean, Ontario

JoAnn Perry, BSN, MSN, PhD
Assistant Professor
School of Nursing, University of
    British Columbia
Vancouver, British Columbia

D. Shelley Raffin Bouchal, RN, BScN, MN,
    PhD (c)
Assistant Professor
Faculty of Nursing, University of Calgary
Calgary, Alberta

Joyce Relyea, RN, BScN, MPH
Public Health Nurse
Capital Health Authority
Edmonton, Alberta

Linda Reutter, RN, BScN, BA, MS (Nursing),
    PhD
Professor
Faculty of Nursing, University of Alberta
Edmonton, Alberta

Janet C. Ross-Kerr, RN, BScN, MS, PhD
Professor
Faculty of Nursing, University of Alberta
Edmonton, Alberta

Carla Shapiro, RN, BN, MN
Lecturer
Faculty of Nursing, University of Manitoba
Winnipeg, Manitoba

Darlene Steven, RN, MHSA, PhD
Professor
Lakehead University
Thunder Bay, Ontario

Continued

Canadian Contributors *(cont'd from previous page)*

Sandra C. Tenove, RN, BScN, MEd, PhD
Associate Professor
Faculty of Nursing, University of Calgary
Calgary, Alberta

Sally Thorne, RN, BSN, MSN, PhD
Professor
School of Nursing, University of
  British Columbia
Vancouver, British Columbia

Ardene Robinson Vollman, RN, BScN, MA,
  PhD
Associate Professor
Faculty of Nursing, University of Calgary
Adjunct Assistant Professor, Department of
  Community Health Sciences
Faculty of Medicine, University of Calgary
Calgary, Alberta

Marilynn J. Wood, RN, BSN, MSN, DrPH
Professor
Faculty of Nursing, University of Alberta
Edmonton, Alberta

•CONGRATULATIONS

You and your students now have access to the Canadian MERLIN Web site for
Canadian Fundamentals of Nursing, Second Edition

Here's how to get "connected" and what you'll find:

sign on at:

www.harcourtcanada.com/potter

what you will receive:

- "Faculty Focus" section offering information for nursing instructors
- Links to related products • Canadian author information
- Canadian content information • Details on related products ... and more

plus:

Canadian Fundamentals of Nursing Weblinks

An exciting new Canadian MERLIN Web site that gives you direct access to hundreds of nursing-related links specifically chosen to complement the content of this book, including many Canadian nursing sites.

Your passcode: CanadianPotter

MERLIN

Mosby

Mosby's **E**lectronic **R**esource **L**inks & **I**nformation **N**etwork

CONTENTS

Health and Wellness

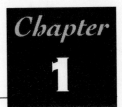

Chapter

1

CLASSROOM DISCUSSION

1. Compare and contrast several conceptualizations of health. Ask students to identify how adherence to these different conceptualizations would influence the scope and nature of nursing practice.

2. Discuss the factors that led to the emergence of each of the three approaches to health: medical, behavioural, and socioenvironmental. Have students provide examples of activities/programs/policies that exemplify each of these approaches in Canada today.

3. Ask students what challenges to Health for All were identified in the Epp Report. Discuss any progress that has been made in meeting these challenges.

4. Discuss the relationship between health promotion and illness prevention. Consider how a nursing practice would differ using a health promotion versus an illness prevention approach.

5. Select a health situation or problem. Have students analyze the determinants of this health problem using the population health promotion model. Then have students identify strategies of health promotion that could be used to address the problem, using the Ottawa Charter strategies.

6. Using the health situation selected above, discuss how the health promotion strategies identified could incorporate empowering elements (using Labonte's empowerment holosphere).

7. Discuss the role of participation within health-promoting nursing practice.

INTERACTIVE EXERCISES

1. Have students interview family and friends to ascertain their perceptions of what it means to be healthy. Students also can ascertain perceptions of what most influences their health. Then have students share their findings with others in the class. Discuss what may account for the similarities and differences in perceptions of health (e.g., age, gender, culture, education, and state of health). Discuss which determinants or prerequisites of health were identified by those interviewed.

2. Identify an article in a newspaper or magazine that addresses a health issue. As a class, analyze the article in terms of the approach to health (medical, behavioural, socioenvironmental) it represents. Consider also: What determinants of health are featured in the article? How would the article be written using another approach to health?

3. Obtain the business plan or annual report of a regional health authority or health department. Have students analyze the goals, objectives, and priorities in terms of the major health determinants. Students should consider which conceptualization of health and approach to health is reflected in the documents.

RESOURCE FOR STUDENT ACTIVITIES

Approaches to health chart

APPROACHES TO HEALTH CHART

	Medical	Behavioural	Socioenvironmental
Health Concept			
Determinants			
Strategies			
Target			

From Labonte R: *Health promotion and empowerment: Practice frameworks. Issues in Health Promotion Series #3*. Toronto, 1993, Centre for Health Promotion, University of Toronto, & ParticipACTION.

CRITICAL THINKING EXERCISES

1. How do you describe your current "health"? What criteria led to this judgement? Which definition of health discussed in this chapter best agrees with your understanding of health? Now, consider another definition of health discussed in this chapter. Would your judgement of your state of health change based on this definition?

2. What do you consider to be the three most important health problems facing Canadians today? What are the major determinants of these issues?

3. Using the three health problems you identified in the previous question, which health promotion strategies would you consider to be most appropriate?

4. You are a community health nurse working in an area where there are many low-income women who smoke. Using a socioenvironmental approach to health, what questions would you need to address to decrease smoking behaviour in your area? How would your approach differ if you were using a behavioural approach to health?

ANSWERS TO CRITICAL THINKING EXERCISES

1. Answers will vary, depending on what definitions are selected. Multidimensional definitions that incorporate both subjective and objective elements may lead to perceptions of being "less" healthy.

2. Answers will vary. Analyze problems and determinants given based on the three approaches to health. Are the determinants physiological risk factors, behavioural risk factors, or psychosocial risk factors and socioenvironmental risk conditions?

3. Analyze the health-promotion strategies in terms of their relationship to the determinants. For example, if poverty is seen as an important determinant, then advocating healthy public policy should be included as a strategy.

4. A socioenvironmental approach would focus on addressing the "causes" of smoking behaviour as they are influenced by the social context of women's lives. Nurses would validate the women's life circumstances and seek to understand how their low-income status influences their lives (e.g., women may smoke to relieve stress resulting from issues arising from low-income situations). The interventions would address the social and economic environment, rather than focussing solely on the health behaviour of smoking. Examples of interventions could include working to change the social conditions and structural barriers that are the "cause" of smoking (e.g., advocate for policies that improve income support, provide supports to cope with stressors) and the barriers to smoking cessation. The women need to be involved as partners in the design of smoking cessation programs that will best meet their needs; the programs must be accessible in terms of location and cost, and there must be adequate support and resources to facilitate their participation. A behavioural approach to health would focus primarily on the behaviour itself, rather than on the context in which the behaviour occurs. A behavioural approach may place greater emphasis on providing information rather than ensuring that supports and resources are in place.

The Canadian Health Care Delivery System

Chapter

2

CLASSROOM DISCUSSION

1. Discuss the current status of the health care system and how it will influence both nurses and consumers. Consider federal and provincial/territorial jurisdictions and the role of professional associations in standard setting and public protection.

2. Discuss methods of financing health care services, including various components of Canada's social safety net and supplementary insurance plans.

3. Discuss some differences in availability/access to health care for clients from different socioeconomic backgrounds and geographic locations. Suggest how technology (e.g., telehealth) might address any concerns raised.

4. Ask students to provide examples of how finances and politics may influence health care delivery.

5. Invite a nurse from a provincial/territorial nurses association to discuss the educational preparation and roles of nurses in Canada and the provinces/territories.

6. Have students access the provincial/territorial government Web site for an organizational chart of the health ministry. Have students name the individuals holding positions within the various portfolios. Speculate on how the organizational structure facilitates or hampers the management of health care services at the local, regional, and provincial/territorial levels.

7. From the Web site mentioned above, determine the provincial/territorial programs that support health promotion, prevention, diagnosis and treatment, and rehabilitation services.

8. Review the levels of care, the variety of nongovernmental health care agencies available, and the types of client services that may be offered in each of the programs determined above.

9. Discuss the current issues in health care delivery:
   a. Emerging professionals
   b. Population-based care
   c. Acute care redesign
   d. Quality health care
   e. Continuum of care
   f. Privatization of services

10. Review the Consumers' Rights to Health Care. Ask students for specific examples illustrating when these rights have been attended to or challenged within the current health care delivery system.

11. Discuss the Canadian Nurses Association's view of nursing in Canada and how it may conform or clash with current overall health care reform measures in your province/territory.

12. Review the concept of the multidisciplinary health team approach and the use of critical pathways.

13. Discuss the emergence of midwives, nurse practitioners, clinical nurse specialists, and community development nurses in your province/territory.

INTERACTIVE EXERCISES

1. Organize a debate on the following issues: Is health a right or a privilege? Is health care a right or a social responsibility?

2. Assign students to attend individual workshops or information sessions on new health care funding. Stimulate a debate on whether health care costs are justified.

3. Arrange for students to visit a variety of health care delivery agencies and report, verbally or in writing, on the following (see Resources for Student Activities, p. 2-3):
   a. Entry into the system and exit from the system
   b. Environment
   c. Type of clients
   d. Nurse's role
   e. Funding: costs to clients
   f. Services offered
   g. Accessibility to clients (e.g., hours of operation)

4. While working in small groups, have students participate in a simulated work redesign project using, if possible, an actual situation from an acute or long-term care facility.

5. Assign students to obtain a journal article or news item on trends or funding in health care from the Internet or another current media source.

6. Have students consider nursing services specific to the health promotion, disease prevention, and safety needs of the following clients:
   a. School-age children at summer camp
   b. Senior citizens at a community centre
   c. Middle-age adults in a work setting

Health agency assessment form

HEALTH AGENCY ASSESSMENT FORM

Student's Name: _____

Name of facility:
Location:
Hours of operation/availability:
Transportation available to the site:
Services provided on-site:
Restrictions/requirements:
Funding source(s):
Cost to clients:
Staffing and responsibilities:
Role of the nurse(s):
Affiliations (hospitals, social services, etc.):
Response of clients:
Student comments:

6   Unit 1: The Client and the Health Care Environment

CRITICAL THINKING EXERCISES

1. Debate the following issues in relation to the future of the Canadian health care system as we presently know it: escalating costs; quality of care; fragmentation; accessibility.

2. Consider and describe how the national economy, changes in the population, and techology have changed the Canadian health care system. Identify what implications these changes have for nursing practice.

3. Consider Mr. Wilson, a 68-year-old client who will have major surgery to replace the joint in his hip. Afterward, extensive therapy will be needed for him to walk normally again. Describe the type of health care agencies that might become involved in the care of Mr. Wilson.

4. Mrs. Ramirez is a 42-year-old client who is employed as an advertising agent for a large corporation. She travels 65 percent of the time. Her business requires her to have a physical examination every two years. During a recent checkup, Mrs. Ramirez was found to have elevated cholesterol and triglyceride levels. Her blood pressure is 134/84, up from two years ago. The nurse who conducted a health history learned that Mrs. Ramirez eats on the go and exercises only when at home. She also smokes two packs of cigarettes a day. What level of health care did Mrs. Ramirez pursue? What level of health care should the nurse initiate, and why?

5. Ms. Yim is a 65-year-old client who experienced a stroke eight days ago. She has lost movement on her left side and is unable to speak clearly. Mr. Rogers is a 60-year-old client who is in the hospital for two days following a total knee replacement operation. Which client would benefit from case management, and why?

ANSWERS TO CRITICAL THINKING EXERCISES

1. Factors debated for each issue should include the following:
   Escalating costs: new technologies (diagnostic as well as treatment) are expensive, aging population is making demands on the system, salaries for trained professionals are rising with inflation and increased costs for education. Escalating costs impact on access to new treatments, drugs, and diagnostic tools; require innovative means of delivering services to growing segments of the population that may not be as mobile; and necessitate fundraising activities to support operational costs.
   Quality of care: practices such as human resources substitution, cross-training, multi-skilling, and use of untrained (or trained on the job) health workers have an impact on quality of services provided.
   Fragmentation: services that are not coordinated and integrated among levels of the health system result in duplication or gaps in services, and have a negative influence on access to services by disadvantaged segments of the population.
   Accessibility: access to health is as important as access to health services. Access is influenced by an awareness of need, an awareness of resources, and the ability to use the services that exist. Cultural competence and physical access, as well as literacy, are important considerations in access to health information and care.

2. Nurses must adapt to new technology through lifelong learning activities, such as specialization, and acquisition of advanced practice skills and credentials.

   Lack of funding influences salaries and job opportunities for nurses; in times of a strong economy, opportunities seem limitless, attracting more people to the profession. When times are leaner, there is a drop in interest in the profession, resulting, over time, in a shortage in the supply of nurses.

   As the population changes, the demands for nurses adapt – in an aging population, more nurses are needed in the geriatric nursing field; in highly ethnic locations, nurses with transcultural skills are needed.

3. Mr. Wilson will need to be involved with restoration/rehabilitation agencies that will assist him to regain his ability to walk normally without pain.

4. Mrs. Ramirez pursued primary prevention for a periodic health examination. Early recognition of her hyperlipidemia will allow her to further take control of her health (health promotion) by modifying her lifestyle habits (i.e., nutrition, activity, and tobacco) and addressing issues of job-related stress. The nurse should initiate health promotion activities such as consciousness raising, education about prevention, and social support for making lifestyle changes.

5. Ms. Yim would best benefit from case management, since she will have multiple disciplines (i.e., nursing, medicine, physiotherapy, speech therapy, occupational therapy) in the acute, home, and/or long-term care settings to coordinate and manage her rehabilitation. Mr. Rogers has a simpler trajectory, with fewer professionals involved and a shorter timeframe for direct care and rehabilitation.

Community Nursing Practice

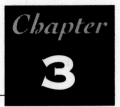

Chapter 3

CLASSROOM DISCUSSION

1. Discuss the historical development of nursing practice in the community.

2. Review the definitions of population and community. Identify important characteristics of a healthy population and a healthy community.

3. Discuss the differences between public health nursing, community health nursing, and community-based nursing. Ask students to identify how nursing practice may be different.

4. Review the human ecology model and its application to community health.

5. Ask students to identify the type of clients who may require community health care and the special needs that may be seen with different age-groups.

6. Invite a nurse or case manager from a public health or home health agency to speak to the class about his or her educational background, experience, and role.

7. Discuss how nursing approaches differ between community and acute care nursing practice. Have students problem solve as to how nursing procedures may need to be adapted.

8. Discuss the roles of the nurse and other professionals and paraprofessionals in community health care settings.

9. Discuss the type of care that may be delegated to ancillary personnel in public health or home care settings.

10. Review the continuum of care as it extends from discharge planning within the acute and restorative care setting to community-based nursing care and, finally, to in-home family-based care.

11. Guide students in the development of a care plan/pathway for a client requiring home care.

12. Discuss the competencies identified by the Canadian Public Health Association for community health nurses, including:
    a. Direct care/Service provider
    b. Collaborator
    c. Educator
    d. Coordinator
    e. Researcher
    f. Community developer

Ask students for specific examples of nursing activities related to each competency.

13. Compare and contrast the implementation of practice innovations in the acute care and community health environments. Examine the different roles and influence of health professionals, clients, and the broader community in implementing change.

INTERACTIVE EXERCISES

1. Have students role play a case study situation for a client requiring home care, with a focus on a case management approach.

2. Assign students to observe nurses at a community agency. Have students report, verbally or in writing, on their observations, including the type of clients seen, services offered, and follow-up established.

3. Obtain a sample public health or home care nurse's caseload, and ask students to determine a schedule for visiting, along with necessary referrals or equipment.

4. Have students report, verbally or in writing, on the changes that have occurred in community-based health care over the past decade, or on current issues and trends.

5. Assign students to complete a community assessment. Have students report, verbally or in writing, about its population/demographics, services, and possible health care concerns.

RESOURCE FOR STUDENT ACTIVITIES

Issues of vulnerable populations in the community

ISSUES OF VULNERABLE POPULATIONS IN THE COMMUNITY

Issue	Health Concerns	Nursing Actions
Low Income and Homelessness		
Violence		
Risk Behaviours		
Chronic Conditions		
Gender and Age		

CRITICAL THINKING EXERCISES

1. As a nurse working with the family of a severely disabled child, you learn that there is an absence of respite services to provide parental support and limited educational resources in your community. What activities or roles of the community-health nurse would be important to establish a special-education daycare service, operated by volunteer educators?

2. Mr. Crowder is a 42-year-old man with emphysema and glaucoma who visits the nursing clinic periodically. Your assessment reveals that he is homeless and that he currently spends nights in a shelter two blocks away. He has been able to acquire medications for his breathing and eyedrops for his glaucoma from clinic funds, but he lost his inhaler three days ago. What factors might you consider in attempting to support Mr. Crowder's efforts to manage his chronic health concerns and promote his general health?

3. Conduct a community assessment of an area that you have visited infrequently. Observe the community locale by driving through the more populated area. Observe the people, their public interactions, and the use of informal meeting places to gain an initial sense of community membership and relationships. Look for the following services: hospital; medical, community health, and alternative care clinics; pharmacy; grocery store; schools, park or playground; community organizations; and emergency services such as police and fire departments.

ANSWERS TO CRITICAL THINKING EXERCISES

1. Facilitator and collaborator roles would be important to establish a special-education daycare service. The community health nurse would work with local agencies, people in the community, and any regulatory agencies to establish a new service. It would be important to be a strong client advocate so that the client's needs are well represented.

2. It would be useful to talk with the staff who maintain the local shelter. Is there a place where the client can safely store his medications during the day? You might try giving the client a small bottle or container to be used for his daily medication doses. Determine where he typically goes for nourishment so that he can establish a routine time to take the medications. Taking eyedrops can be difficult. Does the client have access to bathroom facilities with a mirror? You can teach the client to use eyedrops safely. Talk with Mr. Crowder about his concerns for his health. Discuss with him what helps and what hinders his efforts to manage his health concerns. Consider his own knowledge and skills, his available support network, and his access to needed supports and services. Explore ways to build on available strengths and to overcome existing barriers that influence Mr. Crowder's efforts to manage his health concerns and promote his health. This exploration can occur in discussion with Mr. Crowder as well as with staff at the shelter. Additionally, explore the potential to expand Mr. Crowder's formal support network by identifying other services that can help him manage his health concerns and promote his general health.

3. Report on your community assessment.

Leadership, Delegation, and Quality Management

Chapter 4

CLASSROOM DISCUSSION

1. Compare and contrast the definitions of *leadership* and *management*.

2. Discuss the different management types and their application to nursing.

3. Review and provide examples of leadership styles. Ask students to give examples of nursing situations where the different styles may be implemented.

4. Discuss the current leadership and management roles in nursing. Ask students to identify the leadership opportunities available to student nurses and the skills necessary to assume leadership roles.

5. Invite a nurse executive or manager to speak to the class about his or her role, educational preparation, and experience.

6. Review the process of delegation and ask students to give examples of effective and ineffective delegation they have observed.

7. Review centralized and decentralized management structures. Have students identify the advantages and disadvantages of each type of structure.

8. Discuss the nursing care delivery models:
   a. Total patient care
   b. Functional nursing
   c. Team nursing
   d. Primary nursing
   e. Case management

   Ask students to identify where and in what situations each of the models may be used best.

9. Discuss total quality management (TQM) as a philosophy for change.

10. Discuss the process/components of quality improvement (QI) in health care settings, including the different approaches that may be taken with the process.

11. Invite a nurse, preferably a QI nurse director, to speak to the class about the role of QI in his or her agency in relation to the health care delivery process.

12. Review actual QI projects from an affiliating agency, if possible, and discuss possible rationale for the selection of evaluation measures, criteria, and standards.

INTERACTIVE EXERCISES

1. Provide information on the number and qualifications of staff and the types of clients. Students should work individually or in small groups to develop a staffing pattern and client assignment for an acute care or long-term care facility or home care agency.

2. Assign students to attend a QI meeting in a health care agency or a workshop on the subject, and have them complete an oral or written report on their experience.

3. Assign a small group of students to develop a QI project specific to one area of client care or nursing education.

CLIENT CARE EXPERIENCE

1. Assign students in the clinical area to observe or work with the coordinator, team leader, or regional supervisor and document the leadership characteristics that are demonstrated. Have them share their observations and experiences in a postclinical discussion.

RESOURCE FOR STUDENT ACTIVITIES

Assessment of leadership styles

ASSESSMENT OF LEADERSHIP STYLES

Autocratic Characteristics	Democratic Characteristics
Laissez-Faire Characteristics	**Situational Characteristics**

CRITICAL THINKING EXERCISES

1. It is a busy morning, and Josh has just completed making rounds on his five clients. One of his clients, Mrs. Robinson, is a 60-year old woman who requested that Josh reposition her in bed because of discomfort in her right leg. Mrs. Robinson had surgery on her right leg to repair a fracture and has a dressing that extends along the right thigh. Nancy is a nursing assistant who is working with Josh this morning. Josh approaches Nancy and says, "Would you please go into Mrs. Robinson's room and help turn her?" What, if anything, is inappropriate with Josh's delegation?

2. Linda is the manager of a busy clinic. Her philosophy of leadership has been use of decentralized decision making. In addition to a staff dietitian, pharmacist, and social worker, there are three staff nurses under her supervision: Lisa, Jeff, and Nina. Lisa has worked at the clinic for over ten years and has assisted Linda in managing the clinic when Linda is absent. Jeff just joined the clinic team about six months ago but has shown good progress as a clinician. Nina has been a staff member for one year after having worked in an operating room for five years. Nina has had difficulty in completing her work on time and has received counselling from Linda. The clinic is starting a new service, diabetic education, and Linda wants the nursing staff to be involved as part of the clinic's multidisciplinary team. Linda has been asked by the clinic director to develop standards of care for client and family instruction. What leadership approaches might Linda use? How might she apply situational leadership principles in involving Lisa, Jeff, and Nina in this project?

3. Assume that you are part of a quality improvement (QI) work team. Your team receives a report from the manager that the rate of infection in clients who have in-dwelling Foley catheters is high. The QI team agrees that a problem exists. (Refer to Chapter 44 of *Canadian Fundamentals of Nursing*, Second Edition for the procedure on care and maintenance of an indwelling Foley catheter.) Knowing that the outcome of infection is undesirable, what criteria might your team monitor in determining possible causes for the incidence of urinary infection in your clients?

ANSWERS TO CRITICAL THINKING EXERCISES

1. It is appropriate to delegate trained assistive personnel to turn and reposition clients. However, Josh's communication was not clear or concise. He gave no information about why the client needed repositioning or any guidance as to how turning might be affected by the client's surgical condition.

2. If Linda is an effective leader, she will want all staff to work collaboratively in developing the standards of care. This would involve the nurses, dietitian, pharmacist, and social worker. Since all staff must be able to practise under the standards, a supportive leadership style would help to gain consensus on the standards. Linda might choose to delegate responsibility to Lisa to direct separate meetings of the staff nurses to develop their portion of the standards of care. If staff members were assigned responsibility for different aspects of the project, Linda would want to be sure that Nina received direction and specific expectations on what was to be completed. Jeff is still relatively new and also might require specific instructions and expectations. If Jeff were to show good performance, Linda would coach him in assuming more responsibility.

3. Refer to the procedure for possible factors that might cause infection. These factors become your criteria for data collection. For example, staff would conduct observations of all clients with catheters, looking to see if drainage systems are positioned below the level of the bladder, catheter and drainage tubing are connected securely, and that documentation shows that the client received daily catheter care.

Theoretical Foundations of Nursing Practice

Chapter
5

CLASSROOM DISCUSSION

1. Discuss the following: What is a theory? What constitutes its structure?

2. Distinguish between nursing theory and nursing process. How do they relate to one another?

3. Discuss the utility and comprehensiveness of nursing's metaparadigm (i.e., person, environment, health, and nursing) for organizing thinking about nursing.
   a. Have students consider the following variables that they might encounter in their assessment of an individual client situation. Discuss which aspects of the metaparadigm might help them better understand the following:
      Family
      Socioeconomic status
      Culture
      Rights
      Physical fitness
      Health care policy
      Diagnosis of a chronic illness
      Lifestyle choices
      Religion
      Sexual orientation
      Climate
      The multidisciplinary team
   b. Discuss the following: not all information about all of these variables will be directly relevant to the metaparadigm concepts. If it does not relate directly to a concept, does that mean it is not relevant to nursing?

4. Discuss why it has been so important for the practical profession of nursing to develop an appreciation for its theoretical aspect.

INTERACTIVE EXERCISES

1. In small groups, have students discuss the implications for nursing of various ways of interpreting nursing's four metaparadigm concepts. They should consider how different types of theoretical models provide nursing with different approaches to interpreting each concept (see Resource for Student Activities, p. 17).

2. Have students complete the think-pair-share activity:
    a. Individually, students should identify the professional and the social forces that influenced the development of nursing theory.
    b. Students should then pair up with a partner and discuss their ideas.
    c. Have students share the consensus of their thinking with the class.

3. Assign a one-minute paper:
    a. Students should write for one minute about what they think are the most important things they have learned about nursing theory.
    b. Have students share their thoughts with one other person.
    c. Each pair of students should then combine with another pair and discuss their ideas.
    d. Have each group of four report to the class on their conclusion about the most important aspects of nursing theory and the issues that were debated most strongly.

CLIENT CARE EXPERIENCES

1. Discuss what guides the nursing assessment of a patient. Consider how nurses know what data to seek.

2. Discuss whether patient care is different depending on the theoretical perspective used. Discuss whether patients would notice the difference.

3. There is an old expression: "A man is in some ways like every other man, in some ways like some other men, and in other ways like no other man." Have students consider the implications of this idea for client care. Discuss how nursing theories help nurses identify common and unique aspects of clients.

RESOURCE FOR STUDENT ACTIVITIES

Nursing metaparadigm concept chart

NURSING METAPARADIGM CONCEPT CHART

Metaparadigm Concept	Interpretation	Example of Specific Theoretical Model
Person		
Environment		
Health		
Nursing		

CRITICAL THINKING EXERCISES

1. How do you think that different ways of conceptualizing the client of nursing might influence the kinds of decisions nurses might make in their practice? Consider how understanding the person in terms of needs, system theory, or interaction might lead you to notice certain things and not others.

2. What gaps in information or misunderstandings might occur if nurses failed to use a systematic way of thinking about each individual client in their care?

3. How do you think that conceptual frameworks and nursing theories might be used to generate research questions for developing knowledge for evidence-based practice?

4. Why is it useful for nurses to question how they know what they know?

ANSWERS TO CRITICAL THINKING EXERCISES

1. If you assume that all of the choices and decisions a person makes are based on a set of needs, you might believe that basic or primary urges are more influential in human decision making than are rationality, free will, and a sense of purpose. You would have to assume that some needs were inherently more powerful than others (i.e., the need for food would take precedence over the need for reproduction). Nurses have long struggled with what such ideas might contribute to a larger philosophical understanding of how to interpret the individual differences between people and how to avoid inappropriate judgements about their various decisions. Similarly, subscribing to systems theories can have an impact on your decisions when they lead you to understand all aspects of a person in interaction. Perhaps there are occasions in which it is appropriate and relevant to attend to parts of the whole (i.e., in an emergency, in a specific interaction in which there is already agreement as to why the client needs a nurse).

2. Traditionally, it has been quite common for nurses working in high acuity trauma or critical care units to assume that the emotional or psychosocial aspects of their clients are not as relevant as the physiological and biological. However, there are scenarios in which failure to notice the client's emotional state might actually put that client at risk. Similarly, it is not appropriate to ignore the relevance of physical health aspects of our clients in a community or acute mental health setting. While these are perhaps extreme examples, they help us appreciate the serious errors in clinical judgement that nurses can make if they fail to recognize the advantages of a comprehensive and systematic approach to assessing clients. While they can refine and synthesize these approaches to fit their particular clinical setting over time, expert nurses always retain an awareness of the larger context of what might be happening for their clients, and can respond quickly to relevant variations or unusual clinical manifestations.

3. While the early theorists thought that conceptual frameworks might eventually be tested as a whole to determine their relative effectiveness, later theorists recognized that they were not designed to be service delivery structures, as much as they were tools for the conceptual development of expert nursing reasoning. Conceptual frameworks illuminate theoretical relationships among concepts that are important in nursing practice, and guide us to develop research questions that will generate more substantive knowledge about such relationships. For example, if a conceptual framework tells us that thoughts and feelings are relevant to biological functions, researchers might develop questions that extend substantive knowledge related to how to support people emotionally as they go through cancer chemotherapy, or how to use therapeutic relationships to enhance recovery from traumatic injury.

4. Nursing knowledge will always take the form of important general information that is applied in unique and individual cases. While it is useful to know a lot of general information about diabetes management, every new individual who is diagnosed with diabetes will represent an entirely distinct life experience than did every other person for whom the nurse may have cared. Because of this, general knowledge will always be open to appropriate variations and modifications when we apply it to individual cases. However, as professionals, nurses cannot simply act on a whim or a hunch, they must be able to base their clinical judgements on scientific evidence, professional practice standards, the law of the land, and many other factors, in addition to their knowledge of the individual client and his or her preferences. To reason in this manner, the nurse must be highly knowledgeable about the science, and standards and regulations that should govern any situation, and, at the same time, be able to think critically about the implications of following usual practice in any specific instance. This is the kind of thinking that the conceptual frameworks were designed to promote.

Nursing Healing and Caring

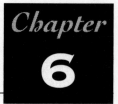

CLASSROOM DISCUSSION

1. Discuss the importance of caring.

2. Compare and contrast the theoretical views regarding caring, including those of Leininger, Watson, and Swanson.

3. Ask students to identify their definitions and perceptions of caring.

4. Discuss the findings regarding clients' perceptions of nurses' caring behaviors.

5. Review what is meant by an "ethic of care."

6. Ask students to describe the advocacy role in nursing as it relates to caring.

INTERACTIVE EXERCISE

1. Arrange role-playing situations of nurse-client interactions that demonstrate caring or non-caring behaviors. Ask students to identify how the non-caring behaviors may be changed.

Caring behaviors in nursing chart

CARING BEHAVIORS IN NURSING CHART

Nursing Behaviors	Specific Examples
Providing Presence	
Comforting	
Listening	
Knowing the Client	
Spiritual Caring	
Family Care	

CRITICAL THINKING EXERCISES

1. Lindsey is a student nurse assigned to care for Mrs. Lowe, a 62-year-old client being treated for lymphoma (cancer of the lymph nodes). The charge nurse informs Lindsey that the nurse who does intravenous procedures will be up shortly to insert a long-term, percutaneous intravascular catheter for Mrs. Lowe's chemotherapy. This is the first day Lindsey has cared for Mrs. Lowe, but she has learned that the client has not had an intravenous line previously. In what way can Lindsay provide presence and be comforting for Mrs. Lowe?

2. During your next clinical practicum, select a client to talk with for at least 15 to 20 minutes. Ask the client to tell you about his or her illness. Review the skills of listening in Chapter 6 and Chapter 22 of *Canadian Fundamentals of Nursing*, Second Edition. Immediately after your discussion, reflect on the discussion with the client and answer the following questions:
   a. What do you believe the client was trying to tell you about his or her illness?
   b. Why was it important for the client to share his or her story?
   c. What did you do that made it easy or difficult for the client to talk with you?
   d. Would you rate yourself a good listener? If not, why not? If so, explain.

3. The next time you are assigned to a clinical agency, ask to read their philosophy and standards of care documents. Does the language in the documents represent a caring ethic?

ANSWERS TO CRITICAL THINKING EXERCISES

1. Lindsey can check with the IV nurse and the procedure manual to learn more about what the actual catheter insertion involves (e.g., what is the procedure, how long does it take, what must the client do). Lindsey should then plan to stay with Mrs. Lowe during the catheter insertion. Lindsey can assure Mrs. Lowe of the IV nurse's expertise and review with her the basic elements of the procedure. Lindsey can make Mrs. Lowe more comfortable before the procedure, meeting any elimination needs and positioning the client. By spending time answering Mrs. Lowe's questions, staying by her side, and offering words of comfort, Lindsay's presence can help to relieve any anxiety that the client may experience.

2. It is important to ask yourself whether you really heard the client's story. Were you listening for the content and meaning of the story? If the conversation failed to proceed to a story, what was the reason? If you were attentive, showing good eye contact, body language, and responsive nonverbal gestures, you were likely being an effective listener.

3. Review an agency's philosophy and standards of care for representation of a caring ethic.

Diversity in Caring

CLASSROOM DISCUSSION

1. Discuss the concept of transcultural nursing and culturally competent care, including the recognition of the cultural identity of both the client and the nurse.

2. Discuss the concepts of culture, ethnicity, and religion.

3. Review efficacious, neutral, and dysfunctional health care practices. Ask students to provide examples of each type of health care practice and the effects on nursing practice.

4. Review the Giger and Davidhizar's transcultural assessment model and its application in nursing. Have students use the model to obtain information from their peers, family members, or clients.

5. Review the current demographics of the local community and larger society and their influence on overall health care needs.

6. Ask students to share personal experiences in regard to traditional health beliefs and practices.

7. Compare and contrast the health beliefs (cause of illness, prevention, and remedies) of Aboriginal peoples, Chinese Canadians, South Asians, Black Canadians, and European Canadians.

8. Invite a nurse who works in a community setting with clients from diverse sociocultural backgrounds to discuss cultural competence.

9. Have students bring in examples from the media and/or Internet of health problems or needs that are specific to one or more sociocultural group.

INTERACTIVE EXERCISES

1. Assign students to investigate the resources that are available in an affiliating agency for promoting communication and education for clients with language differences (i.e., interpreters, multilingual information packets).

2. Have students role play one or more of the following, or similar, transcultural situations:
   a. Teaching a client who has a language difference to give an injection
   b. Explaining to a client how home remedies are interacting with the prescribed medication
   c. Adapting acute or home care routines to avoid conflicts with religious practices
   d. Completing a health history with the client's entire family "camping out" and monopolizing the conversation
   e. Preparing a client, who has always worn a special amulet around her neck, for surgery

3. Assign students to research the health practices of a specific cultural group. Organize a "cultural awareness" class where students share their information on the specific culture with the group. Interest may be stimulated, for example, with the inclusion of traditional foods and music.

4. Assign students to review the demographics of their own communities and begin to determine specific health care practices and needs.

CLIENT CARE EXPERIENCES

1. Conduct preclinical or postclinical conferences for discussion of cultural adaptations that may be or have been implemented for clients of diverse backgrounds. Ask students to share information on possible barriers to and/or resources for transcultural nursing.

2. Working individually or in small groups, have students identify the following for an assigned client and/or a case study situation, specific to sociocultural needs/adaptation:
   a. Nursing diagnoses
   b. Long-term or short-term goals and desired client outcomes
   c. Nursing interventions
   d. Evaluation criteria/measures

RESOURCES FOR STUDENT ACTIVITIES

Giger and Davidhizar's transcultural assessment model
Comparison chart of cultural group beliefs

GIGER AND DAVIDHIZAR'S TRANSCULTURAL ASSESSMENT MODEL

CULTURALLY UNIQUE INDIVIDUAL

1. Place of birth
2. Cultural definition
   What is . . .
3. Race
   What is . . .
4. Length of time in country (if appropriate)

COMMUNICATION

1. Voice quality
   A. Strong, resonant
   B. Soft
   C. Average
   D. Shrill

2. Pronunciation and enunciation
   A. Clear
   B. Slurred
   C. Dialect (geographical)
3. Use of silence
   A. Infrequent
   B. Often
   C. Length
      (1) Brief
      (2) Moderate
      (3) Long
      (4) Not observed

continued

4. Use of nonverbal cues
   A. Hand movement
   B. Eye movement
   C. Entire body movement
   D. Kinesics (gestures, expression, or stances)
5. Touch
   A. Startles or withdraws when touched
   B. Accepts touch without difficulty
   C. Touches others without difficulty
6. Ask these and similar questions:
   A. How do you get your point across to others?
   B. Do you like communicating with friends, family, and acquaintances?
   C. When asked a question, do you usually respond (in words or body movement, or both)?
   D. If you have something important to discuss with your family, how would you approach them?

SPACE

1. Degree of comfort
   A. Moves when space invaded
   B. Does not move when space invaded
2. Distance in conversations
   A. 0 to 50 cm
   B. 50 cm to 1 m
   C. 1 m or more
3. Definition of space
   A. Describe degree of comfort with closeness when talking with or standing near others
   B. How do objects (e.g., furniture) in the environment affect your sense of space?
4. Ask these and similar questions:
   A. When you talk with family members, how close do you stand?
   B. When you communicate with co-workers and other acquaintances, how close do you stand?
   C. If a stranger touches you, how do you react or feel?
   D. If a loved one touches you, how do you react or feel?

   E. Are you comfortable with the distance between us now?

SOCIAL ORGANIZATION

1. Normal state of health
   A. Poor
   B. Fair
   C. Good
   D. Excellent
2. Marital status
3. Number of children
4. Parents living or deceased?
5. Ask these and similar questions:
   A. How do you define social activities?
   B. What are some activities that you enjoy?
   C. What are your hobbies, or what do you do when you have free time?
   D. Do you believe in a Supreme Being?
   E. How do you worship that Supreme Being?
   F. What is your function (what do you do) in your family unit/system?
   G. What is your role in your family unit/system (father, mother, child, advisor)?
   H. When you were a child, what or who influenced you the most?
   I. What is/was your relationship with your siblings and parents?
   J. What does work mean to you?
   K. Describe your past, present, and future jobs.
   L. What are your political views?
   M. How have your political views influenced your attitude toward health and illness?

TIME

1. Orientation to time
   A. Past oriented
   B. Present oriented
   C. Future oriented
2. View of time
   A. Social time
   B. Clock oriented

24   Unit 2: Caring Throughout the Life Span

3. Physiochemical reaction to time
   A. Sleeps at least 8 h a night
   B. Goes to sleep and wakes on a consistent schedule
   C. Understands the importance of taking medication and other treatments on schedule
4. Ask these and similar questions:
   A. What kind of timepiece do you wear daily?
   B. If you have an appointment at 14:00, what time is acceptable to arrive?
   C. If a nurse tells you that you will receive a medication in "about a half hour," realistically, how much time will you allow before calling the nurses' station?

ENVIRONMENTAL CONTROL

1. Locus of control
   A. Internal locus of control (believes that the power to effect change lies within)
   B. External locus of control (believes that fate, luck, and chance have a great deal to do with how things turn out)
2. Value orientation
   A. Believes in supernatural forces
   B. Relies on magic, witchcraft, and prayer to effect change
   C. Does not believe in supernatural forces
   D. Does not rely on magic, witchcraft, or prayer to effect change
3. Ask these and similar questions
   A. How often do you have visitors at your home?
   B. Is it acceptable to you for visitors to drop in unexpectedly?
   C. Name some ways your parents or other persons treated your illnesses when you were a child.
   D. Have you or someone else in your immediate surroundings ever used a home remedy that made you sick?
   E. What home remedies have you used that worked? Will you use them in the future?

F. What is your definition of "good health"?
G. What is your definition of illness or "poor health"?

BIOLOGICAL VARIATIONS

1. Conduct a complete physical assessment noting:
   A. Body structure (small, medium, or large frame)
   B. Skin colour
   C. Unusual skin discolourations
   D. Hair colour and distribution
   E. Other visible physical characteristics (e.g., keloids, chloasma)
   F. Weight
   G. Height
   H. Check lab for variances in hemoglobin, hematocrit, and sickle cell phenomena if Black or Mediterranean
2. Ask these and similar questions:
   A. What diseases or illnesses are common in your family?
   B. Has anyone in your family been told that there is a possible genetic susceptibility for a particular disease?
   C. Describe your family's typical behaviour when a family member is ill.
   D. How do you respond when you are angry?
   E. Who (or what) usually helps you to cope during a difficult time?
   F. What foods do you and your family like to eat?
   G. Have you ever had any unusual cravings for:
      (1) White or red clay dirt?
      (2) Laundry starch?
   H. When you were a child, what types of foods did you eat?
   I. What foods are family favourites or are considered traditional?

Chapter 7: Diversity in Caring   25

NURSING ASSESSMENT

1. Note whether the client has become culturally assimilated or observes own cultural practices.
2. Incorporate data into plan of nursing care:
   A. Encourage the client to discuss cultural differences; people from diverse cultures who hold different worldviews can enlighten nurses.
   B. Make efforts to accept and understand methods of communication.
   C. Respect the individual's personal need for space.
   D. Respect the rights of clients to honour and worship the Supreme Being of their choice.
   E. Identify a clerical or spiritual person to contact.
   F. Determine whether spiritual practices have implications for health, life, and well-being (e.g., Jehovah's Witnesses may refuse blood and blood derivatives; an Orthodox Jew may eat only kosher food high in sodium and may not drink milk when meat is served).
   G. Identify hobbies, especially when devising interventions for a short or extended convalescence or for rehabilitation.
   H. Honour time and value orientations and differences in these areas. Allay anxiety and apprehension if adherence to time is necessary.
   I. Provide privacy according to personal need and health status of the client (NOTE: the perception of and reaction to pain may be culturally related).
   J. Note cultural health practices.
      (1) Identify and encourage efficacious practices.
      (2) Identify and discourage dysfunctional practices.
      (3) Identify and determine whether neutral practices will have a long-term ill effect.
   K. Note food preferences.
      (1) Make as many adjustments in diet as health status and long-term benefits will allow and that dietary department can provide.
      (2) Note dietary practices that may have serious implications for the client.

From Giger JN, Davidhizar RE: *Transcultural nursing: Assessment and intervention,* ed 3, St. Louis, 1999, Mosby.

	Family	Health	Illness	Remedies
Aboriginal People				
Chinese Canadian				
South Asian				
Black Canadian				
European Canadian				

CRITICAL THINKING EXERCISES

1. What impact does culture have on cultural beliefs, illness, and wellness behaviours?

2. In what ways does communication present barriers to culturally competent care, even when the nurse and the client speak the same language?

3. In what ways do time orientation; spatial needs; and efficacious, neutral, or dysfunctional health care practices affect compliance or adherence to a particular treatment regimen?

ANSWERS TO CRITICAL THINKING EXERCISES

1. Health care practices from an individual's culture may work against standard medical practice. The client may be unwilling to blend cultural practices with recommended therapy. Some cultures may believe that disease causation is related to natural and spiritual factors; therefore, some clients may not practise standard screening and disease prevention and control. In some cases, cultural practices may assist with standard therapies.

2. English may be a second language. In times of stress, the client and family may revert back to the original language. Even when the client generally understands the English language, the client, and family, may not understand some idiomatic expressions. Additionally, the care provider may not notice or understand cultural, nonverbal cues, with regard to eye contact, touch, or space.

3. Clients may be unwilling or unable to understand why cultural health practices may not be compatible with the standard medical therapy. Thoroughly assessing the client and obtaining a true understanding of the cultural practices may assist in reaching a compatible compromise between cultural practices and standard treatment.

Caring in Families

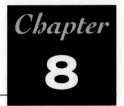

Chapter 8

CLASSROOM DISCUSSION

1. Review the definition of and the different forms of *families*.

2. Stimulate a discussion on current trends and alternative lifestyles associated with families and their influence on nursing and health care.

3. Describe the theoretical approaches to viewing the family, including the application of systems and developmental theories.

4. Discuss the structure and function of the family and the roles that may be assumed by family members.

5. Review the developmental stages of the family.

6. Explain the concepts of family nursing: family as context, family as client, and family as system. Provide examples that demonstrate the difference in these approaches.

7. Ask students to identify what should be included in an assessment of a family.

8. Discuss health promotion activities that may be implemented for families. Ask students to provide examples of specific interventions or teaching/learning plans that focus on family needs and cultural practices.

9. Invite a family practice nurse or counselor to speak to the class about his or her role, educational background, and experiences.

10. Ask students to identify how the following situations may influence the family unit:
    a. A single father has a heart attack (MI) and is no longer able to continue in his current job.
    b. A mother of three young children is in an automobile accident, is paraplegic, and must use a wheelchair.
    c. An adolescent in an extended family demonstrates schizophrenic behavior.
    d. A child in a blended family is having difficulty at school.

See the appendix on page 1716 of *Canadian Fundamentals of Nursing*, Second Edition for The Calgary Family Assessment Model.

11. Guide students in the application of the nursing process using an actual or simulated family case study.

INTERACTIVE EXERCISES

1. Have students bring in an example from the media and/or Internet on changes in the family, or assign students to investigate a current trend or issue in family life (e.g., single parenting, domestic violence).

2. Have students obtain an article from a nursing journal that discusses family-centered nursing care.

3. Assign students to report, verbally or in writing, on the support systems or resources that are available to the family within the affiliating agency or local community.

CLIENT CARE EXPERIENCE

1. Working individually or in small groups, have students identify the following, specific for an assigned family situation and/or case study example:
   a. Nursing diagnoses
   b. Long-term or short-term goals and desired client outcomes
   c. Nursing interventions
   d. Evaluation criteria/measures

RESOURCE FOR STUDENT ACTIVITIES

Family assessment tool

FAMILY ASSESSMENT TOOL

The family assessment tool is used when the beginning student interviews family members and observes family interaction. It is a guideline only and is not meant to be all-inclusive. The student must ensure that individual health histories accompany this assessment.

FAMILY FORM AND STRUCTURE

Names of adults   Ages
_____

Relationship _____
                       (Single, married, divorced, separated, cohabiting)
Names of children   Ages
_____
_____
_____

Others living in home (include age, sex, relationship)
_____

Cultural background (include pertinent health beliefs, child-rearing practices, related health concerns)
_____

Developmental stage _____

Progress toward accomplishment of developmental tasks _____

Concerns related to developmental stage _____

Do family members consider pets a part of the family? What types? How many? Any concerns about their care? _____

RESOURCES

Significant relatives and friends not occupying immediate residence _____

Strengths and coping skills _____

How does the family obtain health services? _____

Membership in community groups (e.g., church affiliation) _____

Education (formal and informal) _____

Finances (ability to meet current and future needs) _____

FAMILY PATTERNS

Persons working outside the home _____

Type of work _____ Number of hours _____

Satisfaction with work _____

How are the housekeeping tasks accomplished? _____

Are family members satisfied with the way tasks are divided? _____

How are child-rearing responsibilities divided? _____

Who makes the major decisions in the family? _____

Who makes day-to-day decisions? _____

Are family members satisfied with the way decisions are made? _____

FAMILY FUNCTION

Goals

Long term _____

Short term _____

Individual family members' goals _____

Are individual and family goals appropriate, considering their current health problem and status? _____

How are individual family members and the family as a whole coping with their current health problem and status? _____

COMMUNICATION

Do husband and wife communicate regularly and effectively with each other?

_____

Are family members able to communicate openly and honestly with each other?

_____

Is conflict openly expressed and discussed? _____

Do family members respect one another's point of view? _____

Do family members offer emotional support to each other? _____

CRITICAL THINKING EXERCISES

1. Saundra is a home health nurse visiting a family consisting of an older adult mother and her daughter. In trying to gain a better understanding of this family and how it functions, Saundra learns about additional family members and the social and religious groups in which they participate. She also assesses the mother and daughter carefully in an effort to understand their personal values, beliefs, and concerns. To understand the caregiving relationship between mother and daughter, Saundra assesses the history of the relationship and the meaning it has for both family members. What theoretical approach is Saundra using in assessing this family?

2. Mr. Lee is a 70-year-old client who is being discharged from the hospital following a broken hip. The nurse determines the level of the client's mobility and the extent to which it will influence his ability to ambulate within his home. The nurse makes recommendations for rearranging furniture and placing extra chairs along Mr. Lee's usual walking path. After learning how dependent Mrs. Lee normally is on the client's ability to assist with daily activities, the nurse makes recommendations to the family for Mrs. Lee to hire a temporary housekeeper. Has the nurse provided care to the Lee family as context, client, or system?

3. Mr. and Mrs. Baillargeron, both in their early 50s, are the youngest members of large Catholic French Canadian families. They are employed full time and have two teenage children of their own. Both sets of their parents are in their 80s and have chronic health problems. All of their brothers and sisters are geographically farther away. How can you assist Mr. and Mrs. Baillargeron in developing extended resources to aid in caring for their parents and at the same time maintain the responsibilities of their own family unit?

ANSWERS TO CRITICAL THINKING EXERCISES

1. The nurse uses the general systems theory. The family is viewed as an open social system that exists and interacts with larger systems. The mother and daughter are members of a caregiving subsystem.

2. The Lee family was cared for as a system.

3. Mr. and Mrs. Baillargeron are "sandwiched" between elder parents and teenage children, while trying to meet the demands and expectations of their full-time jobs and other outside commitments. The nurse can aid this family in finding outside resources for their elder parents. Ideas include the following: Have the teenagers post a Web page and maintain it for the distant family members regarding the parents'/grandparents' needs, concerns, and information. Ask the extended family to send money to help support the inexpensive, community-based, gerontological day care with activities, meals, games, health lectures, and socialization, or pay CNAs at night as their health demands increase. Have the family sign up for rotating weekends to stay with the grandparents (e.g., 1 weekend per month). The family members who live farther away may send more money or cards, letters, pictures, or e-mails. Additional support may be available through the church and community center. Any of these efforts would help relieve the responsibilities of total caretaking by any one person, which creates caregiver role strain and decreased ability to function. These efforts also remind the elders that they are still part of their community and decreases the potential for depression and elder abuse (which is all too common when elders have been isolated from their peers).

Developmental Theories

CLASSROOM DISCUSSION

1. Describe the role of human development theories and their application to nursing practice.

2. Discuss and provide specific examples of the principles of growth and development.

3. Review the four major areas of theory development:
   a. Biophysical development
   b. Psychosocial development
   c. Cognitive development
   d. Moral development

4. Compare and contrast the various theories of human development.

5. Ask the students to identify how the nurse may apply developmental theories to client interactions. Have students provide examples of situations that the nurse may encounter with clients of different ages.

6. Using actual or simulated case studies, guide students in the application of selected developmental theories in the assessment of clients and determination of nurse-client interactions.

CLIENT CARE EXPERIENCE

1. Have students identify the developmental level and requirements of their assigned clients and discuss, verbally or in writing, how the nurse-client interactions may be adapted to meet their client's needs. Review the application of developmental theories to client assignments in post-clinical care conferences.

CRITICAL THINKING EXERCISES

1. A 7-year-old boy has been diagnosed with immune-mediated diabetes. A nurse must begin the educational process for him and his family. What developmental tasks must the nurse determine are already accomplished by the client and his family to design an effective educational program and meet the needs of a family now faced with a chronic illness in one of its members? Based on his cognitive development, how would the nurse approach teaching him about his diabetes?

2. A 76-year-old female has just been diagnosed with breast cancer. She also has severe cardiovascular disease that limits her choices of treatment. Her oncologist has recommended a series of chemotherapy that her cardiologist believes would be fatal. Her family is urging her to do all that is recommended. The client, who is in good spirits despite her diagnosis, chooses palliative care. Based on her developmental stage, how can you help the family adjust to her choice?

3. A 45-year-old executive from a local corporation enters the emergency department with intense chest pain. Upon evaluation, it is determined that he has severe cardiovascular disease and requires open heart surgery. His children, ages 13 and 17, and wife accompany him to the hospital. They live a very expensive lifestyle, and he is the sole wage earner for the family. The oldest son is planning to enroll in an eastern Ivy League school in the fall. After the client settles in his room, he asks for computer access to complete some work before surgery. How will the nurse assist this client in changing his lifestyle while understanding his developmental tasks?

ANSWERS TO CRITICAL THINKING EXERCISES

1. Theoretical developmental guidelines would place this 7-year-old in Piaget's and Kohlberg's punishment and obedience orientation. He may have a hard time understanding that the insulin injections and blood sugar checks are not punishment for something he has done wrong. He is also likely to be more concerned about satisfying his own needs at this time than following routines; dietary requirements that do not include candy and other pleasure foods and that do include consistent meal and snack times may become very difficult and conflict over control may occur. He is at the early Erikson's stage of industry versus inferiority and Piaget's period of concrete operational thought. Achieving competence in the new skills that he is learning is essential, but he recognizes that he is not like his peers. He may judge himself to be a failure in some skill development while learning about self-care for his diabetes management. The nurse must also assess whether his fine motor skills are sufficient for teaching injections. Working with his parents, the nurse must assist the family to normalize this child's life as much as possible, encourage him to be independent and see his diabetes management as a sign of successful achievement, and reinforce that this disease was not caused by something that this child did or said.

2. Developmentally, according to most adult theorists, this 76-year-old client is dealing with reappraisal of the past and shifting to new aspirations and goals while realistically adjusting to decreased strength and health. These are also the years of Erikson's stage of integrity versus despair, related to her life review; she benefits from support as she puts her life into perspective. She sees her choice of palliative care as a way to respectfully end her life. She may not have shared her feelings with her family. Providing grief support for the family as they come to understand this developmental stage may assist them in supporting her choice.

3. This client is in the age of Erikson's stage of generativity versus self-absorption. Theories of adult life cycle acknowledge the importance of sacrificing his needs to meet the needs of his family. His needs for a healthy lifestyle may have been ignored to achieve what is necessary for his family. These are supposed to be his productive years. He is coming to terms with his accomplishments and disappointments. This health crisis will very likely push him into some type of mid-life crisis. He will be required to make lifestyle changes necessary to manage the heart disease, deal with the realization that his body is getting older (accepting and adjusting to the physiological changes of middle age), and come to terms with how he may feel about himself since he has let down those who have been depending on him. The nurse will assess these factors in planning for the emotional support needs of the client during cardiac recovery.

Conception Through Adolescence

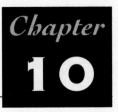

Chapter

10

CLASSROOM DISCUSSION

1. Ask students to identify factors that may influence growth and development.

2. Review conception, intrauterine life, and the transition to extrauterine life. Identify or ask students to identify the following for each trimester of pregnancy and childbirth:
   a. Characteristics of physical, cognitive, and psychosocial development
   b. Specific health concerns and health promotion and safety activities

3. Review growth and development of the neonate, infant, toddler, preschool child, school-age child, and adolescent. Identify or ask students to identify the following for each age-group:
   a. Characteristics (milestones) of physical, cognitive, and psychosocial development
   b. Language development and communication patterns
   c. Specific health concerns and health promotion and safety activities

4. Discuss how perceptions of health and illness are developed in young children.

5. Discuss the effect of hospitalization on children and parents or caretakers. Ask students to provide examples of possible behavior patterns.

6. Discuss and ask students to provide additional examples of implementation strategies for the hospitalized child in relation to the following:
   a. Minimizing separation anxiety
   b. Establishing trust
   c. Reducing fear
   d. Minimizing physical discomfort
   e. Fostering normal growth and development
   f. Incorporating play and diversional activity into daily care

7. Invite a maternal-child nurse or nurse practitioner to speak to the class about his or her role, educational background, and experiences.

INTERACTIVE EXERCISES

1. Assign students to report, verbally or in writing, on the support systems/resources that are available within an affiliating agency or local community for pregnant families, neonates, infants, toddlers, preschoolers, school-age children, adolescents, and parents.

2. Working individually or in small groups, have students design a teaching plan for parents of infants, toddlers, preschool children, school-age children, and/or adolescents, based on a specific health need or concern of this age-group, incorporating cultural practices as appropriate. Have the students present the teaching plan to the class and/or to the target group of parents within an agency or community setting (e.g., school group).

3. Have students obtain an article from a nursing journal that focuses on a specific health need or concern associated with prenatal clients and/or children of this age-group (e.g., home safety, nutrition). Assign students to complete an oral and/or written report on an identified health need or concern for neonates, infants, toddlers, preschool children, school-age children, or adolescents.

4. Have students design activities and/or identify age-appropriate toys for infants, toddlers, preschool children, school-age children, and adolescents. (Piaget's stages of development may be used as a framework.)

5. Organize a role playing activity in which students simulate interactions with parents of newborns and infants, toddlers, preschool children, school-age children, and/or adolescents. Use the following, or similar, situations:
   a. A 3-year-old who is having surgery tomorrow
   b. A 6-month-old who requires numerous diagnostic tests
   c. A 5-year-old who will be having a series of injections
   d. A 2-year-old who has never been away from home and is hospitalized for an indefinite period of time
   e. A 9-year-old who has leukemia
   f. A 15-year-old who is newly diagnosed with diabetes mellitus
   g. An 18-year-old who has suffered extensive burns

CLIENT CARE EXPERIENCES

1. Have students assess and report on the developmental status and activities of clients in one or more of the following settings:
   a. Prenatal clinic
   b. Obstetrician's or pediatrician's office
   c. Day care center
   d. Preschool
   e. Well-baby clinic
   f. Elementary or high school

2. Assign students to observe and/or participate in the nursing care of prenatal clients, newborns, infants, toddlers, preschool children, school-age children, and adolescents in an acute care or community health setting. Discuss the experience with the group, focusing on the specific nursing interventions implemented for these clients and families.

3. Guide students in the application of the nursing process for prenatal clients, neonates, infants, toddlers, preschool children, school-age children, and/or adolescents. Working individually or in small groups, have students identify the following:
   a. Nursing diagnoses
   b. Long-term and short-term goals and desired client outcomes
   c. Nursing interventions
   d. Evaluation criteria/measures

RESOURCES FOR STUDENT ACTIVITIES

Comparative assessment: neonate to adolescent
Assessment of hospitalized child
Lifestyle questionnaire for school-age children

COMPARATIVE ASSESSMENT: NEONATE TO ADOLESCENT

Assessment Area	Neonate	Infant	Toddler	Preschool Child	School-Age Child	Adolescent
Physical Development						
Cognitive Development						
Psychosocial Aspects						
Health Concerns						
Health Promotion Activities						

Chapter 10: Conception Through Adolescence   37

	Assessment Data
Developmental Stage	
Response to Hospitalization	
History of Prior Illness, Hospitalization, Separation	
Medical History	
Perception of Illness (if able to obtain)	
Available Support Systems	

Date _____

Child's first name _____

Child's age _____ Grade _____

Lifestyle Questionnaire for School-Age Children*

Activities that promote health	Yes	No	Sometimes
1. I sleep at least 8 hours every night.			
2. I brush my teeth twice a day.			
3. I visit the dentist every year.			
4. I watch less than 2 hours of TV every day.			
5. I exercise (running, biking, swimming, active sports) one hour every day.			
6. I eat fruits.			
7. I eat vegetables.			
8. I limit my intake of salty snacks and high-sugar snacks.			
9. I have a physical examination every 2 or 3 years.			
10. I stay away from cigarettes.			
11. I stay away from alcohol.			

Injury prevention	Yes	No	Sometimes
12. I wear a seat belt in an automobile.			
13. I look both ways when crossing streets.			
14. I follow bike safety rules.			
15. I stay away from lighters or matches.			
16. I never ride ATVs (all-terrain vehicles).*			
17. I wear a helmet when I go on bike trips.			
18. I swim with a buddy.			
19. I wear a life jacket when I ride in a boat.			
20. I take medicine only with my parent's permission.			
21. I stay away from real guns.			
22. I tell my parents where I am going.			
23. I say "no" to drugs.			
24. Our home has a smoke detector that works.			
25. Our home has a fire extinguisher.			
26. If there is a fire, I know a safe way out of my house.			

Feelings	Yes	No	Sometimes
27. I think it is okay to cry.			
28. I enjoy my family.			
29. It is easy for me to fall asleep at night.			
30. My appetite is good.			
31. I like myself just the way I am.			

*The American Academy of Pediatrics recommends that children do not ride on these vehicles.

From Antwerp CV, Spaniolo AM: Checking out children's lifestyles, *MCN Am J Matern Child Nurs* 16(3):144, 1991.

CRITICAL THINKING EXERCISES

1. Mrs. Kim is attending a health clinic for newly pregnant mothers. A major area for discussion of health promotion is focused on teratogens. How should the nurse explain what a teratogen is and what types of exposure should be avoided? What types of lifestyle changes should be discussed?

2. Two-year-old Jamal has been admitted to the hospital because of pneumonia. His parents wish to participate in his care when they are present but will not be able to be with him continuously. The mother plans to spend the late evening and night at this hospital but will continue to work during the day. The father will visit on his way to work in the morning. Identify nursing measures that will minimize separation anxiety for Jamal.

3. Six-year-old Jackie has been admitted to the hospital for osteomyelitis of her right foot and is receiving intravenous antibiotic therapy. What strategies can the nurse use in her daily care to reduce her fears? How can the nurse establish a trusting relationship with Jackie?

4. Twelve-year-old Elizabeth is brought to the pediatric clinic for a physical examination. She is concerned about her lack of physical development compared to her peers. Discuss ways to educate Elizabeth about puberty and the variations that occur.

5. Fifteen-year-old Daniel is in skeletal traction with a fractured femur. Discuss ways to meet Daniel's needs for diversional activity.

ANSWERS TO CRITICAL THINKING EXERCISES

1. A teratogen is any agent capable of producing an adverse effect in the fetus. Some adverse effects occur only if the fetus is exposed to the teratogen during organ development. Types of exposure to avoid include German measles, herbs, home remedies, selected legal prescription drugs and over-the-counter drugs, and illegal substances. Drugs associated with fetal abnormalities include, but are not limited to, anticoagulants, anticonvulsants, barbiturates, antimicrobials, alcohol, chemotherapeutics, tobacco, LSD, and cocaine. Lifestyle changes to discuss include stopping any medications, remedies, and illegal drugs and quitting alcohol and tobacco use. Caffeine consumption should be limited, and diet should be reviewed.

2. Jamal's parents need to plan with the nurse for any departures. If possible, the nurse should be in the room to provide some support and distraction when the parents leave. The parents should tell Jamal about arrivals and departures based on terms that he can understand, such as "I'll be back before I go to work" or "I'll be back after work and I'll stay until breakfast." Nursing measures and suggestions to minimize separation anxiety include the following: Explain to the parents that protest is normal behavior and demonstrates a strong relationship with the parents. Encourage parents to leave some item that the child knows belongs to them because it will assure the child that they will return. Encourage bringing favorite toys from home or familiar objects such as a "special blanket" that provides comfort. Encourage telephone calls from family members to provide a link between home and hospital. Tape pictures of family members where the child can easily see them, and discuss the photographs with the child. Use cassette tape recordings of family members reading stories, singing, or talking to provide comfort in their absence.

40   Unit 2: Caring Throughout the Life Span

3. Strategies to reduce fears begin with an understanding of the school-age child's development. At this age, fears include physical disability, loss of support systems, and changes in body image. The child can be assisted in coping by allowing her to feel a sense of control. Things such as bed time and bath time may be decided by Jackie in an effort to allow her to feel that she has some control over her situation. Jackie should be helped to sit up for physical assessments. For any procedures that she may be facing, a doll, parent, or staff member, if available, should be used to demonstrate what will happen to her. Jackie should be allowed to hold any equipment such as a stethoscope, and use it on a doll or parent. Any sensations that the child will feel should be described (e.g., the x-ray table will feel cold). Toys such as molding clay, percussion instruments, and pounding toys will allow Jackie an opportunity to release pent-up anger and frustration. Therapeutic play should be allowed, especially in a designated playroom that is safe from any medical procedures. Trust can begin to be established by the child observing friendly interaction between the nurse and parents before she is approached. The child should be approached at eye level, and communication should begin first with a stuffed animal or doll. Extended eye contact and broad smiles should be avoided. The nurse should appear confident and unhurried. If possible, parents should be included in the initial admitting activities.

4. It is important to first establish what changes Elizabeth thinks should be happening to herself at this point. The nurse must understand the importance of being like one's peers at this age. Discussion of the types of changes and the patterns that ensue may be one method of confirming and reassuring her normalcy. Elizabeth may not recognize changes that have already taken place within her own body. Showing Elizabeth her own personal growth curve can help to reassure her about her own changes.

5. Identify areas of interest for Daniel. Diversional activities should be designed around his areas of interest. Cognitive development can be stimulated through reading books of interest. Hand-held computer games also might help. Enlist the help of parents or peers to encourage visits from others. It may be helpful to develop a type of schedule to eliminate times of too many or too few visitors. Provide for time to watch television or videos. Do not forget to ask Daniel if he would like to help plan activities.

Young to Middle Adult

Chapter

11

CLASSROOM DISCUSSION

1. Discuss the theories related to young and middle adulthood and how the nurse may apply them to clinical situations.

2. Ask students to identify how young and middle adults manifest their cultural backgrounds and practices.

3. Review the developmental tasks and health perceptions that may be associated with young and middle adults.

4. Review growth and development of the young and middle adult. Identify or ask students to identify the following for the young and middle adult:
   a. Characteristics of physical, cognitive, and psychosocial development
   b. Specific health and psychosocial concerns
   c. Risk factors and health promotion/safety activities

5. Discuss tasks and concerns associated with the young adult, including career, finances, marriage, parenthood, establishment of a family, and care of older parents.

6. Provide an overview of pregnancy and the development of the childbearing family. Identify and/or ask students to identify specific health needs and concerns for the childbearing family.

7. Stimulate a discussion on different lifestyles of the young adult family, such as single parenting, homosexual relationships/parenting, and dual-income families.

8. Discuss the specific health risks associated with the young and middle adult.

9. Invite an nurse practitioner who works with adults to speak to the class about his or her role, educational background, and experiences dealing with this age-group and their specific health needs.

10. Ask students to discuss the concept of a "mid-life crisis" and how it may affect an individual.

11. Ask students from this age-group to share their own experiences in dealing with families, children, employment, school, and other lifestyle decisions and responsibilities.

INTERACTIVE EXERCISES

1. Assign students to report, verbally or in writing, on selected support services or resources that are available within an affiliating agency or the community for young and middle adults.

2. Have students obtain examples from the Internet, nursing journals, or other media resources related to the stressors that may be prevalent in the lives of young and middle adults, such as industry downsizing and unemployment, and two parents working and managing child care.

3. Assign students to complete an oral and/or written report on an identified health need or risk factor associated with young and middle adulthood (e.g., the need for breast and testicular self-examination).

4. Arrange for students to observe young or middle adults at a health screening, clinic, childbirth class, or community activity (e.g., PTA meeting) and report on the type of interactions and communication patterns that were demonstrated.

5. Working individually or in small groups, have the students design and present a teaching plan based on a specific health need of this age-group.

CLIENT CARE EXPERIENCES

1. Assign students to observe and/or participate in the nursing care of young and middle adult clients in an acute care, rehabilitation, or community health setting. Discuss the experience with the group, focusing on the specific nursing interventions implemented for these clients.

2. Guide students in the application of the nursing process for young and middle adult clients. Working individually or in small groups, have students identify the following, specific for an actual young or middle adult client and/or case study situation (incorporating cultural practices, as appropriate):
   a. Nursing diagnoses
   b. Long-term or short-term goals and desired client outcomes
   c. Nursing interventions
   d. Evaluation criteria/measures

General assessment: young to middle adult

GENERAL ASSESSMENT: YOUNG TO MIDDLE ADULT

| AGE: | HEIGHT: |
| SEX: | WEIGHT: |

	Description/Comparison to Norms
Physiological Development	
Cognitive Development	
Psychosocial Development	
Career/Job-Related Activities	
Health Concerns/Health Promotion Activities	
Leisure Activities	

CRITICAL THINKING EXERCISES

1. Joan K. is a 24-year-old woman who smokes two packs of cigarettes a day. She began smoking when she was 14 years old. Joan complains to the nurse at the clinic, " I just can't seem to kick the habit no matter how hard I try." What information does the nurse need to know to assist Joan in quitting smoking?

2. James D., age 48, married, and the father of 13- and 16-year-old sons has recently had to assume the responsibility of caring for his 78-year-old mother after she suffered a stroke. Describe the nurse's role in assisting James in caring for his mother.

ANSWERS TO CRITICAL THINKING EXERCISES

1. A thorough assessment needs to be conducted by the nurse to determine whether Joan is really determined to quit smoking, what methods Joan has tried in the past to quit smoking, and what resources Joan has to assist her to quit smoking. Young adults are continually evolving and adjusting to changes at home, in the workplace, and in their personal lives. The nurses should consider factors that may affect Joan's compliance with any regimen that may be decided upon to help her quit smoking. These factors include Joan's educational level, socioeconomic factors, motivation to quit smoking, home and work environment (particularly related to others around her that smoke), and what support Joan will have from her family and friends to quit smoking. The nurse should also assist Joan in changing her lifestyle habit of smoking by providing education to Joan about the risk for health problems related to smoking and options for Joan to consider in her efforts to quit smoking. The nurse should also provide support for Joan in her efforts to quit smoking and to remain compliant with the chosen treatment regimen.

2. James, as with many middle adults, is in the "sandwich generation," caught between the responsibilities of caring for dependent children and for aging parents. James will need assistance in his transition to the new role of "caregiver" for his mother, while continuing to provide for his wife and children. The nurse can assist James in identifying the complexity of health needs of his mother and determining the availability of health and community resources. The nurse should also assess family relationships and determine the perceptions of how the responsibility of caring for James's mother will impact existing relationships within James' nuclear family. Provision of support in James decision making regarding the health care needs of his mother is critical for James's own sense of well-being.

Older Adult

CLASSROOM DISCUSSION

1. Discuss the demographics of the aging population and their relationship to health care delivery.

2. Review myths and stereotypes associated with the older adult and the aging process. Have students bring in media examples of how these are perpetuated in society.

3. Discuss the biological and psychosocial theories of aging and how the nurse may apply them in interactions with older adult clients.

4. Ask students to identify the developmental tasks and psychosocial changes specific to the older adult life stage (e.g., retirement, isolation, death).

5. Review growth and development for the older adult. Identify and/or ask students to identify the following:
   a. Characteristics of physical, cognitive, and psychosocial development
   b. Specific health and psychosocial concerns
   c. Risk factors, perceptions of health, and health promotion/safety activities

6. Discuss the differences between normal physiological aging and pathological changes.

7. Invite a gerontologic nurse practitioner to speak to the class about his or her role, educational background, and experiences with older adults.

8. Invite a senior citizen to speak to the class about societal changes and health care concerns.

9. Discuss the experience with the group, focusing on the specific nursing interventions implemented for the older adult (see Resource for Student Activities, p. 48). Stimulate a discussion on the societal influences that currently affect older adults, including changes in the workforce, health care coverage (Medicare), housing, and access to the community and its resources.

10. Discuss specific nursing interventions that may be implemented for older adults, including the following:
    a. Therapeutic communication
    b. Touch
    c. Reality orientation
    d. Resocialization
    e. Validation
    f. Reminiscence
    g. Body image therapy

INTERACTIVE EXERCISES

1. Assign students to report, verbally or in writing, on the support systems and resources and health care services that are available in the affiliating agency or community for the older adult.

2. Working individually or in small groups, have students design a teaching plan for a group of older adults, based on a specific health need or concern. Have the students present the teaching plan to the class and/or to the target group within an agency or community setting.

3. Assign students to complete a brief oral and/or written report on an identified health need or psychosocial change associated with older adults.

4. Organize an "empathetic experience" for the students to simulate the physiological and pathological changes associated with aging. Use the following or other similar ideas:
   a. Place pebbles in the shoes and bind the hands and feet to simulate arthritis
   b. Rub petroleum jelly on eyeglasses to simulate cataracts
   c. Limit mobility with the use of a cane, a walker, or other assistive devices
   d. Apply earmuffs to reduce auditory input and put gloves on the hands to reduce tactile sensation

5. Have students observe and report on the activities and interactions of older clients in a community setting, such as at a senior citizen center or housing complex, health screening agency, or a day care center.

CLIENT CARE EXPERIENCES

1. Assign students to observe and/or participate in the nursing care of older adults in an acute care, extended care or nursing home, rehabilitation, or community setting.

2. Guide students in the application of the nursing process for older adult clients, incorporating cultural practices as appropriate. Working individually or in small groups, have the students identify the following, specific for an older adult client and/or case study example:
   a. Nursing diagnoses
   b. Long-term or short-term goals and desired client outcomes
   c. Nursing interventions
   d. Evaluation criteria/measures

Specific interventions for the older adult

SPECIFIC INTERVENTIONS FOR THE OLDER ADULT

	Interventions
Home Safety	
Nutrition	
Medication Administration	
Exercise	
Socialization	
Access to Resources	

CRITICAL THINKING EXERCISES

1. Mr. Brown, age 73, has come to the clinic for a routine check of his blood pressure and cholesterol level. The policy of the clinic is to review all medications at every clinic visit. What concerns related to safe medication use will you discuss with Mr. Brown?

2. Mrs. Shephard's daughter has come with her to the clinic. She is concerned about her mother's memory. She tells you that although her mother's memory is usually excellent with only occasional forgetting of names or the location of keys, this has suddenly changed. Two days ago Mrs. Shephard phoned her daughter six times in two hours asking where her husband (the late Mr. Shephard) was and when told of his death four years ago denied this fact. When her daughter arrived at her house to check on her, she found that Mrs. Shephard had emptied the contents of all the closets onto the floor and accused her daughter of theft. Mrs. Shephard has spent the last two nights at her daughter's house for safety. Suspecting delirium, what biophysiological areas and conditions should you consider as potentially reversible causes?

3. On her visit to the clinic you note that Mrs. Johnson, a frail 86-year-old, has lost 15 pounds since her visit 1 month ago. Mrs. Johnson lives alone now since the death of her husband 2 months ago. Her children live out of town. What areas will you include in your assessment?

ANSWERS TO CRITICAL THINKING EXERCISES

1. Basic knowledge: Does he know the names and reasons for use of all of his medications?
   Does he have the names of the medications written down (with dosages)?
   Does he take medicine prescribed by more than one doctor?
   Does he take over-the-counter medications in addition to his prescription drugs?

   Use as prescribed: How does he take his medications?
   Why are they not taken as prescribed? (Reasons such as availability or side effects?)

   Knowledge of precautions and warnings: Possible side effects
   When to call the doctor or clinic

2. Metabolic: Electrolyte imbalance (dehydration, hypokalemia)
   Hypoglycemia or hyperglycemia
   Medication side effects

   Structural: Cerebrovascular accident or stroke
   Subdural hematoma (head injury after an unreported fall)

   Infectious: Pneumonia
   Urinary tract infection

3. Nutrition (daily food intake, access to food supplies, ability to prepare meals)
   Dental (condition of teeth/dentures, tongue, gums)
   Depression (possible social isolation, recent death of spouse)
   Memory (forgetting to eat, forgetting how to prepare food)
   Medications (causing anorexia, nausea, vomiting, diarrhea)
   Cancer (ask standard screening questions)

Critical Thinking and Nursing Judgment

Chapter

13

CLASSROOM DISCUSSION

1. Provide a definition for critical thinking, including the inherent skills, aspects (reflection, language, and intuition), and levels (basic, complex, and commitment).

2. Discuss the components and concepts of the critical thinking model presented:
    a. Specific knowledge base
    b. Experience
    c. Competencies
    d. Attitudes
    e. Standards

    Have students give examples of actual activities that may occur with each phase.

3. Share personal nursing situations with the students in which inferences were made about the client and actions taken were based on professional knowledge and experience.

4. Using a case study or actual client situation, have students discuss how they would adapt the environment and nursing care to meet the client's specific individual needs.

5. Using one or more of the following examples, have students identify what the nurse may expect to find and what questions need to be answered for a client experiencing the following:
    a. Acute pain
    b. Incontinence
    c. Dyspnea
    d. A reddened skin area
    e. Hypotension

6. Stimulate a discussion on what resources could be used in health care settings if an emergency situation (e.g., hurricane) existed, and there was no running water or power and supplies were dwindling.

7. Discuss how critical thinking and the nursing process "mesh" together. *Guide students through the steps of the nursing process, providing examples of critical thinking throughout. Demonstrate how the use of clinical inferences and accurate diagnostic reasoning leads to successful clinical decision making.

    * The critical thinking model is used throughout the text, in coordination with the nursing process, as a basis for client care experiences. Practice in its application may help to enhance future learning and clinical problem solving.

INTERACTIVE EXERCISES

1. Have students complete a flow sheet that follows a common decision-making process, such as buying a car (see Resources for Student Activities, p. 54).

2. Have students write about or present the concept of creativity in nursing care using the following, or a similar, situation: A client with frequent memory lapses requires numerous oral medications at home and does not have the financial resources to purchase commercially available assistive devices.

3. Arrange an individual or group exercise for students to use critical thinking skills. Set up stations in classrooms or skill laboratories where the students encounter one of the following, or similar, client situations:
   a. The "client" (student volunteer or mannequin) is found lying on the floor beside the bed.
   b. There are discrepancies in the medication orders and the available supplies.
   c. An incorrect IV solution is hanging, running at the wrong rate, dripping, and/or infusing into an area with phlebitis or infiltration.
   d. The client states a difficulty—discomfort, difficulty breathing, or dizziness.

   Have students identify, verbally or in writing, the nursing actions that should be taken in these situations. Discuss the activity in a "debriefing" session.

CLIENT CARE EXPERIENCE

1. Provide the students with a client assignment in an acute, long-term, or home care setting. Have students prioritize the assignment and discuss the rationale for their decisions.

RESOURCES FOR STUDENT ACTIVITIES

Critical thinking flow chart
Decision-making process
Critical thinking model

CRITICAL THINKING FLOW CHART

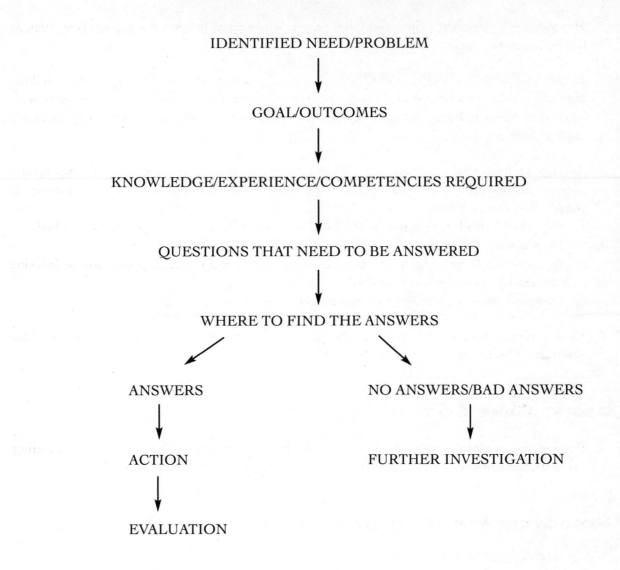

IDENTIFIED NEED/PROBLEM

↓

GOAL/OUTCOMES

↓

KNOWLEDGE/EXPERIENCE/COMPETENCIES REQUIRED

↓

QUESTIONS THAT NEED TO BE ANSWERED

↓

WHERE TO FIND THE ANSWERS

ANSWERS   NO ANSWERS/BAD ANSWERS

↓   ↓

ACTION   FURTHER INVESTIGATION

↓

EVALUATION

Outside influences: time, money, resources, people involved, environment

Steps	Application Examples
1. Recognize and define the problem or situation	
2. Assess all options	
3. Weigh each option vs. criteria	
4. Test possible options	
5. Consider the consequences of the decision	
6. Make the final decision	

CRITICAL THINKING MODEL

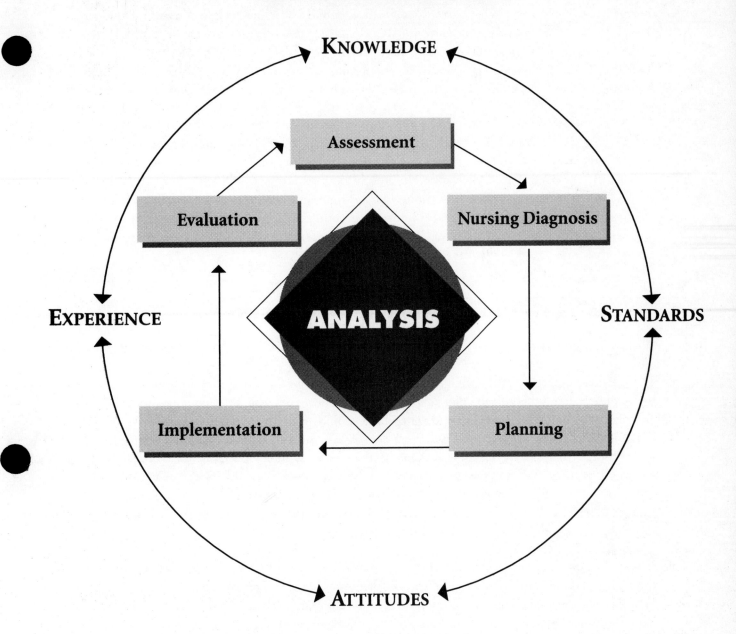

CRITICAL THINKING EXERCISES

1. Select a day and write a journal entry describing any one of the following experiences *that stimulated your thinking:* an interaction you had with a client, an interaction you had with your spouse or one of your children, or an interaction you had with someone you were trying to help. For the entry, discuss each of the following:
   a. Describe, as thoroughly as you can, what you did.
   b. Describe your decision-making process.
   c. Describe what you would do differently when a similar incident occurs.
   d. Describe your strengths and weaknesses in dealing with the situation. Identify your thoughts, perceptions, and feelings.

Chapter 13: Critical Thinking and Nursing Judgment   55

2. Mrs. Stein returns to the clinic for a 1-month follow-up. She was placed on an 1800-calorie diet during her previous visit. Her current weight is 3 pounds over her weight 1 month ago. Mrs. Stein's explanation of her eating pattern reveals that her calorie intake is much too high. The nurse begins to again describe the importance of the 1800-calorie diet and the types of foods that Mrs. Stein should eat. The client seems inattentive as the nurse gives an explanation. What approach to problem solving might the nurse take to better understand Mrs. Stein's situation?

3. Mr. Spicer is a terminally ill client. His wife and son are asking you about the type of pain control he is receiving. Mrs. Spicer is asking that the physician increase her husband's medication, even if it means he will not be responsive. She does not want her husband to suffer. The son is vehemently opposed to too much narcotic, feeling that his father is still able to make decisions for himself. Mr. Spicer remains alert much of the time and is able to talk with you about his feelings regarding death. He seems to appreciate your availability in talking with him. How might you apply the critical thinking attitudes of fairness, responsibility, and creativity in this case study?

ANSWERS TO CRITICAL THINKING EXERCISES

1. Write a journal entry.

2. The nurse assumes that Mrs. Stein has been able to follow her diet and that additional information will help her adhere to the diet. The nurse has made a conclusion quickly. Critical thinking and problem solving go hand in hand. The nurse should consider all possible factors that might influence Mrs. Stein's appetite (e.g., stress, depression, or even planned family activities). The nurse should then do a thorough, systematic assessment with Mrs. Stein. For example, open questions such as "Tell me how you are doing with your new diet," followed by "What do you see as the reason for having difficulty following the diet?" may reveal the true problem. Precision and clarity will help the nurse not only identify the proper cause for Mrs. Stein's overeating but also determine the most appropriate strategy for diet adherence.

3. It is important that you remain an advocate for Mr. Spicer, while at the same time listening to the concerns voiced by both Mrs. Spicer and her son. You are responsible for providing accurate information to the client and family regarding pain medications prescribed for Mr. Spicer. You also must communicate family and client choices to the physician. You should be creative by offering additional comfort options to Mr. Spicer and his family together to discuss the issue of pain control openly.

Nursing Assessment

Chapter 14

CLASSROOM DISCUSSION

1. Review the process and methodology of client assessment.

2. With the critical thinking approach, ask students to think about and identify what follow-up questions are necessary when a client states that he or she has a problem (e.g., pain, difficulty sleeping).

3. Discuss the difference between subjective and objective data.

4. Review the potential sources of data for accurate assessments. Ask students to determine the advantages and disadvantages of the different types of data and data sources.

5. Share personal experiences and techniques with the students about data collection and assessment in the clinical area.

6. Review the components of a nursing history.

7. Discuss the client interview, phases, and techniques. Provide examples of information that may be best obtained with problem-seeking, direct, and open-ended questions. Identify possible barriers and facilitators when conducting an interview.

8. Stimulate a discussion of how internal and external factors may influence nurse and client perceptions.

9. Discuss the purpose of and the techniques used in a physical examination.

10. Using pictures and/or videos of client situations or specific problems (e.g., decubitus ulcers, peripheral edema), ask students to make preliminary inferences and determine how the situations may be further investigated.

INTERACTIVE EXERCISES

1. Using a student "actor" portraying a variety of possible client situations (e.g., abdominal pain, limping, emotional upset), have students quickly assess what they observe. Provide students with a listing of possible client data and have them write or verbally identify which are objective and which are subjective.

2. Videotape or audiotape students conducting interviews with their peers. Individually, or in a group, critique the techniques used. Focus on areas that may have required additional clarification and/or barriers to the communication process. (Save tapes of student interviews for review as they proceed through the educational program.)

3. For the following diagnostic test results (or other selected examples), have students report, verbally and/or in writing, as to whether they are within normal limits and, if not, what the values may indicate:

   WBC = 35,000/mm^3
   RBC = 3.5 million/mm^3
   Hematocrit = 32/100 ml
   Hemoglobin = 11.5 gm/100 ml
   Platelets = 70,000/mm^3
   BUN = 25 mg/100 ml
   Uric acid = 9 mg/100 ml
   Potassium = 4.2 mEq/L
   Urine specific gravity = 1.032

4. Have students work individually or in small groups to complete a written assessment on a student peer or from the case study below. An assessment tool specific to a nursing framework/theorist or health care facility may be used (see Resources for Student Activities, p. 59).
   a. Have students identify objective and subjective data.
   b. Have students cluster the collected data.

Case Study:

A 72-year-old woman has been admitted to the medical center with a diagnosis of congestive heart failure. She states that she came to this country with her son 5 years ago. She lives alone in a second floor apartment. Her son lives about 10 miles away and visits as often as possible, but "he works very hard and has a family of his own." The client has been independent up to this point but indicated that she becomes tired quickly after cleaning and shopping. Sometimes the client feels like her heart is "skipping." She has also been getting up in the middle of the night to urinate. The client speaks and understands both English (somewhat limited) and Spanish (fluent in speech, reading, and writing). The physician has prescribed Lanoxin 0.125 mg q.d., Lasix 40 mg b.i.d., and a 2-gm sodium diet. The client becomes slightly short of breath on exertion, experiences occasional memory lapses, and has 2+ edema of both lower extremities. Her vital signs are as follows: BP=150/94, T=98.4°F, P=68, R=18.

CLINICAL SKILL

1. Demonstrate the techniques, and then have students practice inspection, palpation, percussion, and auscultation on each other.

CLIENT CARE EXPERIENCES

1. Using Gordon's functional health patterns or another nursing framework, have students complete a focused assessment of a particular system or problem for an assigned client.

2. Assign students to do a brief interview with an actual client (with or without an assessment tool), and have them return to discuss their findings and feelings as a group.

Focus on verbal and nonverbal communication patterns.

RESOURCES FOR STUDENT ACTIVITIES

Assessment according to Gordon's functional health patterns
Physical assessment beginning practice tool
Nursing health history
Admission form

ASSESSMENT ACCORDING TO GORDON'S FUNCTIONAL HEALTH PATTERNS

Health Pattern	Client Status
Health Perception – Health Management	
Nutritional – Metabolic	
Elimination	
Activity – Exercise	
Cognitive – Perceptual	
Sleep – Rest	
Self-Perception – Self-Concept	
Role – Relationship	
Sexuality – Reproductive	
Coping – Stress – Tolerance	
Value – Belief	

From Gordon M: *Nursing diagnosis: process and application*, ed 3, St. Louis, 1994, Mosby.

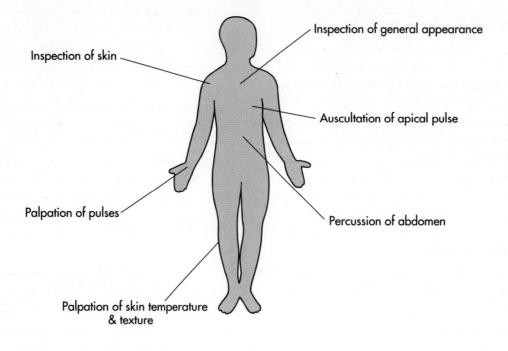

Inspection of general appearance

Inspection of skin

Auscultation of apical pulse

Palpation of pulses

Percussion of abdomen

Palpation of skin temperature & texture

NURSING HEALTH HISTORY

BIOGRAPHICAL INFORMATION

Name _____ Sex _____ Date _____

Address _____

Family member or significant other name _____

Address/phone number _____

Marital status _____ Religious preference/practices _____

Occupation _____

Length of occupation _____

Health care provider _____

Insurance _____

Reason for seeking health care _____

PRESENT ILLNESS

Onset _____ Sudden or gradual _____

Duration _____

Symptoms _____

Precipitating factors _____

Relief measures _____

Expectations of health care providers _____

PAST HISTORY

Illnesses: Childhood _____

            Illnesses & hospitalizations _____

            Operations _____

            Major illnesses _____

Allergies: Type _____

            Reaction _____

            Treatment _____

Immunizations _____

Habits: Alcohol _____ Smoking _____ Drugs _____

            Duration _____

Medications: Prescribed _____

            Self-medicated _____

Sleep patterns _____

Exercise patterns _____

Nutritional patterns _____

Work patterns _____

FAMILY HISTORY

Health of parents, siblings, spouse, children _____

Risk factor analysis: cancer, heart disease, diabetes mellitus, kidney disease, hypertension, mental disorders

_____

Environmental History

Cleanliness ——————————————————————————————

Hazards ——————————————————————————————

Pollutants ——————————————————————————————

Psychosocial/Cultural History

Primary language ——————————————————————————

Cultural activities/social group ———————————————————

Community resources ———————————————————————

Mood ——————————————————————————————

Developmental stage ————————————————————————

Review of Systems

Head:	Headaches ———————	Dizziness ————————
Vision:	Last eye exam —————————————————————	
	Glasses ———————	Contacts —————— (hard, soft, long wearing)
	Blurring ———————	Double vision ————————
	Pain ———————	Inflammation ————————
Hearing:	Impairment ———————	Type of hearing aid ————————
		Date of new batteries ————————
	Discharge/pain —————————————————	
Nose:	Allergic rhinitis ———————	Type of allergen ————————
		Relief measures ————————
	Frequency of colds/year ————————————————	
	History of polyps, fracture, surgery ————————————	
	Sinuses ———————————————————————	
	Nosebleeds ———————————————————————	
Throat & mouth:	Last dental exam —————————————————	
	Dentures ———————————————————————	
	Pain/bleeding —————————————————————	
	Speech disorders ————————————————————	
	Swallowing problems —————————————————	
Respiratory:	Cough ———————	Sputum/hemoptysis ————————
	Dyspnea ———————	Dyspnea on exertion ————————
	Pain —————————————————————————	
	Activity tolerance ———————————————————	
	Last chest x-ray —————————————————————	
Circulatory:	Pain ———————	Palpitations ————————
	Edema ———— Numbness —————	Tingling ————————
	Changes in color/hair of extremities —————————	
	Syncope ———————	Dizziness ————————

Nutritional: Appetite _____

Nausea _____ Vomiting _____

Weight loss/gain _____

Elimination:

Bowel: Pattern _____ Use of laxatives _____

Constipation/diarrhea _____

Bleeding _____ Ostomy _____

Urine: Pattern _____ Medications _____

Incontinence _____ Infections _____

Hematuria _____ Catheter _____

Reproductive: Pregnancies _____ Children _____

Last Pap test _____ Results _____ LMP _____

Bleeding/discharge _____

Self-breast/testicular exam _____

Neurological: Orientation _____ Convulsions _____

Paralysis/paresthesia _____ Weakness _____

Incoordination _____ Headaches _____

Musculoskeletal: Pain _____ Stiffness _____

Deformity _____

Exercise patterns _____

Integument: Color _____ Turgor _____

Texture _____ Temperature _____

Rashes/lesions _____

Vital Signs: Temperature _____ Pulse _____

Respirations _____ BP _____

ADMISSION FORM

BARNES HOSPITAL ST. LOUIS, MISSOURI		
Person to Contact:	Emergency Phone:	

Why you came to the hospital?

Allergies (food, drugs, latex, environment)?

Items brought in from home? ☐ Medications ☐ Dentures ☐ Contacts ☐ Glasses ☐ Hearing Aid	Did you bring: ☐ Money ☐ Jewelry ☐ Credit Cards ☐ Checkbook/Checks ☐ Other _____ *(These need to be locked up with security or sent home. Hospital will not be responsible for valuables left in room)*

	MEDICINE NAMES	Dose & How Often Taken	Reason You Take Medicine	Time of Last Dose
Prescribed by a Doctor				
Non-Prescription				

Do you have any problems with your medicines?

Do you smoke? ☐ Yes ☐ No Do you chew tobacco? ☐ Yes ☐ No	Do you use "street" drugs? ☐ Yes ☐ No How much alcohol do you drink? _____	How much caffeine do you drink or eat? _____

Medical History: ☐ Epilepsy ☐ Cancer ☐ Chicken Pox/Shingles ☐ Menstrual Disease
☐ Heart Disease ☐ Stroke ☐ Hepatitis ☐ Fainting/Dizzy Spells ☐ Circulation Problems
☐ Lung Disease ☐ Diabetes ☐ High Blood Pressure ☐ Stomach Problems ☐ Swelling
☐ Liver Disease ☐ TB ☐ Rheumatic Disease ☐ Bladder Problems ☐ Bleeding
☐ Immune Disorders ☐ Sexually Transmitted Disease: _____
☐ Other _____

HISTORY COMMENTS:

Could you be pregnant? ☐ Yes ☐ No	When was your last period? _____

What surgeries or procedures have you had? (Date)

Family Health History: ☐ Hypertension ☐ Diabetes ☐ Heart Disease ☐ Stroke ☐ Cancer ☐ Other _____

Which of the following have you had in the past 12 months?
☐ Self Breast Exam ☐ Prostate Check ☐ Glaucoma Check ☐ Rectal Check (over 40) ☐ Dental Exam
☐ Mammogram (over 40) ☐ Testicular Check ☐ Pelvic Exam ☐ Hearing Check ☐ Vision Check

Are your immunizations current? ☐ Yes ☐ No ☐ Unknown
(Call ID Specialist)

(Courtesy Barnes-Jewish Hospital, St. Louis, MO.)

64 Unit 3: Critical Thinking in Nursing Practice

Are you on a special diet?	How is your appetite?
Any foods you can't eat and why?	Any difficulty eating or swallowing?
Nutritional supplements/or diet substitutions (e.g., vitamins, artificial sweeteners, salt substitutes)	Weight loss/gain (amount) in the last 12 months?

How often do you have a BM?
Do you have any difficulty having a bowel movement?
☐ use laxatives   ☐ hemorrhoids
☐ use stool softeners   ☐ black/tarry

Do you have any difficulty urinating?

☐ burning   ☐ blood   ☐ leaking   ☐ frequency

Do you tire easily?   ☐ Yes   ☐ No

Do you get regular exercise?   ☐ Yes ☐ No
What kind? _____   How often? _____

Have you fallen recently?   ☐ Yes   ☐ No

What activities do you need help with?
☐ Feeding/eating   ☐ Meal preparation   ☐ Walking on level surfaces
☐ Dressing   ☐ Transportation   ☐ Walking on stairs
☐ Grooming/bathing   ☐ Housework   ☐ Paying for medicines
☐ Taking medications   ☐ Handling finances
☐ Toileting   ☐ Grocery shopping
☐ Moving/positioning   (RN consider appropriate consults)

Aides used at home:
☐ Eye glasses   ☐ Contact lenses
☐ Hearing aid   ☐ Cane
☐ Walker   ☐ Wheelchair
☐ Prosthesis: _____
DENTURES: ☐ Upper   ☐ Lower
PARTIALS: ☐ Upper   ☐ Lower

Is it difficult for you to carry out prescribed health care regimens (Diet, Activity, Medications)?   ☐ Yes   ☐ No
If YES, explain:

How much sleep do you normally get?

What helps you fall asleep?

Who do you live with?   ☐ Alone   ☐ Spouse only   ☐ Family   ☐ Friends   ☐ Nursing Home

Who helps you at home?   ☐ Spouse   ☐ Family   ☐ Friends   ☐ Home Health   ☐ Visiting Nurse

Do you have concerns about your family while you are in the hospital?

What major changes have you had in your life in the past 12 months?

Do you feel you deal successfully with stress?   ☐ Yes   ☐ No   Would you like additional resources?   ☐ Yes   ☐ No

Do you have concerns that your illness/hospitalization will affect:
☐ appearance   ☐ job   ☐ male/female roles   ☐ how you feel about yourself

Is religion important in your life?   ☐ Yes   ☐ No   Will this illness/hospitalization interfere with any religious beliefs/practices?   ☐ Yes   ☐ No

What do you expect from us while in the hospital?

Do you have a Living Will?   ☐ Yes   ☐ No   Do you have a Power of Attorney?   ☐ Yes   ☐ No
Do you have a copy with you?   ☐ Yes   ☐ No

Patient/Significant Other Signature: Relationship:	Date	Staff Signature: Title:	Date

☐ REVIEWED BY REGISTERED NURSE   SIGNATURE: DATE:

TO BE COMPLETED BY STAFF ONLY

Patient provided: ☐ Admit kit   ☐ ID band   ☐ Sensitivity/Allergy band on patient   ☐ Allergy sticker on chart
Patient instructed: ☐ Valuables policy   ☐ Waiver signed   ☐ Smoking   ☐ Visitation
☐ Nursing call/Emergency   ☐ TV/phone   ☐ Fall precautions/band on wrist
☐ Patient's rights/responsibilities   ☐ Received copy of Personal Directions for My Healthcare

Time patient arrived on Division: _____   SIGNATURE: _____

Chapter 14: Nursing Assessment   65

CRITICAL THINKING EXERCISES

1. Mrs. Kinsey is a 61-year-old woman who is being seen at home following hospitalization for her arthritis. She greets you at the door, and you enter the home. The two of you sit down at the kitchen table. You notice many unwashed dishes in the sink, and the counter is covered with stacks of mail. On the kitchen table are six bottles of medication. What inferences might you make from your observations? How might you assess the client to gather more objective information about her health status?

2. Miss Fong has been assigned to your care for the first time. The nurse from the previous shift tells you she had surgery on her left lower leg and has a very large bandage. During the night she required an analgesic to help her sleep. She is able to drink liquids without nausea. You know that one of your responsibilities is to do an assessment of the client's condition. What are three priorities you would focus assessment on?

3. Mr. Rossi comes to the clinic with the following history: for the last 3 days he has had ringing in his ears and dizziness. Within the last 24 hours he has experienced nausea and headache as well. Identify three different open-ended questions that will prompt Mr. Rossi to discuss his condition.

ANSWERS TO CRITICAL THINKING EXERCISES

1. The client may be having trouble with activities of daily living, excessive fatigue, and some memory impairments. You may want to begin by obtaining information about the client's usual activity status. The client may be very active but does not like to do dishes or housework. You may want to ask questions about pain and mobility in relation to arthritis. It may be difficult for her to open mail.

2. Pain: presence, intensity, factors that relieve pain, effect of analgesia, factors that worsen pain

   Left lower leg: circulation, color, surgical site integrity

   Adequacy of sleep: does the client feel rested?

3. "What can you tell me about your dizziness and ringing in the ears?"

   "Tell me about your headache."

   "What makes these symptoms worse or better?"

Nursing Diagnosis

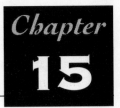

CLASSROOM DISCUSSION

1. Discuss the evolution of nursing diagnosis and the development and role of NANDA.

   Review how nursing diagnoses are developed and added to the NANDA listing and how those general diagnoses may be used with clients.

2. Present the process by which the collection, clustering, and analysis of data leads to nursing diagnosis.

3. Demonstrate the correct format for nursing diagnoses.

4. Ask students to identify the difference between medical and nursing diagnoses.

5. Identify possible sources of diagnostic error and ways in which the nurse may avoid such errors.

6. Have students identify possible assessment data and related factors for sample nursing diagnoses.

INTERACTIVE EXERCISES

1. Provide examples of properly and improperly formulated nursing diagnoses, and have students critique and correct the statements, if indicated.

2. Working individually or in small groups, have students formulate nursing diagnoses based on an assessment of a student peer, assigned client, and/or case study situation (see Chapter 14, p. 58). Have students record and select the nursing diagnoses on actual health care agency documentation forms.

CLIENT CARE EXPERIENCE

1. For an assigned client, have students complete an assessment and identify one or more nursing diagnoses. Discuss the assessment findings and diagnoses in the postclinical conference.

NURSING DIAGNOSIS WORKSHEET #1

Assessment Data	Samples of Nursing Diagnoses	Related Factors
	Fluid volume deficit	
	Nutrition, altered: less than or more than body requirements	
	Knowledge deficit	
	Impaired skin integrity	
	Constipation	
	Pain, chronic	

NURSING DIAGNOSIS WORKSHEET #2

Assessment Data	Diagnostic Label	Related Factors

CRITICAL THINKING EXERCISES

1. Your client's nursing Kardex contains a care plan for bathing/hygiene and toileting self-care deficit related to decreased mobility of right arm. What data do you need from the assessment database to determine whether the nursing diagnosis is relevant?

2. Using a client's assessment cluster data from the history and physical examination components, identify which trends are fully supported by data and which trends need more data. (Using multicolored highlighters can assist with this exercise.)

3. How do you organize assessment data to derive nursing diagnoses that reflect client response to illness, hospitalization, and lifestyle changes?

ANSWERS TO CRITICAL THINKING EXERCISES

1. You need a history of previous upper arm strength and mobility, history of injuries, chronic illnesses, and surgeries to affected area.

2. Obtain a completed assessment from clinical area or previous assignment and highlight data clusters.

3. Organization can be through a systems approach or functional patterns, or you can follow the organization of an assessment form from a clinical agency. Be sure that the organization includes all dimensions of the client and not just the physiological aspects.

Planning for Nursing Care

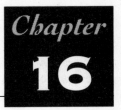

Chapter

16

CLASSROOM DISCUSSION

1. Discuss how planning follows from assessment and nursing diagnosis and what is incorporated in the planning stage of the process.

2. Discuss prioritizing and its importance. Have students prioritize a series of client experiences according to Maslow's hierarchy of needs.

3. Present information on client-centered goals and outcomes:
   a. Involvement of client and family
   b. Focus in different health care settings
   c. Difference between long-term and short-term goals
   d. Difference and relationship between goals and expected outcomes
   e. Format for documenting goals and outcomes

4. Discuss what difficulties may be encountered in developing client goals and outcomes.

5. Explain nurse-initiated, physician-initiated, and collaborative interventions, and provide examples.

6. Ask students to identify what the nurse needs to be aware of or possible questions on a physician's order.

7. Discuss how the Nursing Interventions Classification (NIC) project may be used in nursing education, practice, research, and costing.

8. Review the different formats for documenting the nursing process, including nursing care plans, critical pathways, and patient-focused care. Discuss the differences and similarities that may be found in varied health care settings.

9. Present the components that are included in the documentation of nursing interventions.

10. Guide students, using overheads, the blackboard, or handouts, through the process of assessment, nursing diagnosis, and planning with an actual or case study client situation. Focus on the factors involved in the selection of nursing interventions.

11. Discuss the role of consultation and the use of a consultant as part of the nursing process.

   Invite an actual or potential nursing consultant (e.g., an ostomy nurse or pediatric nurse specialist) to speak to the class about his or her role.

INTERACTIVE EXERCISES

1. Provide students with properly and improperly written client goals and outcomes, and have them critique and correct them, if indicated.

2. Have students identify types of interventions (nurse-initiated, physician-initiated, or collaborative) from a list that includes examples of each type.

3. Organize a debate or discussion on the advantages and disadvantages of standardized forms and care plans.

4. Assign students to attend a workshop, program, or demonstration of a computerized nursing care plan documentation system, as available.

5. Provide students with properly and improperly written nursing interventions, and have the students critique and correct them, as indicated.

6. Working individually or in small groups, have students identify long-term and short-term client-centered goals, expected outcomes, and nursing interventions based upon the nursing diagnoses that were formulated for a student peer assessment and/or case study situation.

CLIENT CARE EXPERIENCE

1. Have students identify long-term and short-term client-centered goals, expected outcomes, and nursing interventions based upon the nursing diagnoses that were formulated for the client assignment.

RESOURCES FOR STUDENT ACTIVITIES

Multi disciplinary critical pathway sample form
Kardex care plan
(Refer to Chapters 14 and 15 for additional tools.)

Medical Diagnosis (Code): **Expected Length of Stay:**

Nursing Diagnosis/Client Need:

Expected Outcomes:

Interventions	1st Day (Date)	2nd Day (Date)	3rd Day (Date)
Nursing			
Treatments			
Medications			
Diagnostic Tests			
Diet Therapy			
Consults/Referrals			
Teaching/Discharge Needs			

Nursing Diagnosis/Client Problem	Expected Outcomes	Nursing Interventions

CRITICAL THINKING EXERCISES

1. How do you link goals and expected outcomes of nursing care from nursing diagnoses?

2. What criteria do you use to determine expected outcomes for a given set of client-centered goals?

3. What criteria do you use to select interventions?
   a. What client cultural information is needed?
   b. What health care resource information is needed?
   c. What assessments do you make regarding your competency to perform a specific skill?

ANSWERS TO CRITICAL THINKING EXERCISES

1. Measurable criteria are used to determine when the client's need or problem that generated the nursing diagnosis is resolved. Nursing diagnoses form the basis for the goals of care. Return to the nursing diagnosis developed for Mr. Brown (Table 15-4, p. 319 of *Canadian Fundamentals of Nursing*, Second Edition), and develop goals and expected outcomes.
   Diarrhea related to irritation:
       Goal: Return to normal bowel function by 1 month
       Expected outcomes: Stool formed and soft
                                Stool color within normal limits
                                No pain with defecation
                                No abdominal distention

   Altered nutrition: less than body requirements related to inability to absorb nutrients because of chronic diarrhea for 3 weeks:
       Goal: Client returns to presurgical weight by 3 months
       Expected outcomes: Client returns to regular diet within 3 days
                                Client has no GI signs or symptoms
                                No food intolerance

2. Expected outcomes are the measurable responses of the client to nursing care. Expected outcomes are directed toward goal attainment. When written, expected outcomes should be client-centered, singular, observable, measurable, time limited, mutual, and realistic.

3. Resources available:
   a. Client's cultural background and practices
      Experience with the health care delivery system
   b. Client's resources
      Client's level of care
      Preparation of nursing assistance
      Client's assessment
      Changes in client's status
      Discharge planning activities
   c. Knowledge about agency's policy for delegation
      Reassessment of client to determine that delegation is still appropriate
      Evaluation of caregiver's competence in performing delegated activity
      Feedback from caregiver

Implementing Nursing Care

Chapter **17**

CLASSROOM DISCUSSION

1. Discuss what is included in the implementation phase of the nursing process.

2. Review protocols and standing orders. Discuss the differences between the two and how they may be implemented in acute, long-term, and outpatient/home care settings.

3. Discuss the components of the information-processing model for decision making.

4. Discuss the role of reassessment in the nursing process and the revision of the care plan or pathway, including the following:
   a. Introduction of new data
   b. Alteration/addition/deletion of nursing diagnoses
   c. Adaptation/alteration of nursing interventions

5. Share situations in which assessment of the situation indicated the need for assistance from another nurse or ancillary personnel. Ask students if they can think of other instances in which assistance may be required.

6. Discuss what should be done when the nurse is not familiar with treatments, medications, or other agency policies and procedures.

7. Ask students to think about the knowledge and skills that are necessary for the implementation of nursing care.

8. Discuss delegation from a nursing perspective. Ask students to share how they feel about delegating certain activities to other professionals or paraprofessionals (e.g., medication administration or catheterization).

9. In the following situations (or other examples), have students identify what information is required before carrying out the intervention:
   a. Clients with medication orders for laxatives, antihypertensives, and diuretics
   b. An older client who has had a stroke and is scheduled to ambulate

10. Discuss the differences and relationship between cognitive, interpersonal, and psychomotor nursing skills.

INTERACTIVE EXERCISES

1. Have students identify, verbally or in writing, specific nursing interventions required in the following areas:
    a. Assistance in performance of ADLs
    b. Counseling or educating
    c. Giving care to achieve goals
    d. Giving care to facilitate achievement of goals
    e. Supervision or evaluation of other staff members

2. Have students work in small groups to determine what adaptations may be made in nursing care for clients (of different ages) with the following conditions:
    a. Visual or hearing impairments
    b. Strong cultural ties—rituals and practices
    c. Language barriers
    d. Altered perceptions—memory lapses, loss of contact with reality

3. Assign students to research and report on an article from a nursing journal that supports a specific nursing intervention.

4. Working individually or in small groups, have students adapt or revise the plan of care for a student peer, an assigned client, and/or a case study situation. Provide possible changes in status that may occur, which would require the revision.

    For the case study in Chapter 14 (p. 58), have students revise the plan of care based on the following information:
    a. Increasing edema in the client's lower extremities
    b. Loss of appetite and desire for personally prepared foods
    c. Increased dyspnea upon exertion
    d. Son's recent unemployment and loss of income

CLIENT CARE EXPERIENCES

1. Assign students to observe or participate in communicating nursing activities at a change of shift report, conference, or staff meeting.

2. Have students adapt or revise the plan of care for an assigned client. Discuss the changes in status that required the revision in the clinical postcare conference. Focus on the use of the critical thinking model in client interactions.

RESOURCES FOR STUDENT ACTIVITIES

Student care plan
Flow chart
(Refer to Chapters 14 through 16 for additional tools.)

STUDENT CARE PLAN

Supporting Data	Nursing Diagnosis	Goals/ Outcomes	Nursing Intervention	Scientific Rationale	Evaluation Measures

FLOW CHART

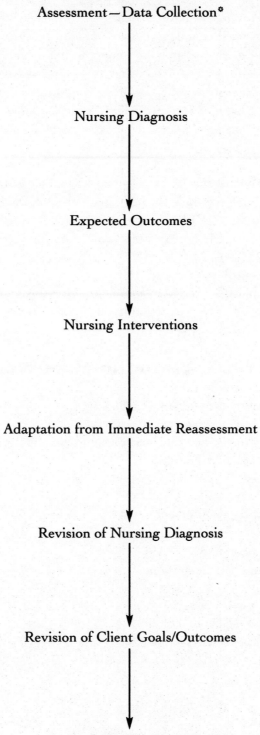

Assessment — Data Collection*

↓

Nursing Diagnosis

↓

Expected Outcomes

↓

Nursing Interventions

↓

Adaptation from Immediate Reassessment

↓

Revision of Nursing Diagnosis

↓

Revision of Client Goals/Outcomes

↓

Revised Nursing Strategies

*Looking and listening all the time

CRITICAL THINKING EXERCISES

1. Mrs. Allen has a long-term history of osteoarthritis. At present, she plans to move into an older adult assisted living retirement complex. She voices sadness at leaving her home and neighbors; however, most of all she worries about maintaining her independence. Although she knows she can get assistance with daily activities, she wants to be able to learn how to accomplish her personal care and conserve energy. What types of nursing interventions are appropriate for direct care activities for Mrs. Allen or a care provider? What activities do you think Mrs. Allen may need assistance with? What are important areas of teaching for Mrs. Allen? How will you design interventions to counsel Mrs. Allen?

2. You are assigned to ambulate Mr. Clay, who had abdominal surgery 24 hours ago. Mr. Clay weighs 270 pounds and is 6 feet tall. He has a patient-controlled analgesia (PCA) system for pain control. His intravenous (IV) fluids are running at 100 mL/hr, and he has two IV antibiotics scheduled to run every 6 hours. What questions do you need to answer before you attempt to ambulate this client?

3. Your client needs a complicated wound irrigation and dressing change. What measures will you take to reduce the risk of an adverse reaction to this intervention?

ANSWERS TO CRITICAL THINKING EXERCISES

1. Direct care activities: grooming, hygiene
   Assistive care activities: ambulating, energy conservation
   Teaching: medications, range-of-motion exercises, mobility aids, and diet
   Counseling: adapting to chronic illness

2. Knowledge of medications
   Determination of appropriate equipment
   Patency of IV
   Assessment for medication allergy
   Five Rights of Medication Administration

3. Knowledge of skin and wound care
   Knowledge regarding hazards of immobility
   Determination of personnel needed to turn and position client
   Time management skills to plan for assistance with care

Evaluation

Chapter 18

CLASSROOM DISCUSSION

1. Review standards for evaluation that are used in a health care agency, such as JCAHO.

2. Discuss the Nursing Outcomes Classification (NOC) project.

3. Discuss the process and aspects of evaluation in respect to client focus and health care delivery.

4. Review the relationship between client goals and expected outcomes.

5. Present the steps of the evaluation process. Discuss observations that need to be made and questions that need to be asked or answered to determine attainment of goals.

6. Discuss specific evaluation measures in relation to expected outcomes. Relate the discussion to continuity of care, discharge planning, and documentation. Provide examples of how evaluative measures may vary in different health care settings.

7. Ask students to identify the process that occurs when client goals are not met.

8. Review the process/components of quality improvement (QI) in health care settings, including the dimensions of performance and types of approaches. Relate quality improvement to the evaluation component of the nursing process. Discuss rationale for the selection of evaluation measures, criteria, and standards.

9. Stimulate a discussion on how the nursing process is realistically used in a managed care environment with earlier discharges.

10. Have students determine possible evaluative measures for the following client goals:
    a. Client will maintain a low-fat diet
    b. Client will self-inject insulin
    c. Client will have a diminished amount of pain (below 3 on 1–10 scale)
    d. Client will evidence decreased anxiety and a greater attention span

INTERACTIVE EXERCISES

1. Working individually or in small groups, have students document client responses and evaluate attainment of goals for a student peer and/or case study situation care plan. For the simulated case study (see Chapter 14, p. 58), have students decide the client outcomes and whether goals were met. Ask students to identify how the plan of care may need to be revised to assist the client to attain goals.

2. From the following situation, have students identify assessment versus evaluation measures and data:

   The nurse is preparing to document on a client who had abdominal surgery this morning.

   Vital signs were within acceptable limits. The surgical incision was intact with no drainage noted. Coughing and deep breathing were done according to schedule.

   The client experienced a moderate degree of pain at the incisional site, which was relieved after administering the prescribed analgesic. Family members have expressed an interest in learning client care activities.

CLIENT CARE EXPERIENCES

1. Have students document client responses and evaluate attainment of goals for an assigned client. Ask students whether the client outcomes and goals were met. Ask students to identify how the plan of care may need to be revised to assist the client to attain goals.

2. For an assigned client, have students develop and submit an entire plan of care for at least one nursing diagnosis.

RESOURCES FOR STUDENT ACTIVITIES

Agency care plan sample
Steps in the evaluation process
(Refer to Chapters 14 through 17 for additional tools.)

Client Name:

Date/ Initials	Nursing Diagnosis	Short-Term Goals/Outcomes	Resolved/Revised (Date/Initials)	Nursing Actions/Orders

Discharge Planning:

Steps	Examples
Examine the Goal	
Assess Client's Response/Behavior	
Compare Established Outcome Criteria	
Judge the Degree of Agreement Between Established Outcome and Response	
Possible Reasons for Partial or Lack of Goal Achievement	

CRITICAL THINKING EXERCISES

1. Mr. Vicar has been visiting the clinic for more than a month. He visits weekly for follow-up care for a chronic venous stasis ulcer of the left leg. The nurse's note at the time of his first visit contained the following information: "Ulcer with irregular margins, 4 cm wide by 5 cm long, approximately 0.5 cm deep, draining foul-smelling purulent yellowish drainage. Only subcutaneous tissue visible. Skin around ulcer, brownish rust in color. Zinc oxide and calamine gauze applied to the ulcer; elastic wrap bandage applied to gauze. Client instructed to return in 2 weeks." As the nurse who is caring for the client on the follow-up visit, what expected outcomes would you anticipate for the goal of "wound will demonstrate healing within 4 weeks"? What evaluative measures would you use to determine if the wound was healing?

2. Ms. Acad is a 55-year-old woman who experienced a heart attack and is now recovering on a medical cardiology unit. Her primary care nurse has identified the need to teach Ms. Acad about activity restriction, diet, stress management, and medications. Ms. Acad will likely be in the hospital for 3 more days. Explain why evaluation is important in this case. How will the nurse's evaluation of Ms. Acad's learning influence the plan of care at discharge?

3. As a nurse on a neurological unit, you care for a number of clients with parkinsonism, a disorder that causes an unsteady gait, muscle weakness, and muscular rigidity. Over the last month five clients with parkinsonism have fallen. Develop a quality indicator and monitoring criteria to measure this practice problem.

ANSWERS TO CRITICAL THINKING EXERCISES

1. Expected outcomes: ulcer is no bigger than $4 \times 5 \times 0.5$ cm; skin surrounding ulcer shows signs of healing; no drainage; no pain; remaining tissues are pink and healthy.

   Evaluative measures: observation of wound; measurements of wound; olfactory assessment of any drainage; palpation of underlying tissue.

2. Importance of evaluation:
   Ensure that care meets the client's current needs.
   Short hospital stays require that care be efficient and client-centered.
   Evaluation will keep the teaching program for Mrs. Acad on target, rather than each health provider teaching the same concepts.
   Evaluation will also document client learning.

3. Quality indicator: Clients' falls will remain at 2% or less of total client population per month.

Professional Nursing Roles

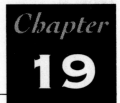

Chapter

19

CLASSROOM DISCUSSION

1. Review and discuss the historical evolution of the nursing profession within the context of the society of the era. Provide students with a chronological outline to facilitate discussion and note taking.

2. Using a selected nursing journal as a reference, present a broad overview of the development of nursing practice through the twentieth century by highlighting the changes in the focus of articles, advertisements, etc.

3. Discuss the similarities and differences of the various conceptual nursing models and theories. Guide students in the application of one or more models to an actual or simulated case study example.

4. Present various philosophies of nursing. Ask students to relate their own personal philosophy.

5. Review the different pathways to becoming a registered nurse (see Resources for Student Activities, p. 89).

6. Ask students to each identify one person they have met who is their ideal of a professional. Students should then outline why this individual fulfills their concept of a professional.

7. Discuss the legal concepts associated with nursing practice, including licensure, standards of practice, and nursing practice acts.

8. Ask students to identify the goal of graduate nursing education in the preparation of professional nurses. Discuss the health care settings or situations in which a nurse would require this level (master's or doctoral) of nursing education.

9. Review the differences between continuing and in-service education programs. Ask students to identify possible topic areas that may be presented in both types of programs.

10. Ask students to provide examples of actual activities associated with the varied roles of the nurse (see Resources for Student Activities, p. 89). Use available educational media that portray nurses in various roles and settings.

11. Ask students to share their individual nursing career goals and interests, and discuss the education and experience required for that particular career avenue.

12. Invite a nurse practitioner to class to discuss his or her role, educational preparation, and experience.

13. Have the students participate in a multidisciplinary team meeting and observe the roles and responsibilities of various team members. Have the students share their experience with others in the class.

14. Review the characteristics of a profession, and ask students to determine how nursing fulfills each one.

15. Have the students attend a professional association meeting in their area and then share their experiences with others.

16. Discuss the political influences that interact with nursing with particular emphasis on health care policy, the nursing shortage, and cost constraints in health care. Ask the students how they can be involved in health care reform and lobbying.

INTERACTIVE EXERCISES

1. Assign students to write about a major event that is having an impact on nursing.

2. Assign students, either individually or in a group, to write a letter to a politician concerning a current issue affecting nurses (e.g., increasing tuition fees for university, shortage of faculty, shortage of nurse, overcrowding of emergency rooms) and suggesting ways to improve the situation.

3. Assign students to various agencies where nurses are employed. Students are to observe the roles and responsibilities of nurses and other members of the multidisciplinary team.

4. Have students attend a meeting or convention of a professional association to observe activities. Have students share their experience and discuss particular issues.

5. Have students bring in examples from the Internet or other media sources (e.g., newspapers and magazines) that reflect current changes or trends in nursing practice or societal influences on nursing.

Comparative chart of nursing education
Nursing roles chart

COMPARATIVE CHART OF NURSING EDUCATION

	Diploma	Baccalaureate	Master's Degree	Doctorate
Average Number of Years				
Degree or Credential Received				
Primary Focus of the Graduate				
Preparation for RN Licensure				
Specialized or Generalized Study				
Usual Setting				

Role	Actual Clinical Examples
Caregiver	
Clinical Decision Maker	
Protector/Client Advocate	
Case Manager	
Rehabilitator	
Comforter	
Communicator	
Teacher	

CRITICAL THINKING EXERCISES

1. You are assigned to teach a male client who lives in a northern outpost and speaks Ojibwa about his hypertension, diabetes, medication regimen, diet, and exercise. What must you consider in developing a plan of care?

2. You are part of a selection team to hire a nurse practitioner for five cardiovascular physicians who will be working in a community health centre. Based on your knowledge of advanced practice nurses, what role would you recommend, and why?

3. Part of your education includes experiences in different types of health care settings. How would your role in the primary care setting be different from your role in the acute care setting?

ANSWERS TO CRITICAL THINKING EXERCISES

1. In planning to teach the client about his hypertension, diabetes, and medications, you assume the role of a teacher or educator. You must consider the differences in culture when planning for the Aboriginal client. These differences may include his role in the family, how he is perceived by the family and community if he is seen as being ill, and how he establishes priorities for his personal care over the needs of his family and community. Socialization in these small communities often entails the "sharing of food," and, therefore, it may be difficult to maintain a low fat, diabetic diet. Also, fruits and vegetables are difficult to obtain during the winter months. Special Canadian diabetes plans focus on the needs of the Aboriginal population and give values for food often served at various functions.

2. The nurse practitioner (NP) would be expected to demonstrate a comprehensive knowledge base in cardiovascular nursing. The NP would have advanced assessment skills; leadership responsibilities; and advanced knowledge in therapeutics, health promotion and disease prevention, family health, and community development and planning. The NP would be expected to undertake specific duties, including (1) comprehensive patient assessment, (2) development of a care plan through collaboration with members of the multidisciplinary team, (3) prescribing of therapeutic interventions according to legislation and medical directives, and (4) liaising with cardiologists and staff to communicate important information, provide individual counselling and assessment, and meet the needs of health promotion, and illness prevention, cure, and rehabilitation.

3. In the acute care setting, your role would focus on providing care that would help the acutely ill client improve his or her current state of health and return home. As a primary care nurse, you would focus on helping the client maintain his or her level of health, and promote an ongoing healthy lifestyle. Although nurses in both settings have a responsibility to provide the client and family with an education about the illness and self-care, the perspective and focus of care differs considerably.

Ethics and Values

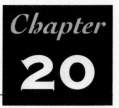

Chapter 20

CLASSROOM DISCUSSION

1. Discuss the definition of *values* and *value systems* from a nurse and client perspective.

2. Discuss individual perceptions regarding values and how they are learned and changed.

3. Review the formation of values, including the advantages and disadvantages of different modes of value transmission, and sociocultural influences.

4. Ask students to explore their personal definition of caring and how the value of caring may influence their nursing practice.

5. Review the Canadian Nurses Association Code of Ethics for Registered Nurses. Provide personal observations and experiences that demonstrate the presence or absence of these values.

6. Ask students to discuss how the nurse incorporates values into his or her personal and professional practice.

7. Stimulate a discussion on client advocacy and the promotion of individual values.

8. Discuss the values clarification process, incorporating the concepts of being nonjudgemental and that there are no right or wrong answers.

9. Provide students with the following situations (or other actual or simulated situations) in which values clarification may be implemented. Ask them for their responses and how their own values may coincide or conflict with those of the client.
   a. A client elects not to continue with possible lifesaving therapy
   b. A client elects to have an abortion or chooses to give the child up for adoption
   c. An adult places his or her parent in a nursing home

10. Discuss the definition of *ethics*. Ask the students to share their thoughts about the relationship between values and ethics.

11. Review the concept of caring with respect to values and ethics in nursing practice.

12. Discuss and identify the purpose of the Code of Ethics for nursing practice.

13. Have students identify the role of the ethics committee in ethical decision making and how the nurse may be involved in the process.

14. Discuss the concept of moral reasoning, including the impact of emotions, the law, religious faith, and culture.

15. Review and provide examples for the philosophical constructions of deontology, utilitarianism/teleology, feminist ethics, and the ethics of care.

16. Discuss ethical principles.

17. Ask students to speak about financial resources that may have an impact on ethical decision making. Have them identify areas that they believe are most at issue in various health care settings and/or specialties.

18. Discuss the legal and ethical implications associated with informed consent and advance directives (personal care directives).

19. Use an actual or simulated client experience as a stimulus for a discussion on ethics in practice. Guide students in the application of a model for ethical decision making for an actual or simulated client situation.

20. Ask students to verbalize how ethics and ethical principles are interwoven in the nursing research process.

21. Using case studies, have the students identify the most common issues in bioethics that occur for nurses.

INTERACTIVE EXERCISES

1. Stimulate a debate on whether caring and caring behaviours may be learned by all individuals.

2. Have students complete a cultural values exercise (see Resources for Student Activities, p. 36) or list and prioritize ten values that guide their daily interactions.

3. Organize a debate on one of the following issues (or a similar topic):
   a. Withholding care from a client who has religious beliefs that forbid the treatment versus overriding his or her wishes through a court order
   b. Honouring a family's request to withhold information from a loved one versus respecting the patient's right to know
   c. A do not resuscitate (DNR) order versus a "slow code" and a full code
   d. A nurse who refuses to care for certain clients (e.g., those with AIDS or having abortions) versus the agency's needs and the clients' right to health care

4. Provide students with actual or simulated client situations and ask them to identify, verbally or in writing, where ethical principles are applied appropriately (e.g., providing client dignity during procedures) or not applied (e.g., calling a client "dearie").

5. Have students discuss issues that are currently of concern to the Canadian Nurses Association (CNA) and the provincial and territorial nursing associations.

6. Assign students to attend an ethics committee meeting, if possible, to observe the functions and procedures, or invite a representative to speak to the class about the role of the committee.

7. Have students bring in examples from the media and/or Internet on actual or possible ethical dilemmas for health care providers.

CLIENT CARE EXPERIENCES

1. Have students identify possible ethical concerns for assigned clients in preclinical or postclinical conferences. Ask students to determine what resources are available within the agency or community to assist in working through an ethical dilemma.

2. Have students determine a client's values and identify how they compare with their own value systems.

RESOURCES FOR STUDENT ACTIVITIES

Cultural values exercise
Ethical decision making worksheet

CULTURAL VALUES EXERCISE

If persons from a variety of cultures were given this questionnaire, some would strongly agree with the beliefs listed on the left and others would strongly agree with the opposite viewpoint listed on the right. Circle 1 if you strongly agree or 2 if you moderately agree with the statement on the left. Circle 3 if you moderately agree or 4 if you strongly agree with the statement on the right.

1. Preparing for the future is an important activity and reflects maturity.

   1 2 3 4

   Life has a predestined course. The individual should follow that course.

2. Vague answers are dishonest and confusing.

   1 2 3 4

   Vague answers are sometimes preferred because they avoid embarrassment and confrontation.

3. Punctuality and efficiency are characteristics of a person who is both intelligent and concerned.

   1 2 3 4

   Punctuality is not as important as maintaining a relaxed atmosphere, enjoying the moment, and being with family and friends.

4. When in severe pain, it is important to remain strong and not to complain too much.

   1 2 3 4

   When in severe pain, it is better to talk about the discomfort and express frustration.

5. It is self-centered and unwise to accept a gift from someone you do not know well.

   1 2 3 4

   It is an insult to refuse a gift when it is offered.

6. Addressing someone by their first name shows friendliness.

   1 2 3 4

   Addressing someone by their first name is disrespectful.

7. Direct questions are usually the best way to gain information.

   1 2 3 4

   Direct questioning is rude and could cause embarrassment.

8. Direct eye contact shows interest.

   1 2 3 4

   Direct eye contact is intrusive.

9. Ultimately, the independence of the individual must come before the needs of the family.

   1 2 3 4

   The needs of the individual are always less important than the needs of the family.

Modified from Renwick GW, Rhinesmith SH: *An exercise in cultural analysis for managers*, Chicago, 1995, Intercultural Press.

Is this an ethical dilemma?
Relevant information:
Examination of own values:
Identification of the problem:
Courses of action:
Negotiation of the outcome:
Evaluation of the action:

CRITICAL THINKING EXERCISES

1. Complete the "cultural values" exercise (Box 20-7 in *Canadian Fundamentals of Nursing*, Second Edition) with your classmates or with members of another class of professionals. Compare the answers and discuss the differences.

2. You are caring for a 17-year-old client who has been admitted for treatment of sickle cell crisis. She needs fluid management and comfort management. Even though she is receiving narcotics around the clock, she continues to complain of pain. She also complains about her roommate, the food, and the intravenous line. She comes from a community far from the hospital, and her mother cannot visit every day. She has an older brother who has been convicted of possession of illegal drugs. Discuss your approach to this client. Rank her needs. What is your priority action, based on what you know so far? Examine and describe your opinions about pain, pain management, and addiction.

3. You are a clinic nurse in a small community clinic. A 45-year-old male client has been coming to the clinic for several years for treatment and support of his acquired immunodeficiency syndrome (AIDS). During recent months he has lost his long-term companion to AIDS. In addition, both his parents died many years ago. His clinical condition has deteriorated. His vision is failing, his nutritional status is difficult to maintain, and he has been hospitalized three times in the past three months for pneumonia. He asks for your help in planning his suicide. Discuss your response to his request. Begin by examining your personal feelings about suicide. Include a discussion about your understanding of AIDS: Where does it come from? Who gets the disease? Why? What are your feelings and opinions about people with AIDS? Construct your response, keeping in mind the ethical principles of fidelity, autonomy, beneficence, and non-maleficence. Since all of these principles collide in this example, it will be important to identify each and to recognize personal responses to the role that each plays in this narrative. Just as important is the role that one imagines they play for the client, especially as they differ from one's own. For the sake of this discussion, it is illegal in your province for nurses to prescribe medicines. What are your possible courses of action?

ANSWERS TO CRITICAL THINKING EXERCISES

1. No *right* answers exist to this exercise. The goal is to provide a structured experience that illustrates how variable personal values can be. A second goal is to encourage the practice of tolerance, even in the presence of difference. It would be helpful to guide discussion toward the differences that exist within the group, even if many similarities exist.

2. Clients who live with sickle cell disease experience acute exacerbations of pain. Management of the pain requires large doses of narcotics, in addition to other management modalities. Especially in large metropolitan communities, the fact that sickle cell clients are mostly from an African American culture renders them vulnerable to being stereotyped as poor or addicted. The goal of this exercise is to understand how easy it is to classify clients in error, and how the consequences of the error might include inadequate care. A common misconception about pain management includes the idea that too much medication will result in drug addiction. This idea and other about pain, narcotics, cultural biases, and stereotyping should be expressed. Discussion of this common event, in which sickle cell clients are mislabelled as malingering or manipulative, provides an excellent opportunity for exploration of values, values clarification, ethical standards of care, and critical thinking.

3. The goal of this discussion is to challenge you with a situation in which caring and compassion may conflict with personal philosophy. You should try to articulate personal opinion about suicide, quality of life, the role of "family," and the value of a network of loved ones. In addition, your answer should explore personal opinion about persons with AIDS, a client population that has experienced marginalization and discrimination, which are unacceptable in a health care setting. In the end, the answer should include some reference to hospice care or other kinds of comfort and support, regardless of personal opinion about suicide. In answering these questions, you have the opportunity to use an ethic of care to construct both a personal and professional plan of management.

Legal Implications in Nursing Practice

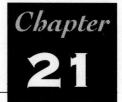

Chapter 21

CLASSROOM DISCUSSION

1. Discuss the various sources of law that influence nurses and nursing practice.

2. Review the role of provincial/territorial nursing bodies in regulating nursing practice, licensure, and disciplinary measures.

3. Review registered nurse versus student nurse liability. Ask students to identify possible situations in which the student nurse may be held liable.

4. Discuss torts that may be committed by nurses.

5. Explain the criteria for professional negligence/malpractice. Describe several scenarios, and ask students to respond to the situations, giving their rationale as to whether the nurse may be held liable for negligence.

6. Discuss and provide examples of acts of omission and commission.

7. Review the legal implications of nursing documentation.

8. Discuss standards of care and their application to nursing practice.

9. Review some of the case studies in the text (e.g., *Granger* v. *Ottawa General Hospital*), and ask students to provide their opinions on how each situation could have been avoided.

10. Invite a nurse who has appeared as an expert witness to speak to the class about court procedures and actual cases.

11. Review confidentiality and informed consent with respect to legal and ethical guidelines.

12. Discuss the responsibilities of the nurse in relation to informed and implied consent for the following, or similar, situations:
    a. An unconscious client
    b. Parents refusing treatment for a child
    c. A sedated client
    d. A 16-year-old parent
    e. An adult client involved in a research study
    f. An older client being prepared for surgery

13. Discuss the concept of shared liability of the nurse and physician, and the nurse's legal relationship with other members of the health care team. Ask students to provide examples of situations in which shared liability may occur.

14. Have students respond to the action to be taken by the nurse when there is short staffing or they are "floated" to another unit or client assignment.

15. Stimulate discussions as to the legal implications for nurses that may be associated with the following areas:
    a. Abortion
    b. AIDS or communicable diseases
    c. Assisted suicide
    d. Euthanasia
    e. Living wills/advance directives
    f. Organ donation

16. Invite a psychiatrist or someone from a mental health advocacy group to review the provincial/territorial Mental Health Act and discuss the unique issues that surround the care of individuals with mental health problems.

17. Invite a risk manager and/or nurse lawyer to speak to the class about his or her role, educational preparation and experience, and the concepts of nursing accountability, liability, and malpractice.

INTERACTIVE EXERCISES

1. Have the students role play examples of torts in client situations.

2. Provide students with examples of documentation, and have students critique and correct them according to legal guidelines.

3. Have students participate in role playing a courtroom experience in which a nurse must face negligence charges. Assign students to the various roles, including judge, jury, prosecutor, and defendant. Provide the students with background information from an actual or simulated experience. Have students develop the questions to be asked and the documents (possibly both good and bad examples) to be presented as evidence.

4. Assign students to attend a meeting of their provincial/territorial regulatory body or a legislative session (if possible) to observe the procedures involved in establishing regulations, statutes, and legislation.

Worksheet on torts
Criteria for professional negligence/malpractice

WORKSHEET ON TORTS

Torts	Definition	Nursing Example
Assault		
Battery		
Defamation		
Invasion of Privacy		
Professional Negligence/ Malpractice		

Criteria	Explanation	Examples
1. The nurse (defendant) owed a duty to the client (plaintiff).		
2. The nurse did not carry out that duty.		
3. The client was injured.		
4. The cause of the client's injury was a result of the nurse's failure to carry out that duty.		

CRITICAL THINKING EXERCISES

1. Mrs. Lee has leukemia and has been hospitalized for acute and extreme anemia. She is married and has two young daughters. The physician has ordered blood transfusions to assist Mrs. Lee over her crisis. Unfortunately, Mrs. Lee's religion prohibits her from receiving blood transfusions. The husband has stated that although he does not share her religion, he will concur with her wishes. Without the transfusion, Mrs. Lee will die. The physician has told you that he will declare a medical emergency and order you to initiate the transfusions as soon as Mrs. Lee slips into a coma from lack of oxygen. He has told you that if you do not comply, he will report you to the nursing supervisor and make sure that you are fired.
   A. What risks do you face if you administer the transfusion?
   B. What should you do?
   C. Would your answer change if this woman had been admitted in a coma and you had no information regarding her wishes concerning blood transfusions?

2. Mr. Andrews is an 80-year-old man admitted for gallbladder surgery. He is recuperating. On the day that the physician allows him to walk down the hall with assistance, he asks you to help him do so. Mr. Andrews is wearing antiembolism hosiery, and he has slippers in the closet in his room. You get Mr. Andrews out of bed and assist him in walking down the hall, which has a newly buffed linoleum floor. You forget to put on his slippers, although you know about them. While walking down the hall, you turn to look at a very good-looking resident who has just begun to make rounds for the morning. As you are looking around, Mr. Andrews's foot slips out from under him and he falls to the floor, breaking his hip. Identify the elements of negligence, and use this scenario to apply those elements.

ANSWERS TO CRITICAL THINKING EXERCISES

1. A. This is a question of informed consent. If Mrs. Lee is mentally competent at this time, it is her choice as to whether she wishes to receive or refuse a blood transfusion. The law allows any mentally competent adult to refuse medical treatment, even if it is potentially life saving. If, due to her illness, Mrs. Lee is no longer capable of making an informed decision, consent must be obtained from her legal guardian or designated substitute decision maker. Mrs. Lee may have legally delegated medical decision-making authority to her husband in a proxy directive. The law in Canada does allow physicians and other health care professionals to administer treatment in an emergency situation when the patient's consent cannot be obtained. However, this inferred or presumed consent can only occur in the absence of some previous non-consent by the patient. If you administer this transfusion (against her wishes or those of a legally empowered surrogate decision maker), you may be found liable for battery.

B. In a situation such as this it would be prudent to document any pertinent communications you have had with the patient and her husband. You should check for the presence of an Advance Directive for Health Care or proxy directive in the medical record. If there is such a document, this should be brought to the attention of the physician. If it is clear that the transfusion is in direct opposition to the previously expressed wishes of Mrs. Lee and the current direction from her spouse, you should refuse to hang the blood. Finally, *you* should contact your nursing supervisor to inform her or him of the situation and seek support from your administration.

C. Yes. The law then presumes that the woman would wish to be treated. This is in keeping with the emergency doctrine.

2. Elements of negligence are as follows: (a) The nurse owed a duty of care to the client. The duty was to assist the client in walking safely down the hall. (b) There was a breach of duty. The nurse failed to ensure that the client had on appropriate footwear, and also turned away from the client. (c) The client was injured. He fell and broke his hip. (d) The nurse's failure to carry out the duty caused the injury. The nurse's acts of not using appropriate footwear (especially on a slippery floor), and looking away, caused the client to fall and injure himself.

Communication

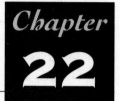

Chapter 22

CLASSROOM DISCUSSION

1. Discuss the different levels of communication: intrapersonal, interpersonal, transpersonal, small group, and public. Provide examples of each level.

2. Explain the elements of the communication process: referent, sender, message, channels, receiver, feedback, interpersonal variables, and environment.

3. Discuss the aspects inherent in verbal and nonverbal communication, symbolic communication, and metacommunication. Demonstrate situations in which the nurse may obtain assessment data from verbal and nonverbal communication.

4. Discuss the concept of perceptual bias as it relates to the process of communication. Ask students to share personal experiences in which they have been the sender or recipient of perceptual bias in an interaction.

5. Identify the factors that may influence communication. Ask students to identify how the use of space or distance between communicators (intimate, personal, social, or public) may be different depending upon the type of nurse-client interaction.

6. Review the elements of professional communication and how the nurse communicates with other members of the health care team.

7. Discuss the techniques involved in therapeutic communication. Provide the students with examples of possible client statements and questions, and ask the students to give appropriate responses.

8. Discuss the dimensions of a helping relationship, giving examples of the nurse's role in establishing an effective rapport.

9. Provide examples of how the communication process is integrated within the nursing process. Ask students to give examples of situations in which the opportunity for communication is available.

10. Invite a psychiatric nurse clinician and/or an interpreter to discuss specific elements of communication.

INTERACTIVE EXERCISES

1. Have students observe a live or videotaped role playing situation to identify barriers to communication and methods that could have been used to facilitate communication.

2. Working individually or in small groups, have students determine how communication is influenced by the following: language, sensory abilities, neurological impairment, medication, mental status, and age or developmental level.

3. Assign students to investigate available resources within an affiliating agency for enhancement of communication (e.g., interpreters, speech therapy).

4. Ask students to identify how communication may be adapted for the following clients:
   a. 5-year-old child
   b. Hearing-impaired older adult
   c. Primarily Spanish-speaking adult
   d. Aphasic client (post-CVA)
   e. Extremely anxious adolescent

5. Have students follow through on a plan of care for a client with a nursing diagnosis related to ineffectual or impaired communication.

6. Videotape or audiotape students completing a basic health history with a peer. Review the tape individually or as a class, and ask students to critique the interaction and provide suggestions to enhance communication.

7. Have students demonstrate their response in dealing with the following:
   a. A client who is angry
   b. A client who is disoriented
   c. A client who is unresponsive
   d. A client who is silent or withdrawn
   e. A client who is sexually inappropriate

CLIENT CARE EXPERIENCES

1. Assign students in the clinical setting to complete a basic health admission history on clients of different ages and cultural backgrounds. Have the students self-evaluate the experience in relation to therapeutic verbal and nonverbal communication techniques.

2. Have students report on their clients' status to their peers and other members of the health care team.

RESOURCES FOR STUDENT ACTIVITIES

Facilitators of communication
Barriers to communication

FACILITATORS OF COMMUNICATION

Techniques	Examples and Nursing Behaviors
Active Listening	
Sharing Observations	
Sharing Empathy	
Sharing Hope	
Sharing Humor	
Sharing Feelings	
Using Touch	
Using Silence	
Asking Relevant Questions	
Providing Information	
Paraphrasing	
Clarifying	
Focusing	
Summarizing	
Self-Disclosing	
Confronting	

Ineffective Techniques	Examples
Asking Personal Questions	
Giving Personal Opinions	
Changing the Subject	
Automatic Responses	
Offering False Reassurance	
Sympathy	
Asking for Explanations	
Approval or Disapproval	
Defensive Responses	
Passive or Aggressive Responses	
Arguing	

CRITICAL THINKING EXERCISES

1. Mrs. Maria Ramirez, an American of Puerto Rican descent, is faced with the difficult decision of whether or not to continue chemotherapy in the face of a rapidly spreading malignancy. What communication techniques could the nurse use to help her at this point, and what traps must the nurse avoid in such a situation?

2. Jan, a nurse colleague, is having difficulty standing up to a physician who has an abrupt, intimidating communication style. She often ends up with a lot of unspoken anger, developing tension headaches and easily becoming tearful. What could the nurse do to help?

3. Mr. Hess, a client with Parkinson's disease living at an extended care facility, has a stiff, expressionless face. He sits slumped in a recliner chair all day and seems lost in his own world, rarely looking at or interacting with anyone. When he does talk, he mumbles in a soft voice and his words are difficult to understand. What kinds of things could the nurse do to establish a helping-healing relationship with Mr. Hess?

4. Jennifer Hughes, a new graduate, is very discouraged. In school, she had felt a great deal of anxiety about her own performance, and even now she finds it difficult to be positive about herself or her job. What knowledge about communication could she use to help improve her situation?

ANSWERS TO CRITICAL THINKING EXERCISES

1. The nurse could use several basic therapeutic communication techniques that will help Mrs. Ramirez feel safe and accepted, and identify and understand her own values. These might include giving general openings ("Tell me about..."), paraphrasing and clarifying, acknowledging feelings with empathy statements, using caring touch, and using presence and silence. Helping her anticipate the consequences of her decision options would be useful. It is important for the nurse to avoid the trap of sympathy rather than empathy, so that he or she is not overwhelmed by Mrs. Ramirez's plight. The nurse should avoid trying to influence Mrs. Ramirez to make the decision that is closest to the nurse's own values or beliefs and avoid giving personal opinions, approval, or disapproval. The nurse should stress that Mrs. Ramirez has the right to make her own decision but should be aware that in her culture the husband is often a primary decision maker and needs to be included in discussions.

2. The nurse could help his or her colleague in several ways: First, provide a safe, private place away from clients and staff for Jan to talk, reassure her of confidentiality, listen empathetically, and encourage her to express her feelings. Offer to help her try out some assertive communication techniques through role play, and try to provide support by being present the next time the physician interacts with her. Adopt an optimistic stance and voice faith and hope that Jan will learn to cope well with future situations. Suggest some relaxation techniques to help her release muscle tension after such an encounter, and try a dose of humor.

3. The nurse could start building trust by getting to know Mr. Hess as an individual, including whether he is uncomfortable being called by his first name. Family members could be asked to provide information about his likes, dislikes, and personal history. The nurse could take opportunities to visit Mr. Hess for a few minutes just to say hello, comment on what is going on in his environment, and share social conversation. Touch could be used to communicate that he is accepted, and the nurse should realize that he or she cannot rely on Mr. Hess's facial expressions to make sure messages are understood. It is important to minimize environmental distractions, focus concentration when he talks, and patiently ask him to repeat his words if they are not understood.

4. Jennifer could use intrapersonal communication techniques to build her self-confidence. She needs to identify her negative thoughts and replace them with positive assertions. She needs to find positive, caring colleagues who will support her through this period of role adjustment. She could also use transpersonal communication to find additional sources of strength and hope. Practicing positive intentionality and centering herself so that her worries about herself do not intrude also will help her feel more comfortable and competent.

Client Education

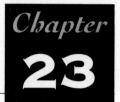

CLASSROOM DISCUSSION

1. Discuss the purposes and standards established for client education. Review the distinction between teaching and learning.

2. Explore how client education fits with *Nursing's Agenda for Health Care Reform*, including the maintenance and promotion of health, restoration of health, and coping with impaired functioning.

3. Discuss teaching and learning in respect to the communication process.

4. Identify the aspects associated with the domains of learning. Provide and/or ask students to give examples of the type of information that may be conveyed with each domain.

5. Discuss the basic principles of learning, including the concepts of motivation, ability to learn, and learning environment.

6. Stimulate a discussion on how the learning environment may be adapted to facilitate the teaching-learning process.

7. Discuss the development of and demonstrate the format for learning objectives.

8. Review the basic principles and methods of teaching, and provide examples of their implementation in client situations.

9. Discuss available teaching tools.

10. Using the following example, or another simulated or actual situation, have students determine how they would approach and organize materials for a client with hypertension who needed information on medications, diet, activity, and recognition of complications.

11. Discuss the areas that are usually included in a teaching plan: topic(s), resources, recommendations for involving others, objectives, and strategies.

12. Ask students to consider which approaches they feel the most and least comfortable with in providing client education.

13. Discuss the use of reinforcement with individuals of varying ages.

14. Explain how teaching-learning principles and strategies are integrated into the nursing process. Ask students to identify nursing diagnoses associated with teaching and learning (e.g., knowledge deficit), related objectives, and strategies. Have students give examples for which the opportunity for teaching may arise during daily client care activities.

15. Compare and contrast individual and group teaching-learning approaches.

16. Provide examples of agency documentation of client education.

17. Invite a nurse educator (e.g., a diabetic educator or an ostomy nurse) from an agency to speak to the class about client education.

18. In accordance with the teaching-learning approach used, explain how the methods of evaluation are determined by the nurse.

INTERACTIVE EXERCISES

1. Have students identify verbally or in writing the factors that may influence the client's ability to learn.

2. Have students investigate and report on the resources available within an affiliating agency for client education (e.g., preoperative instruction or a diabetic educator).

3. Provide examples of learning objectives for students to critique and correct according to the criteria.

4. Assign students a simple physical task that they will teach to another student or group of students. Have them identify the steps involved in demonstrating the procedure.

5. Using the following, or other actual or simulated situations, have students develop a possible teaching plan that specifies the learning need or topic, available resources, objectives, and teaching strategies (see Resources for Student Activities, p. 116):
   a. A new mother going home with her first child
   b. A group of teenagers who sunbathe frequently
   c. School-age children who ride bicycles in a heavy traffic area
   d. Adult women and men in a community group who are unaware of breast and testicular self-examination techniques
   e. Older adults who inquire about diet and exercise

CLIENT CARE EXPERIENCE

1. Have students identify the learning needs of their assigned clients and prepare and present a teaching plan based on the assessment of these needs.

Learning domains and teaching strategies worksheet
Teaching plan form

LEARNING DOMAINS AND TEACHING STRATEGIES WORKSHEET

Client Situation	Learning Domain	Teaching Strategies
Diagnostic testing tomorrow and the client has never had the test before		
Self-injection of medication required		
Noncompliance with the treatment regimen demonstrated		
Need for physical hygiene information demonstrated		
Label reading of foods and/or over-the-counter medications required		

TEACHING PLAN FORM

Learning Need/Topic	Available Resources	Significant Others	Learning Objectives	Teaching Strategies

CRITICAL THINKING EXERCISES

1. Susan, a manager of a preschool, has noticed that many of the children in the preschool are missing days because of illness. Susan states, "These kids always seem to be sick. They seem to get the same thing over and over again." The teachers at the preschool have asked Susan to contact you to educate the 3- and 4-year-olds about the need to use tissues and proper hand washing in hopes of keeping the children healthier. What teaching methods would you employ while teaching these children?

2. Kay, who is a 50-year-old nurse, has recently had a myocardial infarction (heart attack). Her medical history reflects that she has a family history of heart disease and has had hypertension and high serum cholesterol levels for 15 years. She reports eating a diet high in fat and says that she does not exercise regularly. Kay experienced chest pain for 2 days that worsened with activity before she sought medical attention. She states, "The reason why I can't change my diet is because my husband won't eat low-fat food, and I had a heart attack because I have been worried about my husband's health." List your teaching priorities for this client.

3. Anne, who is 20 years old, has just delivered a healthy baby boy. According to her CareMap, now that she is on the mother-baby unit, you are to review her teaching plan with her and individualize it to meet her needs. You ask Anne to review the teaching plan with you. You ask her to read the medical center's baby care pamphlet and discuss its content with you. You discover that although the pamphlet is written at a fifth-grade level, Anne is unable to comprehend the information in the brochure. When you ask her how well she can read and write in English, she responds, "I can read and write well." Describe how you would individualize Anne's teaching plan to effectively teach her how to care for her baby.

4. George, who is 70 years old, has had a cerebrovascular accident (CVA). Before his CVA, he was very active socially, went to work 2 days a week, and golfed 3 to 4 days a week. He is about to start the rehabilitation process. Although he appears to have limited cognitive deficits, he will need to use a walker at home. He states, "Walkers are for old people." Describe how you will approach George and what factors you will consider as you teach him how to use his walker.

ANSWERS TO CRITICAL THINKING EXERCISES

1. You would want to teach the children as a group instead of individually because it will provide you with the most effective use of your time and resources. Teaching the children in their own room will provide them with a comfortable, nonthreatening setting. Reading stories and coloring pictures of people using tissues and washing their hands will make this topic fun and easier to understand. Because children this age may have difficulty comprehending meanings of words, the use of pictures and stories will enhance their understanding of the information. Demonstrating the correct use and disposal of tissue and appropriate hand-washing techniques offers the children behaviors to imitate. Having the children pretend to use tissues, throw them away, and wash their hands while you watch them provides the children with a chance to role play and provides you the ability to give immediate feedback to the children and evaluate the effectiveness of your teaching plan.

2. First, you must deal with Kay's denial. Her statement that blames her husband for her poor health behaviors, her heart attack, and her denial of chest pain for 2 days indicates that she is not prepared to accept or deal with her heart disease. Therefore you should provide support and empathy to Kay and her family. Let her know that you are available for discussion whenever she needs you. Because of her denial, you should provide only information that Kay absolutely requires. Therefore your main teaching priority should center around unstable angina, including causation, signs and symptoms, how to use nitroglycerin, and when to seek medical attention. Information about her diet and exercise routine will have to wait until Kay is ready to accept her illness.

3. Anne is one of the 90 million Americans who are functionally illiterate. Clients who have low literacy skills rely heavily on what is spoken to them. Therefore what you explain becomes very important. Be sure to use language that Anne can understand; she probably has a limited vocabulary as well. Keep teaching sessions short and to the point, and include the most important information first. Be sure to reinforce important information at the end of each session. Allow for repetition of instructions and ask Anne to repeat what she has heard in her own words to enhance retention. Ask Anne to perform return demonstration of required care, such as bathing her baby, and umbilical cord and circumcision care. This will increase Anne's confidence in caring for her baby and will provide you with the chance to give immediate feedback and evaluate the effectiveness of your teaching plan. If possible, personalize teaching sessions by providing a story or relating an experience of your own to help explain the care of her baby. Providing Anne with a baby care pamphlet that has pictures and is printed with a large font will probably be more effective than the standard pamphlet given to new mothers at the medical center. Finally, helping Anne either find a support group for new mothers or encouraging her to attend parenting classes may enhance her ability to care for her baby. Group activities such as these will give Anne opportunities to interact with other new moms and may promote compliance with the care of her baby.

4. First, you need to assess George for any sensory deficits. For example, if he wears glasses or hearing aids, be sure that he uses them while you teach. To facilitate teaching, be sure that you are facing George and that you speak slowly and clearly. Before you can begin to teach George how to use the walker, you will have to help him accept the need to use it. Not dealing with his negative feelings about the walker will impede successful education. After George accepts that he needs to use the walker, provide instructions in short, frequent sessions. Simulate real-life experiences, such as climbing stairs, getting in and out of the car, and walking on carpeted and grassy surfaces. Establish realistic, short-term goals that are mutually set. Basing information that applies to current situations and involving George in the educational process will enhance his achievement of the learning objectives. Be sure that any written instructions you give George use large print that contrasts well with background colors. Finally, determine whether a family member or significant other will be involved in George's care at home. If someone else will be helping George after discharge, be sure to include that person in the teaching process.

Documentation and Reporting

Chapter 24

CLASSROOM DISCUSSION

1. Review and discuss different methods of communicating and reporting a client's status.

2. Ask students to identify what may be included in a client's record and how it varies depending on the health care agency.

3. Discuss the purpose of documentation and reporting.

4. Have students determine the role of accrediting agencies (i.e., JCAHO) in setting standards for documentation.

5. Review general criteria and guidelines for documentation and reporting.

6. Provide examples of nursing and multidisciplinary documentation.

7. Discuss the legal implications associated with client documentation, including confidentiality of records. Use video resources, if available, to highlight this concept.

8. Stimulate a debate on the concepts of "charting by exception" versus "care not documented is care not done."

9. Provide examples of client records or forms from a variety of different health care agencies for students to review.

10. Discuss the following methods of recording, including similarities and differences, and the advantages and disadvantages of each:
    a. Problem-oriented medical records
    b. Source records (narrative recording)
    c. Charting by exception and/or variances
    d. Focus charting

11. Review the use of a multidisciplinary critical pathway in a case management approach.

12. Ask students to identify the specific documentation needs in acute care, home care, and long-term care agencies.

13. Discuss the positive and negative aspects of the computer-based client care record and computerized nursing documentation.

14. Review the information that should be included in the various types of nursing reports.

15. Ask students to identify what situations may warrant the completion of an incident report.

16. Discuss the nursing responsibilities associated with a telephone order.

17. Invite a quality assurance nurse and/or attorney to discuss the legal implications of nursing documentation.

INTERACTIVE EXERCISES

1. Have students critique and correct sample documentation entries according to the guidelines.

2. Assign students to observe or participate in the use of a computerized documentation system, or have students attend a workshop on available systems.

3. Provide an example of an incident report forms along with a case study, and have students practise completing the necessary documentation for the simulated occurrence.

4. Working individually or in small groups, have students write their responses to the following, or similar, situations that may be encountered in the documentation of client care:
   a. Another nurse asks you to chart for him or her
   b. Mistakes are made when writing notes on the record
   c. Coffee is spilled over a whole page of the record
   d. Each entry on the record does not begin with the time and end with a signature and title

5. Using the following simulation, have students document in POMR (SOAP/SOAPIE), PIE, and/or focus charting (DAR) formats:

   A client, newly diagnosed with diabetes mellitus, was admitted to the acute care agency. The client was anxious about learning the technique for self-injection of insulin. The nurse discussed and demonstrated the procedure to the client and his wife. Self-injection technique improved after the first three attempts. A dietary referral was made for the client as he expressed minimal knowledge about necessary restrictions.

CLIENT CARE EXPERIENCES

1. Assign students to observe and/or participate in an end-of-shift report or client conference at an affiliating agency.

2. In actual client care situations, have students maintain an index card with accurate times of nursing assessments and interventions. Use the cards to facilitate practise of documentation and to stimulate postcare discussions of daily experiences.

3. Have students complete written or computerized documentation for their assigned clients, according to expected guidelines. Critique their documentation before actual entry, and provide recommendations for improvement, as indicated.

Problem-oriented documentation form (SOAPIE)
Focus charting form (DAR)

PROBLEM-ORIENTED DOCUMENTATION FORM (SOAPIE)

Subjective Data	
Objective Data	
Assessment (Nursing Diagnosis)	
Plan	
Interventions	
Evaluation	

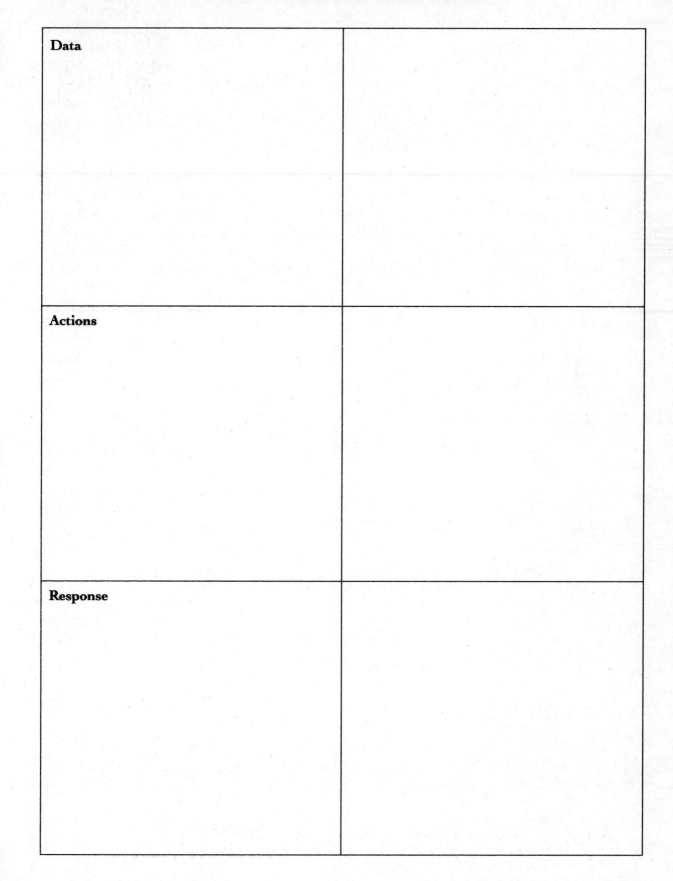

Data	

Actions	

Response	

CRITICAL THINKING EXERCISES

1. Joseph Vojnovic is an 80-year-old man admitted with a diagnosis of possible pneumonia. He complains of general malaise and a frequent productive cough, worse at night. Vital signs are as follows: blood pressure, 150/90 mm Hg; pulse rate, 92 beats per minute; respirations, 22 breaths per minute; and temperature, 38.5°C. During your initial assessment, he coughs violently for 40–45 s without expectorating. His lungs have wheezes and rhonchi in both bases and are otherwise clear. He states, "It hurts in my chest when I cough." Differentiate between objective and subjective data in this case example.

2. The nurse positions Mr. Vojnovic in a semi-Fowler's position, encourages increased fluid intake, and gives Tylenol 650 mg PO as ordered for fever. One hour later, the client is resting in bed. Vital signs are as follows: blood pressure, 130/86 mm Hg; pulse rate, 86 beats per minute; respirations, 22 breaths per minute; and temperature, 37.7°C. He states he has been unable to sleep. His fluid intake has been 200 mL of water. Use the given information to write a nurse's progress note, using each of the following formats: SOAPIE, PIE, and DAR.

3. At the end of your shift 6 h later, you have identified fluid volume deficit as a nursing diagnosis for Mr. Vojnovic. Since his admission he has had fluid intake of about 600 ml, and his urine output was 300 mL of dark, concentrated urine. His temperature is back up to 38.4°, his mucous membranes are dry, and he states he feels very weak. Using the nursing care records, (see Figure 24-2, p. 509, *Canadian Fundamentals of Nursing*, Second Edition), record significant data. List what should be included in the change-of-shift report.

4. Several days later, following treatment with intravenous antibiotics, Mr. Vojnovic is feeling much better and preparations are being made for discharge. He is to take Keflex 500 mg q6h for the next 10 days, continue to drink extra fluids, and get extra rest. He lives alone. Although he is generally cooperative, he does not like drinking water or taking pills. He is to make an appointment with his physician for one week from today and should call the physician if he develops symptoms of recurrence. Write a discharge summary that is concise and instructive.

ANSWERS TO CRITICAL THINKING EXERCISES

1. Objective data include vital signs and an observed nonproductive cough for 40–45 s, sneezes, and rhonchi. Subjective data include general malaise, frequent productive cough (worse at night), and the client's statement of chest pain during coughing.

2. SOAPIE:
   S: States "unable to sleep"
   O: BP 150/90; P 92; R 22; and T 37.7°C
   A: Altered sleep pattern related to frequent productive cough
   P: Enhance comfort by positioning with HOB elevated; monitor for fever
   I: At 07:00 gave Tylenol 650 mg PO for fever; encouraged to drink at least 1,000 mL q4h while awake
   E: Needs to be encouraged to drink more; still unable to sleep

PIE:

P: Altered sleep pattern related to frequent productive cough

I: At 07:00 gave Tylenol 650 mg PO for fever; encouraged to drink at least 1,000 mL q4h while awake

E: Needs to be encouraged to drink more; states he is still unable to sleep

DAR:

D: States he is "unable to sleep"

A: At 07:00 gave Tylenol 650 mg PO for fever; encouraged to drink at least 1,000 mL q4h while awake; vital signs BP 130/86; P 86; R 22; and T 37.7°C

R: Fluid intake has been 200 mL in the past hour; states he is still unable to sleep

3. The change-of-shift report should include the following:

Background information: Joseph Vojnovic, 80-year-old male with diagnosis of possible pneumonia

Assessment: Fluid intake has been 600 mL since admission; urine output 300 mL dark, concentrated urine; temperature now back up to 38.4° C after Tylenol given 6 h ago; mucous membranes dry; complains of feeling "very weak"

Nursing diagnosis: Fluid volume deficit related to fever and inadequate intake

Teaching plan: Encourage to drink 120 mL of fluid at least every 20 minutes and explain/inform him that fluid will help liquefy secretions in the lungs and therefore help rid the lungs of mucus

Treatments: Tylenol 650 mg given at 07:00

Family information: None stated

Discharge plan: He will need to avoid exposure to crowds and maintain increased fluid intake; since he lives at home, he may need some follow-up by a home health nurse to make sure he takes prescribed antibiotics as ordered

Priority needs: Continue to encourage liquids; he is due for Tylenol for fever now

4. Discharge summary for Mr. Vojnovic:

Admitted 4 days ago with possible pneumonia. Treated with IV antibiotics. Increased fluid intake. Lungs clear with productive cough. Afebrile: 24 hours. Follow up to include Keflex 500 mg q6h for 10 days, rest, and increased fluids. Home health to follow up with reinforcement of fluid intake and medication. To see Dr. X in one week. Accurately stated signs and symptoms of pneumonia to report to physician and that he will call if any develop.

Research as a Basis for Practice

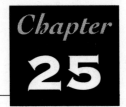

Chapter
25

CLASSROOM DISCUSSION

1. Discuss the historical background and role of research in nursing.

2. Explain how research is used to acquire knowledge and predict phenomena.

3. Ask students to identify how nursing research relates to the determination of the effectiveness of client care.

4. Discuss and provide examples of the different types of research that may be conducted.

5. Identify the role of nurses prepared at different educational levels in the research process.

6. Ask students to identify how nurses, including students, may participate in data collection for and the care of clients participating in research studies.

7. Discuss the ethical considerations associated with the research process, including informed consent, confidentiality, and anonymity.

8. Invite a nursing researcher to speak to the class about roles in research as well as educational preparation and experience needed to undertake research.

9. Discuss how the development of questions regarding clinical nursing problems may stimulate nursing research studies.

10. Provide examples of the ways in which nursing research has been used to enhance and improve nursing practice.

INTERACTIVE EXERCISES

1. Have students investigate and report on how nursing research may coordinate with quality improvement studies within an agency.

2. If possible, have students attend a research ethics review committee to observe topic areas and procedures.

3. Assign students individually or in small groups to develop a research question pertinent to an area of practice. Have students explain how the answer to this question could affect practice.

4. Provide students with a nursing research article and ask them to identify the type of information that is presented by the author(s). Assign students to obtain their own research articles on an area of interest and report the following on an index card: topic area, methods used, ethical considerations, results and application to practice (see Resource for Student Activities, p. 126).

CLIENT CARE EXPERIENCE

1. If possible, have students participate in limited data collection for an actual clinical study in an affiliating agency.

RESOURCE FOR STUDENT ACTIVITIES

Nursing research article worksheet

NURSING RESEARCH ARTICLE WORKSHEET

Topic Area	Methods Used	Ethical Considerations	Results	Application to Practice

CRITICAL THINKING EXERCISES

1. The nurse is concerned about learning to properly treat a pressure sore. Explain the benefits to the client if the nurse learns how to treat it drawing on information from the research literature rather than the scientific method.

2. The research literature reflects many different methods for treating pressure sores. If you wished to determine the best method for doing this, what type of research design would you use?

3. The nurses working on an orthopedic unit decide to study the factors that commonly result in client falls on their unit. How could they design a study to answer their questions?

ANSWERS TO CRITICAL THINKING EXERCISES

1. The client receives interventions that have been proven successful. Measures are more cost effective and time efficient. The client receives the most current type of care.

2. You would use an experimental design that compares two or more treatments.

3. The nurses would need to identify their research question, carry out a review of the literature to determine current knowledge of factors producing falls, identify what type of research method is best suited to the question, and select appropriate design and data analysis techniques. They would need to seek approval from the appropriate research ethics committee.

Self-Concept

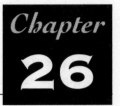

Chapter

26

CLASSROOM DISCUSSION

1. Ask students what self-concept is, what it means to them, and how it may be associated with nursing care.

2. Discuss the components of self-concept (identity, body image, self-esteem, and role performance) and how each component may be positively or negatively influenced. Using a case study example, identify how the components of self-concept are manifested and how they may be affected.

3. Review the role of stressors in relation to self-concept and how the nurse may determine the presence of stressors. Bring multicultural considerations into the discussion.

4. Review how self-concept is developed and changes throughout the life span. Use a theorist's ideas (e.g., Erikson, Piaget, Freud) as a reference framework.

5. Discuss the assessment of a client's self-concept.

6. Ask students to provide specific examples of how the nurse may be a positive or negative influence on a client's self-concept and how a supportive environment may be established to promote self-exploration, self-awareness, and self-evaluation.

7. Guide students in the application of the nursing process for an actual or simulated client who is experiencing an altered self-concept.

INTERACTIVE EXERCISES

1. Assign students to investigate and report on resources that are available in the school, community, or affiliating agency to support and promote self-concept. Have students attend a meeting of a self-help group in the community and share with the class how the group supports individual self-concept.

2. Working individually or in small groups, have students identify nursing diagnoses, client goals and outcomes, nursing interventions, and evaluation criteria for the following client experiencing stress and an altered self-concept:

Maria is 40 years old, has been married for 15 years, and is the mother of an 8-year-old boy. Maria provides the sole financial support for the family, as her husband has been unemployed for 2 years with no immediate job prospects. She is currently concerned about the status of her company and the possibility of losing her income and medical coverage. Maria has returned to school to acquire additional knowledge and skills in the event that she loses her position. Although she enjoys the classes, the work is time consuming and tiring, especially with the long hours she puts in at work. Maria also feels guilty about not being as involved as she would like to be in her son's activities. She is currently experiencing severe headaches and gastric distress and has a tendency to cry easily.

CLIENT CARE EXPERIENCES

1. Have students assess their clients' self-concept and report their findings in postclinical conference. Discuss possible interventions to promote or maintain their clients' self-concept.

2. Have students incorporate interventions to promote and support self-concept, as indicated, into their clients' plan of care.

RESOURCE FOR STUDENT ACTIVITIES

Stressors affecting self-concept assessment form

Self-Concept Components	Examples of Stressors	Health Promotion Activities
Identity		
Body Image		
Self-Esteem		
Role Performance		

CRITICAL THINKING EXERCISES

1. You are assigned to care for a 23-year-old Asian-American client who was in a motor vehicle accident and sustained multiple fractures to his face and a fractured femur (which was fixated through surgery on the eve of admission 4 days ago). He has grown up in the United States; he and his mother came to the United States when he was a young child. He works as a janitor for a local university. He lives with his girlfriend and their 7-month-old daughter. You have been with him for most of the morning and found that he is in moderate pain, which has been treated with morphine. The morphine has decreased his pain rating from a 6 to a 3 but has left him somewhat drowsy. During the morning he has shared with you some of his concerns about when he will be able to return to work. You are in the room when the surgeon tells him about his upcoming surgery. A temporary tracheotomy is planned because of the extensive work needed in the nasal and throat area. After the surgeon leaves, the client tells you he does not want the tracheotomy. He indicates that he is unclear about what it actually entails, even though the surgeon explained it in fairly simple terms. He says to you, "I just want to get back to my normal self." How would you address his comment regarding "get back to normal" and his lack of understanding regarding the tracheotomy?

2. A 51-year-old man has been transferred to the rehabilitation unit following 2 weeks of hospitalization resulting from an industrial accident in which his pelvis was crushed by a hydraulic press. His pelvis was stabilized with an external fixator. Initially he was paralyzed from T12 down. During the 2 weeks since the accident, feeling and movement have begun to return in his lower extremities. With the return of function there have also been spasms that occur with movement and increase in severity if movement is continued. With the gradual return of functioning, the physicians have been hesitant to give the client a prognosis and have told him that waiting and seeing is what will reveal his returning functioning. The client seems satisfied with this explanation at this point. His main focus is on directing his personal care to minimize risk of infection and to ensure that whoever is caring for him understands the importance of waiting for a muscle spasm to subside before continuing with care. A student is assigned to care for the client for a 4-week rotation. The student will be there once a week for 4 hours. How might the student establish trust and assess the client's concerns about the future?

3. As part of your community health experience, you are assigned to visit an 85-year-old woman who has gone to her daughter's home after being hospitalized for a fractured hip. The hip was internally fixated, and the client was discharged using a walker. When you go to the home, you find the 65-year-old daughter near tears. She says, "I just don't know if I can do this. She doesn't like anything I cook. She calls me two or three times during the night to help her to the bathroom. And now my husband has been diagnosed with lung cancer." What additional assessment data would you want to gather?

ANSWERS TO CRITICAL THINKING EXERCISES

1. There are several areas to consider here. First is the establishment of a therapeutic relationship so that the client can develop trust in you. Establishing trust can be facilitated by genuine caring and empathy on your part, honesty about what is known and not known, and carrying through with planned care (e.g., seeing that pain medication is administered within a reasonable time frame). Second is his concern about when he will get back to normal. You might acknowledge his sudden change from being a healthy young person who was able to do whatever he wanted, to someone who is in pain, dependent on others for assistance, and facing surgery. Acknowledging these major changes may help to convey empathetic understanding. Each person would say this in his or her own words, but the essence might be something such as, "You have undergone major changes since the accident. You are in pain, in the hospital, and facing surgery. I think most people would feel somewhat overwhelmed by so much happening in such a short time." You might continue to convey that after such an injury it often takes several months to get back to all of one's previous activities, but that there will be progress on a day-to-day basis. In regard to his concern about the tracheotomy, you might ask the client what he understood. From here you can then assess what is needed (e.g., consulting with the surgeon and requesting that he speak with the client again and finding pictures to illustrate the procedure or clarify areas of misunderstanding) and make plans based on this information.

2. Because the student will have a period of time with the client, there will be time to establish trust. Taking care to listen to the client describe how to carry out procedures related to his wound and pin care would be important. After his routine, if it does not violate significant principles of sterile technique or standards of care, the student could establish caring and trust. Discussing with the client the importance of allowing time for spasms to subside before proceeding could help to alleviate fear. Following through in this discussion with appropriate actions could further contribute to the development of trust. In regard to the future, as the student establishes rapport with the client, the student could inquire if the client has thought about how his rehabilitation will progress. If the client is still focused on the current situation, the student might allow the topic to drop and watch for clues over the next four weeks that the client has begun to think about the future. When clues appear, the student could explore and encourage client sharing.

3. The daughter is experiencing both role strain and role conflict. You would want to explore the mother-daughter relationship; where the mother was living before the fracture; the mother's overall health status; how much help the mother needs; further information about the husband's diagnosis (e.g., how long since the diagnosis was made, and his need for assistance); the husband-wife relationship; and available supports (including their current involvement), such as neighbors, family, and community resources.

Sexuality

Chapter

27

CLASSROOM DISCUSSION

1. Discuss concepts of sexuality. Ask students to share their perceptions of sexuality and its relation to nursing care.

2. Discuss the dimensions of sexuality in relation to the past and current society.

3. Using examples from today's media and societal culture, discuss the concept of sexual identity.

4. Ask students to share their perceptions and/or those perceptions common in society about different sexual orientations. Provide examples of variations in client sexual orientation that the nurse may encounter.

5. Have students review, identify, and describe male and female sexual anatomy and physiology and sexual response.

6. Discuss sexual development throughout the life span and strategies for health promotion that may be implemented with parents, children, and clients at each stage (see Resource for Student Activities, p. 135).

7. Discuss issues related to sexuality, the role of the nurse, and the resources and referrals that are available to the nurse and client.

8. Have students identify how illness may affect sexuality and sexual functioning.

   Use the following or similar examples:
   a. A 56-year-old male after a myocardial infarction
   b. A 16-year-old female client receiving chemotherapy
   c. A 38-year-old woman after a mastectomy
   d. A 25-year-old paraplegic male
   e. An 85-year-old female in a nursing home

9. Discuss how the nurse may recognize sexuality issues in the health care environment. Provide or ask students to give examples of possible situations that may occur with clients in the acute or long-term care environment. Ask how they should respond to each situation.

10. Guide students in the application of the nursing process for a simulated situation in which a client is experiencing an alteration in sexuality.

11. Provide specific examples of and interventions for male and female psychological and physiological sexual dysfunction.

12. Discuss how physical, relationship, lifestyle, and self-esteem factors may influence an individual's sexual behavior.

13. Invite a nurse therapist or counselor who deals with sexuality to speak to the class about the role of the nurse and client care.

INTERACTIVE EXERCISES

1. In a small group, ask students to share their feelings about sexuality and the role of the nurse.

2. For discussion, have students bring in examples from the media of sexual issues that may influence nursing and health care.

3. Organize a debate on a controversial issue relating to sexuality and the role of the nurse, such as a nurse's participation in abortion procedures versus refusal to participate in abortion procedures.

4. Assign students to visit available community agencies (e.g., Planned Parenthood or a fertility or woman's health clinic) and report back to the class on the services offered to clients.

5. Organize a role-playing situation in which the student is the nurse who must complete a sexual health history and/or physical assessment.

6. Working individually or in small groups, have students identify nursing diagnoses, client goals and outcomes, nursing interventions, and evaluation criteria for an actual and/or simulated client who is experiencing alterations in sexual health.

CLIENT CARE EXPERIENCES

1. Have students identify possible sexual health needs for assigned clients. Discuss interventions that may be incorporated into the plan of care to meet these needs.

2. Have students document identified sexual health needs in the client's record and/or student care plan.

RESOURCE FOR STUDENT ACTIVITIES

Health promotion for sexuality chart

HEALTH PROMOTION FOR SEXUALITY CHART

Life Stage	Sexual Development	Health Promotion Strategies
Infant		
Toddler/Preschooler		
School-Age		
Adolescent		
Adulthood		
Older Adult		

132   Unit 5: Psychosocial Basis for Nuring Practice

CRITICAL THINKING EXERCISES

1. Your current clinical experience is in a family practice office. You are conducting the initial interview with a 48-year-old man who started taking antihypertensives 2 weeks ago. You take his blood pressure and find it to be 136/74. You ask him how he has been doing since his last visit. He looks down at the floor and says, "Oh, OK I guess. Seems like I'm just getting old now." What kind of follow-up would be indicated based on this information?

2. You are assigned to care for a 15-year-old girl who was admitted after a motor vehicle accident. Yesterday she had an internal fixation of a fractured ankle. In gathering her nursing history, you explore sexuality and learn that she has just recently become sexually active with her boyfriend of 3 months. When you ask about safe sex and the use of birth control, she tells you that she knows she does not have to worry about STDs with him because he is just not one of those kinds of boys. In regard to birth control, she says that her boyfriend has reassured her that because he is pulling out before ejaculation, there is no risk of her becoming pregnant. How would you proceed, given this assessment data?

3. You are working on a rehabilitation unit and caring for a 67-year-old man who had a stroke 3 weeks ago. He shares a room with another man who is recovering from a stroke. He has been progressing in his self-care skills and now is able to get around with a cane, feed himself, and do most of his bath. His wife is in fairly good health, and the plan is for him to return home within the next 1 to 2 weeks. As you work with him one morning, he says to you, "You know, one of the things that is hardest about being here is not being able to sleep in the same bed as Greta. I miss her so much. Even though she visits everyday, it is just not the same." How would you explore his comment, and what planning would you consider?

ANSWERS TO CRITICAL THINKING EXERCISES

1. The client's verbal response and nonverbal behavior (looking down at the floor) suggest that he may have concerns. You might want to make an opportunity for him to discuss any concerns. Possible openings could be "You sound kind of discouraged" or "Sometimes when people begin antihypertensive medications they notice various side effects. Have you noticed anything different since you began the medicine?"

2. There are two issues evident here. One issue is her assumption that she is not at risk for STDs and the second is her misconception about pregnancy risk. Because she has shared this information with you, she likely trusts you enough to continue with some discussion regarding sexuality. There is no one way to approach this situation. Several approaches may be successful. One approach would be to inquire about her knowledge of STDs. When you have a sense of her background, you could either provide information to clarify or fill in missing information regarding her possible risk for STDs. Another valuable intervention would be to inquire about sexual history, safe sex, and/or contraception with her partner. Often adolescents are uncomfortable discussing sexually related issues with a partner. Providing her with an opportunity to role play how she might ask these questions (if she has not) or negotiating for a reliable method of contraception could be very helpful to her. Finding the words to say it and the concern about how the conversation might flow are often the most difficult aspects of bringing up a sexually related topic with a partner. Once the topics are openly discussed, you can provide information and referral, as appropriate.

3. First, you would want to gather more information to determine what aspects of sleeping with his wife he misses. You might say something like "What part of sleeping with her do you miss most?" or something that acknowledges more clearly a possible sexual concern such as "Many couples are sexually active after one partner has had a stroke. Is sexuality part of your concern?" The tactic that you use will likely depend upon several factors: your own comfort with discussing sexuality; the amount of assessment data that you have gathered thus far; trust and comfort level; and observations that you have made about the couple's relationship (e.g., presence of touching and closeness). If privacy for physical intimacy (whether it is touching or more intimate sexuality) is part of what he misses, you will want to explore the possibilities for privacy within the facility. In a rehabilitation situation, privacy for sexual expression is likely an issue for clients. The facility may have made arrangements for private space. If a private space is unavailable, exploring how to make his room available while providing an acceptable space for the roommate may be a viable option.

Spiritual Health

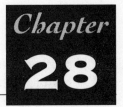

Chapter 28

CLASSROOM DISCUSSION

1. Discuss the concepts of spirituality, faith, religion, and hope.

2. Ask students to share their own meaning of spirituality and how it may be incorporated into nursing practice and a holistic approach to health.

3. Ask students to determine how critical thinking may be used to meet the client's spiritual needs.

4. Review the development of spirituality across the life span in relation to overall health and well-being.

5. Ask students to identify situations that may result in spiritual distress and the behaviors and responses that may be exhibited by the client.

   Use the following or similar examples to discuss possible client reactions and spiritual needs:
   a. A 40-year-old man who has had a heart attack
   b. A 20-year-old client who has been paralyzed after an automobile accident
   c. A 32-year-old mother of two children who has been diagnosed with breast cancer
   d. A 70-year-old client with severe, painful arthritis

6. Discuss religious needs, problems, and conflicts that the nurse may encounter in working with clients.

7. Ask students to share their own religious practices and how they may relate to or interfere with health care delivery.

8. Ask students to identify how recognition of spiritual needs may be viewed outside of specific religions.

9. Discuss how caring and compassion may be incorporated into interventions designed to meet clients' spiritual needs.

10. Identify and/or ask students to identify how illness and hospitalization may interfere with an individual's spirituality and religious practices.

11. Review the association of cultural and religious beliefs and practices. Compare and contrast the differences and similarities in spiritual practices of different ethnic and cultural groups.

12. Guide students in the application of the nursing process for an actual client or simulated case study situation in which there is evidence of spiritual distress.

INTERACTIVE EXERCISES

1. Assign students to report, verbally or in writing, on the support systems and resources that are available within an affiliating agency or the community for clients experiencing spiritual needs.

2. Have students identify examples of specific nursing interventions that will enhance a client's spirituality. Ask students to determine how the routine of an acute or restorative care facility may be adapted to meet a client's spiritual needs.

3. Working individually or in small groups, have students identify nursing diagnoses, long-term and short-term goals and client outcomes, nursing interventions, and evaluation criteria and measures for the following, or similar, case study situation:

   The client is a 28-year-old homosexual male who is terminally ill with AIDS. He was raised in a Catholic home by parents who have maintained a strong belief in their religion and its practices. Although he has denied being a practicing Catholic, the client has made occasional statements that may indicate a conflict in his beliefs and a desire for spiritual assistance.

CLIENT CARE EXPERIENCES

1. Have students identify possible spiritual needs for their assigned clients in a variety of health care settings. Discuss how the clients' spiritual needs may be met by the nurse or spiritual counselor in preclinical and/or postclinical conferences.

2. Have students incorporate the clients' identified spiritual needs into the plan of care or critical pathway.

RESOURCE FOR STUDENT ACTIVITIES

JAREL spiritual well-being scale

JAREL SPIRITUAL WELL-BEING SCALE

DIRECTIONS: PLEASE CIRCLE THE CHOICE THAT **BEST** DESCRIBES HOW MUCH YOU AGREE WITH EACH STATEMENT. CIRCLE ONLY **ONE** ANSWER FOR EACH STATEMENT. THERE IS NO RIGHT OR WRONG ANSWER.

		Strongly Agree	Moderately Agree	Agree	Disagree	Moderately Disagree	Strongly Disagree
1.	Prayer is an important part of my life.	SA	MA	A	D	MD	SD
2.	I believe I have spiritual well-being.	SA	MA	A	D	MD	SD
3.	As I grow older, I find myself more tolerant of others' beliefs.	SA	MA	A	D	MD	SD
4.	I find meaning and purpose in my life.	SA	MA	A	D	MD	SD
5.	I feel there is a close relationship between my spiritual beliefs and what I do.	SA	MA	A	D	MD	SD
6.	I believe in an afterlife.	SA	MA	A	D	MD	SD
7.	When I am sick I have less spiritual well-being.	SA	MA	A	D	MD	SD
8.	I believe in a supreme power.	SA	MA	A	D	MD	SD
9.	I am able to receive and give love to others.	SA	MA	A	D	MD	SD
10.	I am satisfied with my life.	SA	MA	A	D	MD	SD
11.	I set goals for myself.	SA	MA	A	D	MD	SD
12.	God has little meaning in my life.	SA	MA	A	D	MD	SD
13.	I am satisfied with the way I am using my abilities.	SA	MA	A	D	MD	SD
14.	Prayer does not help me in making decisions.	SA	MA	A	D	MD	SD
15.	I am able to appreciate differences in others.	SA	MA	A	D	MD	SD
16.	I am pretty well put together.	SA	MA	A	D	MD	SD
17.	I prefer that others make decisions for me.	SA	MA	A	D	MD	SD
18.	I find it hard to forgive others.	SA	MA	A	D	MD	SD
19.	I accept my life situations.	SA	MA	A	D	MD	SD
20.	Belief in a supreme being has no part in my life.	SA	MA	A	D	MD	SD
21.	I cannot accept change in my life.	SA	MA	A	D	MD	SD

Copyright 1987 by J Hungelmann, E Kenkel-Rossi, L Klassen, R Stollenwerk, Marguette University College of Nursing, Milwaukee, Wisc.

CRITICAL THINKING EXERCISES

1. A client with degenerative joint disease tells you he is afraid he will soon be unable to walk. His affect is blunted, and he often looks away in the distance. His wife tells you that the pain her husband has during walking prevents him from going to church. At one time both husband and wife were very active in church activities. What might you want to learn about the client during your spiritual assessment?

2. Mrs. Stills has been hospitalized with cancer of the ovaries. Her disease has progressed, but she expresses a satisfaction with her life and a faith that God will guide and protect her. She asks you about meditation exercises. In the acute care environment, how might you arrange a teaching session on meditation?

3. Critical thinking is an ongoing process. When you learn that you are assigned to Julio Gonsaga, you note that the Kardex information includes his religion, Catholic, and his place of birth, Cuba. A colleague tells you he can speak some English. The client is 80 years old and reportedly has a bit of a hearing deficit. What knowledge might you wish to reflect on critically before beginning a spiritual assessment of this client?

ANSWERS TO CRITICAL THINKING EXERCISES

1. It would be valuable to first learn about the client's faith and whether his illness has threatened or diminished his beliefs in any way. In addition, assess the degree of the client's hope. It is likely that his hope may be diminished because of the chronic nature of the disease and the ongoing pain he experiences. You need to consult with the physician to learn whether there is a promising treatment for the client's discomfort and mobility restriction. If so, instructing the client on this information may instill realistic hope. You should also assess the significance that friends and associates play as members of this client's community of faith. You may be able to arrange to have taped church services provided or have friends visit more regularly.

2. Meditation exercises would be ideally taught in a private room. If the client shares a semi-private room, arrange a time when the roommate is out for a procedure or is asleep. Close the room doors and close the window shades. Turn off any TV or radio. If the client has a cassette or CD player with a relaxation tape or CD, that can be helpful. Be sure that the client is in a comfortable position, and, if the client receives an analgesic, have her receive a dose about 30 minutes before beginning the instruction. Sit down with the client and coach her through the deep breathing and meditation exercise. This will require planning with other staff members so that you are not interrupted.

3. To apply critical thinking for this client, you should consider the knowledge that you have regarding therapeutic communication, sensory disorders and their effect on communication techniques, the client's culture, and the importance of spirituality to older adults. In addition, a review of typical Catholic rituals might prove useful.

Responding to Loss, Death, and Grieving

Chapter

29

CLASSROOM DISCUSSION

1. Discuss the concept and categories of loss. Have students give examples for each of the categories, using personal experiences whenever possible.

2. Discuss the terms and meanings of grief. Review the tasks associated with "TEAR."

3. Review the possible multicultural differences that may be seen in response to loss and grieving. Ask students to share their own or family experiences.

4. Discuss and provide examples of dysfunctional, anticipatory, and disenfranchised grief responses.

5. Compare and contrast the theories of grief and how the nurse may utilize each one to respond to clients.

6. Review what is included in the assessment of a client's response to loss (see Resource for Student Activities, p. 144).

7. Provide the students with the following or similar client situations, and ask them to identify how the individuals may progress through the grieving process. Encourage students to apply the theories of grieving.
   a. A 50-year-old male who has been laid off from his sales position of 20+ years (he is the sole income earner in the family)
   b. An 86-year-old woman who has just lost her pet cat that she has owned since her husband died
   c. A 20-year-old woman who just had a miscarriage
   d. A 5-year-old child who has experienced the death of a parent or grandparent
   e. The middle-age parents of a young adult male who was killed as an innocent bystander in a robbery

8. Discuss the specific approach and goals of hospice care.

9. Invite a nurse who is employed in a hospice to discuss his or her role, the challenges of the position, client and family reactions, and the needs of the nursing staff.

10. Guide students in the application of the nursing process for an actual or simulated client who is experiencing or having difficulty experiencing grief.

11. Discuss nursing measures to promote comfort for the terminally ill client.

12. Describe postmortem care. Have students discuss their feelings about the procedure, and identify what adaptations may be made according to religious or cultural beliefs.

13. Use popular or educational media (e.g., films or television) to stimulate a discussion on loss and grieving.

14. Discuss legal and ethical issues associated with death and dying (e.g., organ transplants, DNR orders).

INTERACTIVE EXERCISES

1. Assign students to investigate the resources available in the affiliating agency and community to assist clients, families, and nurses to deal with loss and the grieving process.

2. Ask students to specify nursing interventions that will assist clients and families to work through loss and the grieving process. Incorporate creative strategies for clients of different ages and sociocultural backgrounds.

3. Videotape students in a role-playing situation where they are to apply therapeutic communication skills in an interaction with a client who is terminally ill. Have students critique the interaction and offer suggestions to their peers for improvement.

4. Working individually or in small groups, have students identify nursing diagnoses, client goals and outcomes, nursing interventions, and evaluation criteria for an actual or simulated client who is experiencing loss, grieving, or dysfunctional grieving.

CLINICAL SKILL

1. Demonstrate postmortem care in a simulated or actual client situation.

CLIENT CARE EXPERIENCE

1. Assign students to participate in the care of clients who are experiencing loss and grief. In preconference or postconference, discuss the nursing care approach and the feelings of the students in working with the clients.

RESOURCE FOR STUDENT ACTIVITIES

Response to loss—assessment tool

Criterion	Assessment Data	Health Promotion Activities
Personal Characteristics		
Nature of Relationships		
Social Support System		
Nature of Loss		
Cultural/Spiritual Beliefs		
Loss of Life Goals		
Hope		
Phase of Grieving		
Family's Grief		
Risk Factors in Survivors		
Nursing Role Perceptions		

CRITICAL THINKING EXERCISES

1. A Hispanic 28-year-old woman has no living children, and she has just lost her third premature infant. Complications of the pregnancy resulted in a hysterectomy to save her life. She remains very stoic in her responses to the entire loss experience. She states that she has a strong, religious belief system that examines death as part of the greater scheme of mankind, in which "all things work together for the good..." Identify the types of loss and the stage of loss that she has experienced. How can the nurse offer hope and closure? What resources are available in your area to assist the grieving process?

2. While in the grocery store, a former neighbor is seen wandering around lost with a very sad face. The woman explains that her husband of 50 years was recently placed in an institution for late stages of Alzheimer's disease and that he does not recognize her at all anymore. Financially, it has cost her everything to put him into the facility, and now she is living with family. How can you begin to rank the priorities of losses that she is experiencing to identify the most urgent need? What coping strategies or interventions might be suggested to assist her? Should you assess the risk for self-harm?

3. A nursing student has experienced a series of actual and perceived personal losses. On the first day of clinical, her client suddenly dies. She starts crying hysterically in the client's room. The instructor pulls the student aside to talk privately with her. In addition, the student failed her examination the day before the clinical experience because she was unable to focus on her studies. What signs/symptoms would indicate the stage of grieving and the success (or lack thereof) of her present coping strategies? What types of questions might be asked to help her do some critical thinking and problem solving for self-management? What do the American Nurses Association *Standards of Clinical Nursing Practice* say about the roles of the educator and the student?

ANSWERS TO CRITICAL THINKING EXERCISES

1. The Hispanic culture is based upon a strong matriarchal society and the deeply embedded ties to the Catholic religion. Both of these cultural and religious influences value the family as a source of strength and the foundation for their faith. Having children is the basis for the family unit. Therefore, with problems such as the inability to have or carry children, the young female is experiencing losses from several perspectives. One developmental loss is that she is failing her family responsibilities by not carrying on the next generation of the family unit. Another aspect of the loss is the inability to follow through on the church's mission of a family unit, thus creating a sense of loss of self. Despite a loss of self, her religious heritage may be strength in her belief that "death is a part of the scheme of life." Some of the losses that are involved in this situation include the following: (a) categories—loss of a significant other and loss of an aspect of self and (b) types of loss—personal, maturational (developmental), actual, perceived, and anticipated. The stage of grief (loss) that is represented in the CT skill situation reflects possibly Kübler-Ross's first stage of denial, Engel's first phase of the loss of reality, or Rando's first grieving response of avoidance. You should offer a listening ear and allow the young woman to reflect her thoughts when she is ready (not when you or family thinks it is time). Affirmation of worth will be difficult to accept in these early stages. Only time and progression to other phases will allow a more honest assessment of one's value. Your acknowledgment of the loss is very

important to show value of both the young woman and the child that was lost. Closure will come much later in the grieving process but suggestions for grief resolution need to be discussed early to allow time to let the concepts sink in. What resources are available in your area? Some examples of resource persons may include the following: an official person at the local hospital, someone at hospice, a local nursing group, or a single resource person who deals frequently with this type of loss (e.g., a minister or a priest).

2. This woman has experienced the following losses: loss of a significant other, financial/personal independence, anticipated future relationship and social status, and aspects of self. The top priority should be to identify issues of her awareness of dangers to herself that are self-defeating or self-destructive in nature. The risk for self-harm must be very high; many spouses die within 6 months of one another despite their apparent good health. Independence can be maintained by encouraging dignity and respect by the helping family. Open communication will assist in averting any potential problems from misunderstandings of expectations of one another. Often, adult children think that they know what is best for the parent, but often it is not what the parent wants. Some strategies for coping include the following concepts: deal with one issue at a time; identify strengths that can be used to encourage problem-solving skills; encourage open communication between the staff and the spouse; support her spiritual needs; encourage the family to show reliance and valuing of her skills; get the family actively involved in the process; demonstrate techniques of collaboration that will be needed for future success in their relationship; reflect on better times; set up a schedule that is convenient and practical for her to visit with her spouse; allow the staff to work with the spouse and avoid burnout; and identify other friends and relatives who also need her attention. Using the TEAR acronym demonstrates the goals expected with accommodation.*

(*Reference: Harper JM: Plateaus of acceptance: pits of pain. In Corr CA, Stillion JM, Ribar MC, editors: *Creativity in death education and counseling*, Hartford, Conn, 1983, Forum for Death Education and Counseling.)

3. a. Behavioral signs/symptoms of dysfunctional grief would include the following (see Box 29-2, p. 614 of *Canadian Fundamentals of Nursing*, Second Edition): overactivity without a sense of loss; alteration in relationships with family or friends; hostility against a specific person; agitated depression with tension, feelings of worthlessness, and extreme guilt; inability to discuss the loss without crying; and false sense of well-being. Further assessment should include the following areas: activity levels, performance of expected roles, goals, hopes, congruency of verbal and nonverbal behaviors, and her understanding of the loss as she sees the situation. Questions should be specific and reflect hope in improvement of the situation. Leading questions should clarify problems and start the critical thinking of what actually has occurred, which, in turn, will identify what can be done to help. Critical analysis of the situation should be based upon realistic insights to the degree and depth of the losses felt and perceived by the individual. Familiar coping strategies have failed with this new loss. New strengths need to be identified to help establish a problem-solving process that is individualized and based upon her perception of the problem. The priority of questions should start with questions about self-destructive behaviors. Identify past successful strategies used by the student and try to adapt these skills to the current problem. The instructor should encourage the student to prioritize and then approach each problem area separately, rather than trying to solve everything at once. By working on smaller parts, and achieving smaller successes, she can gain hope for success over the whole situation.

b. According to BNE Professional Guidelines, a report to the Board of Nurse Examiners is required whenever practice is questioned within the level of understanding of the student and practitioner. The reporting is limited to serious errors in judgment that are exhibited while in the student's role, clinical practitioner's role, or educator's role. The following are only a few of the issues that might be involved with this situation: (1) there is reasonable cause to suspect the ability of a professional nursing student who might be impaired by chemical dependency or mental illness that puts the patients at harm and/or is unable to safely perform services of the nursing profession; (2) role expectations of nursing educators should not include personal counseling of students, and boundaries should be clearly stated to avoid involvement in personal problems beyond the learning setting; (3) professional conduct of the instructor for privacy, confidentiality, and duty to the student should be a part of the established relationship between the educator and the student without bias or prejudice on either part; (4) failure of the educator to assess risks of potential dangers in the student's behaviors or accepting an assignment when the student is not emotionally prepared for the assignment is a serious threat to professionalism; and/or (5) inappropriate delegation of assignments by the educator and clinical staff will also put clients at risk.

Stress and Adaptation

Chapter 30

CLASSROOM DISCUSSION

1. Discuss the concept of stress, and provide examples of stressors.

2. Describe the physiological adaptation to stress and its limitations.

3. Discuss the different models that the nurse may use to understand and respond to stress (see Resources for Student Activities, p. 150). Guide students in the way these models may be applied to an actual and/or simulated personal or client situation.

4. Review adaptation to stressors in relation to the five dimensions. Ask students to provide other specific examples of adaptation and outcomes.

5. Compare Selye's LAS and GAS, providing examples for each syndrome (see Resources for Student Activities, p. 151).

6. Discuss the psychological responses to stress. Ask students to provide examples and/or share with the group their personal responses to stress.

7. Ask students to provide specific examples of how the following indicators may be assessed in an individual experiencing stress: physiological, psychological, developmental, emotional-behavioral, intellectual, sociocultural, family, lifestyle, and spiritual.

8. Guide students in the application of the nursing process for an actual or simulated client who is experiencing stress.

9. Invite a psychiatric nurse practitioner and/or psychologist from an employee assistance program to speak with the class about stress and responses particular to nurses.

10. Describe stress reduction techniques that the nurse may implement for himself or herself and clients. Have students participate in a stress reduction and/or relaxation exercise.

11. Discuss methods of avoiding or reducing stressful situations and responses. Ask students to provide examples or share personal experiences with improving responses to stress.

12. Invite a student who is close to graduation, or who has recently graduated, to speak to the class about strategies to reduce stress while enrolled in nursing school.

13. Discuss crisis (situational and developmental) and crisis intervention strategies.

14. Stimulate a discussion on student perceptions of job-related stress for nurses (burnout).

15. Review the relationship of stress to illness. Provide examples of specific illnesses that have been directly linked to stress.

INTERACTIVE EXERCISES

1. Assign students to report verbally or in writing on available support systems and resources within the school or an affiliating agency for students, nurses, and clients.

2. Have students develop a questionnaire or use an available tool to assess lifestyle and stressors for themselves, their peers, or assigned clients.

3. Working individually or in small groups, have students identify nursing diagnoses, client goals and outcomes, nursing interventions, and evaluation criteria for one of the following or similar client situations:
   a. A 48-year-old professional man who has been laid off from his job after 20 years with the company
   b. A 14-year-old newly diagnosed diabetic who requires dietary adjustment and insulin injections
   c. A 21-year-old first-time mother of a 4-month-old infant who has just moved to a community far from her family and friends
   d. A 70-year-old woman who has experienced increasing difficulty with activities of daily living as a result of arthritic changes in her arms and legs
   e. A 30-year-old student who is trying to balance school assignments, a full-time job, and family responsibilities with her husband and school-age daughter

CLINICAL SKILL

1. Demonstrate stress reduction techniques that the nurse may implement for himself or herself and clients. Have students participate in a stress reduction and/or relaxation exercise.

CLIENT CARE EXPERIENCES

1. Have students assess assigned clients for indications of stress. Discuss how stress reduction activities may be incorporated into the plan of care for the clients.

2. Assign students to prepare and present a teaching plan for a small group of clients on the recognition and reduction of stress.

Models of stress chart
Comparison of local and general adaption syndromes (LAS/GAS)

MODELS OF STRESS CHART

Model	Stress/ Stressors Defined	Responses	Nursing Interventions
Response-Based			
Adaptation			
Stimulus-Based			
Transaction-Based			

LAS	GAS
General Characteristics	**General Characteristics**
Reflex Pain Response	**Alarm Reaction**
Inflammatory Response	**Resistance Stage**
	Exhaustion Stage

CRITICAL THINKING EXERCISES

1. You are a nurse working at a community health fair. A man stops by your health assessment booth and tells you that he has been apathetic and lethargic since he lost his job 2 months ago. He has begun drinking every evening, and his wife is constantly angry with him. What additional areas would you assess? What social supports would be available in your community for him?

2. John Morgan, who has no family history of heart disease, had a myocardial infarction 3 days ago. What risk-factor assessments do you make? What are some lifestyle issues that will need to be assessed?

3. Lu Chen is a Chinese immigrant who is hospitalized following an automobile accident for a possible concussion and broken finger. What cultural barriers might increase her stress? What can you, as the nurse, do to help alleviate some of that stress?

ANSWERS TO CRITICAL THINKING EXERCISES

1. You should assess for current coping mechanisms and support systems. You should explore how drinking affects his mood (e.g., abusive behavior). Assess for the presence of children and how the loss of a job has affected the family. Social supports include Alcoholics Anonymous, spiritual counseling, and community counseling. It is important to involve his wife in the plan of care since the client has a problem that is affecting the entire family.

2. Assess for smoking, obesity, hypertension, job intensity, support systems, and traumatic life events. Smoking cessation, diet, exercise patterns, and current coping mechanisms will all need to be assessed.

3. Language difficulties, unfamiliarity with Western medicine practices, and possible loss of support if the family is unable to remain at bedside are some of the major stressors. Obtaining an interpreter as necessary, using pictures when explaining care, and involving the family of the client in all aspects of care are ways to alleviate stress.

Vital Signs

CLASSROOM DISCUSSION

1. Discuss general guidelines for taking vital signs, including frequency and parameters.

2. Ask students to identify what information is important before the assessment of vital signs and how the findings are correlated with other assessment data.

3. Explain the documentation of vital signs, providing examples of records from different agencies.

4. With the aid of educational media (e.g., videos, models), review the physiology and regulation of body temperature.

5. Discuss factors that affect body temperature: age, exercise, stress, hormone levels, circadian rhythm, and environment. Have students identify how each factor may increase or decrease body temperature.

6. Discuss potential changes in body temperature that the nurse may encounter, including their causative factors and the client's physiological responses.

7. Ask students to identify the following:
   a. How body temperature may differ from one site to another
   b. Advantages and disadvantages of different types of thermometers

8. Review the conversion of Fahrenheit to and from Celsius temperatures.

9. Discuss the assessment of, and interventions that may be implemented for, increases and decreases in body temperature. Have students identify specific examples of client responses and nursing interventions for situations involving significant increases and decreases in body temperature.

10. With the aid of educational media, review the physiology and regulation of the pulse.

11. Discuss factors that affect the pulse: fever, anxiety, blood loss, exercise, pain, and medications. Have students identify how each factor may influence the pulse.

12. Discuss the assessment of, and nursing interventions that may be implemented for, alterations in a client's pulse. Have students identify specific indications of pulse alterations and the resultant nursing responsibilities.

13. With the aid of educational media, review the physiology and regulation of respiration and the mechanics of breathing.

14. Discuss factors that may influence the rate, rhythm, and depth of respirations. Have students identify how each factor may alter respiration.

15. Discuss the assessment of and interventions that may be implemented for alterations in respiration. Have students identify specific indications of respiratory alterations and the resultant nursing responsibilities.

16. With the aid of educational media, review the physiology of blood pressure.

17. Discuss factors that affect blood pressure: age, stress, race, medical conditions, diurnal variation, and gender. Have students identify how each factor may increase or decrease blood pressure.

18. Discuss potential changes in blood pressure (hypertension/hypotension) that the nurse may encounter, including their causative factors and the client's physiological response.

19. Ask students to identify how vital signs change in accordance with growth and development (see Resources for Student Activities, p. 157).

20. Review the parameters for assessment of blood pressure and subsequent referral when screening is conducted in a community setting or health fair.

21. Ask students to determine the following:
    a. How the environment may influence the measurement of vital signs or the assessment findings
    b. How the environment may be manipulated to promote accurate findings and enhance client comfort

22. Discuss how the measurement and evaluation of vital signs may be incorporated into a client's care plan or critical pathway.

23. Have students identify how the assessment of vital signs may be influenced and adapted in the following, or similar, situations:
    a. Client has just finished drinking coffee
    b. Client returned a few minutes ago from a rigorous physical therapy session
    c. Client has evidence of a dysrhythmia
    d. Client states that he or she feels lightheaded when getting out of bed
    e. Client is currently taking a medication for a cardiac or respiratory condition
    f. Client is 6 months old
    g. Client is experiencing rectal bleeding
    h. Client is an obese adult
    i. Client has a history of seizure activity
    j. Client was in an automobile accident and has casts on both upper extremities

INTERACTIVE EXERCISES

1. Provide practice Fahrenheit and Celsius temperatures for students to convert.

2. Provide a list of clients of various ages and their vital signs, and ask students to determine whether the findings are within expectations.

3. Working individually or in small groups, have students design a teaching plan for a client's self-measurement of pulse and/or blood pressure.

CLINICAL SKILLS

1. Assessment of body temperature:
   a. Explain and demonstrate, using different body sites and equipment, the assessment of body temperature. (Use simulation mannequins or models and/or volunteers to demonstrate the assessment of the vital signs.)
   b. Have small groups of students practice on mannequins and/or their peers the assessment of body temperature using the following:
      Electronic, glass, and disposable thermometers
      Oral, rectal, axillary, and tympanic sites
   c. Evaluate the students' ability to accurately assess and record body temperature through return demonstration and skill testing before clinical experiences.

2. Assessment of the pulse:
   a. Explain and demonstrate, using different sites, the assessment of the pulse, including the correct use of the stethoscope. Use audiotapes, if available, and a dual earpiece stethoscope to facilitate the explanation and demonstration of apical pulse and blood pressure assessment.
   b. Have small groups of students practice on simulation mannequins and/or their peers the assessment of the pulse using the following:
      Temporal, carotid, brachial, radial, ulnar, femoral, popliteal, posterior tibial, and dorsalis pedis sites (see Resources for Student Activities, p. 157).
      A stethoscope for apical pulse determination
   c. Evaluate the students' ability to accurately assess and record the pulse through return demonstration and skill testing before clinical experiences.

3. Assessment of respirations and oxygen saturation:
   a. Explain and demonstrate the assessment of respirations, identifying how the assessment is integrated into the procedure to avoid altering the findings.
   b. Explain and demonstrate the assessment of oxygen saturation through the use of the pulse oximeter.
   c. Have small groups of students practice the assessment of respirations and use of the pulse oximeter.
   d. Evaluate the students' ability to accurately assess and record respirations and use the pulse oximeter through return demonstration and skill testing before clinical experiences.

4. Assessment of blood pressures:
   a. Explain and demonstrate, using different sites and equipment, the assessment of blood pressure.
   b. Have small groups of students practice the assessment of blood pressure using the following:
      Aneroid, mercury, and electronic sphygmomanometers
      Ultrasound and palpation
      Upper and lower extremity sites
   c. Evaluate the students' ability to accurately assess and record blood pressure through return demonstration and skill testing before clinical experiences.

CLIENT CARE EXPERIENCES

1. Assign students to assess, report, and record vital signs for clients of different ages in the clinical setting. Discuss expectations beforehand and the students' findings and interventions after the experience. Ask students how the client's status was reflected in the vital signs assessed.

2. Have students participate in a community blood pressure screening.

3. Have students complete a care plan or pathway for an assigned client, incorporating the measurement and evaluation of vital signs.

4. Have students present a teaching plan on self-measurement of pulse and/or blood pressure to a client within an agency or community setting.

RESOURCES FOR STUDENT ACTIVITIES

Pulse measurement form
Comparison chart—vital signs across the life span
Vital signs assessment form

PULSE MEASUREMENT FORM

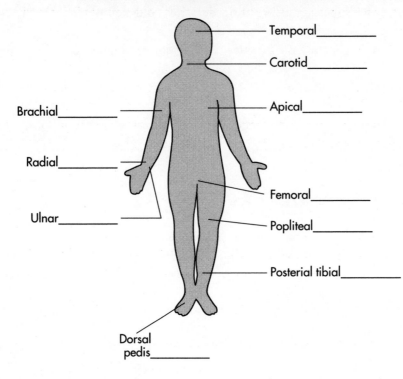

Temporal_____

Carotid_____

Brachial_____

Apical_____

Radial_____

Ulnar_____

Femoral_____

Popliteal_____

Posterial tibial_____

Dorsal pedis_____

COMPARISON CHART—VITAL SIGNS ACROSS THE LIFE SPAN

	Temperature	Pulse	Respiration	Blood Pressure
Infant				
Toddler				
Preschool Child				
School-Age Child				
Adolescent				
Adult				
Older Adult				

154   Unit 6: Scientific Basis for Nursing Practice

VITAL SIGNS ASSESSMENT FORM

Age:		Height:
Sex:		Weight:

Known Medical Conditions:

Vital Signs	Findings	Comparison to Norms
Temperature Site		
Pulse Site(s) Rate Rhythm Strength Equality		
Respiration Rate Depth Rhythm		
Blood Pressure Site Sitting/Standing/Supine		

CRITICAL THINKING EXERCISES

1. A 47-year-old African-American man is coming to the health clinic for a physical examination by the nurse practitioner for a routine employment physical. The nursing assistant obtains the following routine vital signs: tympanic temperature, 36.9° C (98.4° F); right radial pulse rate of 96 and irregular; BP, sitting, right arm 162/82, left arm 150/70; SpO₂, 95% on room air; respiratory rate 22.

   a. As the admitting nurse, what questions would you ask this client to evaluate his risk for hypertension?

   b. Based on these vital signs, what actions should you take?

2. A teenage mother brings her 3-year-old child to the walk-in health center. She notes that he has been fussy, has not had much of an appetite, and is not his active self. The boy is crying and struggling to get out of his mother's lap during your interview. You note that he is small for his age, but otherwise well developed.

   a. Describe the sequence you would use for obtaining vital signs.

   b. When selecting the appropriate equipment for obtaining the vital signs, what, if any, special considerations are needed?

   c. The unlicensed caregiver reports she has obtained a temperature of 37.7° C (99.8° F). What additional information do you request from the caregiver?

3. A 52-year-old woman is admitted to the medical unit for chronic dyspnea and discomfort in her left chest with deep breathing and coughing. She has been smoking for 35 years and has a 20-year history of emphysema. Over the past 4 months she has lost 10 pounds and currently weighs 110 pounds.

   a. When delegating the vital signs to the unlicensed assistant what information and directions should you provide?

   b. The blood pressure and heart rate are within acceptable ranges. The temperature is 37.5° C (99.5° F) tympanic, the respiratory rate 32 and shallow, the SpO₂ 89%. Based on these results, list your actions in priority.

4. An 82-year-old resident in your subacute extended care facility is being treated for pneumonia with antibiotics. She has been on bed rest for the past 2 days. She has a history of hypertension, treated with diuretics, but is otherwise healthy. She has been afebrile for the past 24 hours and is eager to walk to the activity room. She has activity orders "up ad lib."

   a. Should you delegate the ambulation assistance to an unlicensed caregiver?

   b. What places this client at risk for fainting?

   c. Explain to this patient the reason you are obtaining orthostatic measurements.

Answers to Critical Thinking Exercises

1. a. Information that would elicit this client's risk for hypertension includes the following: activity such as work and exercise; typical diet; salt consumption; tobacco use; alcohol use; and family history of cardiovascular disease, high blood pressure, and stroke.

   b. Actions should include reassessment of heart rate and blood pressure. Heart rate should be obtained over 60 minutes using apical count and evaluated for pulse deficit. The blood pressure should be reassessed as the values are outside acceptable range. Attention should be paid to proper size cuff and technique. If the blood pressure is still outside the acceptable range, the health care provider is notified immediately. The client should be counseled to return for follow-up visits for blood pressure checks. Risk-factor modification education is indicated.

2. a. Suggested sequence for vital signs: tympanic temperature, SpO_2, brachial pulse, respirations, with blood pressure last.

   b. When selecting a blood pressure cuff, an appropriate size should be selected based on the child's arm circumference.

   c. Questions of the caregiver should include the type of thermometer used and, if tympanic, which ear was used.

3. a. The unlicensed assistant should be directed not to obtain an oral thermometer. If a tympanic thermometer is not available, axillary temperature is indicated, because to place the client in a supine position would be difficult. The respiratory rate and SpO_2 measurements should be obtained with the client upright. The UAP should be instructed to report a RR >20, SpO_2 <90%, HR >100, immediately.

   b. You should reassess the respiratory rate and include a complete respiratory assessment. The SpO_2 is also repeated. If a prn oxygen order has been written, the parameters should be noted and oxygen applied appropriately. The physician or nurse in charge should be notified immediately. The client should be instructed to maintain bed rest.

4. a. Ambulation out of bed for the first time in 2 days should not be delegated, as you need to evaluate the client's response to assuming an upright position.

   b. The client is at risk for postural hypotension related to bed rest, hypertension medication, and possible fluid volume deficit following pneumonia and fever.

   c. Explanation is given to client for the orthostatic measurements.

Health Assessment and Physical Examination

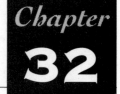

Chapter

32

CLASSROOM DISCUSSION

1. Discuss the purposes of the physical examination and health assessment.

2. Review the importance of determining baseline information to compare findings from the physical examination/assessment.

3. Ask students to identify how cultural awareness and sensitivity may be incorporated into the physical examination/assessment. Have students provide specific examples of how client preparation and the performance of the examination may be amended by the nurse.

4. Review general concepts of growth and development in relation to the approach taken in the performance of the physical examination for different age-groups. Have students provide specific examples of how client preparation and the performance of the examination may be adapted to meet the needs of clients of different age and developmental levels.

5. Stimulate a discussion on how physical assessment may be incorporated into nursing interactions with clients in the health care setting.

   Ask students what information may be obtained during the following or similar nursing activities:
   a. Taking the health history
   b. Providing hygienic care
   c. Assisting the client to dress
   d. Administering medications

6. Identify infection control measures that should be implemented in the performance of a physical assessment (refer to Chapter 33 of *Canadian Fundamentals of Nursing,* Second Edition).

7. Discuss the arrangement of the environment in preparation for the physical assessment.

8. Stimulate a discussion on how the physical assessment may be made more comfortable for the client and the nurse. Have students provide specific examples of nursing interventions that should promote overall comfort for clients of different ages and backgrounds.

9. Review the role and importance of communication with the client throughout the procedure. Ask students to specify possible points in the assessment in which an opportunity for client teaching may arise.

10. Discuss the general organization and sequence of the assessment. Have students identify situations in which the usual sequence may be altered (e.g., client in severe pain).

11. Describe the documentation of the findings from the physical assessment, focusing on the utilization of appropriate terminology. Provide examples of documentation from different agencies or resources.

12. Invite a nurse practitioner to speak to the class about the implementation of the physical examination/assessment and the application of findings into the care of the client.

13. Discuss the responsibilities of the nurse upon completion of the physical examination/assessment.

14. Ask students to identify how the physical assessment may be adapted for the following clients:
    a. A 4-year-old child
    b. A 16-year-old anxious female
    c. An adult male with abdominal pain
    d. An older adult female with arthritis
    e. A client who does not speak or understand the nurse's language
    f. A young adult regaining consciousness after an automobile accident

15. Discuss how the physical assessment and resultant findings may be integrated into the client's care plan or critical pathway.

16. Review the recommended preventive screenings for adults.

INTERACTIVE EXERCISES

1. Organize a role-playing experience with the students simulating the client's physical and psychological preparation for the assessment.

2. Have students identify the expected norms and possible alterations that may be found during the physical assessment.

3. Working individually or in small groups, have students design a teaching plan for adult clients on breast or testicular self-examination or another preventative health measure.

4. Have students practice recording and reporting physical assessment findings.

5. Provide students with a list of physical assessment findings, and have them identify the expected and unexpected findings (e.g., cloudy pupils, transparent conjunctiva, rebound tenderness).

CLINICAL SKILLS

1. Explain and demonstrate (using a simulation mannequin or volunteer) the skills of physical assessment: inspection, palpation, percussion, auscultation, and olfaction.

Ask students to identify where and when each skill would be used best and what information each skill elicits (see Resources for Student Activities, p. 164).

Use educational media, such as audiotapes and videotapes, to reinforce the skills and the assessment findings that are expected.

2. Have students prepare a simulated setting for a client assessment.

3. Describe and demonstrate using simulation mannequins/models or volunteers client positioning during the physical assessment.

4. Explain and demonstrate (using simulation mannequins/models, volunteers, or videotapes/ computer programs) the systematic approach to the physical assessment as follows:
>   General survey
>   Skin, hair, nails
>   Head and neck
>   Thorax and lungs
>   Heart
>   Vascular system
>   Breasts
>   Abdomen
>   Female genitalia (speculum examination, if appropriate for class)
>   Male genitalia
>   Rectum and anus
>   Musculoskeletal system
>   Neurological system

Review normal anatomy and physiology, as indicated.

5. Explain and demonstrate the use of specific equipment (as appropriate to the class) used in the physical assessment: ophthalmoscope/otoscope, speculum, reflex hammer, etc.

6. Working in pairs or small groups, have students practice selected areas and/or the entirety of the physical assessment, with supervision.

7. Evaluate students' ability to perform and document selected areas and/or an entire physical assessment through return demonstration and skill testing before clinical experience.

CLIENT CARE EXPERIENCES

1. Have students present a teaching plan on breast and/or testicular self-examination to a client group in an acute care or community setting.

2. Assign students to observe and/or perform a physical assessment (as appropriate to the class) for a client in a health care setting; provide supervision, as indicated. Have students record and report their findings. Discuss the expectations with the group before the experience and their findings and personal observations and feelings after the assessment.

3. Have students complete a care plan/pathway for an assigned client, incorporating the physical assessment and evaluation of findings.

RESOURCES FOR STUDENT ACTIVITIES

Physical assessment skills chart
Comparison form—physical assessment findings

PHYSICAL ASSESSMENT SKILLS CHART

Assessment Skill	Area(s) Assessed	Information Obtained
Inspection		
Palpation		
Percussion		
Auscultation		
Olfaction		

COMPARISON FORM—PHYSICAL ASSESSMENT FINDINGS

Assessment Area	Expected Findings	Unexpected Findings
General Appearance/ Behavior		
Vital Signs		
Skin, Hair, Nails		
Head, Neck		
Thorax, Lungs		
Heart		
Vascular System		
Breasts		
Abdomen		
Female/Male Genitalia		
Rectum, Anus		
Musculoskeletal System		
Neurological System		

CRITICAL THINKING EXERCISES

1. A 32-year-old client entering a neighborhood clinic has the following symptoms: frequent productive cough, fatigue, decreased appetite, and persistent fever. What focused assessment should the nurse conduct?

2. The nurse is performing an abdominal assessment and observes a pulsating midline abdominal mass. What is the nurse's next line of action?

3. A 75-year-old black man is being visited 1 week postoperatively by the home health nurse to assess his peripheral vascular status following a femoral-popliteal bypass graft for arterial insufficiency. What assessment data need to be obtained by the nurse?

4. Develop a teaching plan for a female client (age 40) with a family history of breast cancer who acknowledges that she does not perform a monthly breast self-examination (BSE).

5. What physical examination techniques does the nurse use during assessment of the following clients?
   a. A client suspected of having a head injury
   b. A client with a cast on the lower leg
   c. A client reporting abdominal pain

ANSWERS TO CRITICAL THINKING EXERCISES

1. The nurse should perform a detailed history, identifying that this client is at risk for lung disease (e.g., tuberculosis, HIV pulmonary disease, and pneumonia). All techniques of respiratory assessment should be completed, such as inspection, palpation (excursion, tactile fremitus, percussion, auscultation), pulse, blood pressure, and temperature.

2. The nurse must not palpate the abdominal mass; the physician should be notified.

3. Assessment criteria: color, temperature, pulse, edema, and skin changes

   Systems assessed: skin and neurovascular

   Client's history: especially pain, helps to identify occlusion (3 Ps: pain, pallor, pulselessness)

   Pallor in the dark-skinned client: normal brown skin appears yellow brown and normal black skin appears ashen gray

4. The teaching plan should include the following: review and educate client about why BSE is important; provide literature from the American Cancer Society regarding breast cancer; discuss risk factors for breast cancer; discuss ACS's recommendations for early detection of breast cancer; demonstrate how to perform BSE and have client demonstrate BSE; and schedule an appointment with client's primary caregiver for examination.

5. Physical examination measures:
   a. Head injury—client's history, complete neurological examination (most importantly Glasgow coma scale and cranial nerves II, III, IV, VI)
   b. Cast on lower leg—inspection and palpation of skin and neurovascular assessment
   c. Abdominal pain—client's history and palpation of affected area

Infection Control

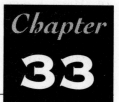

Chapter 33

CLASSROOM DISCUSSION

1. Discuss the chain of infection, including factors that contribute to the development of an infection.

2. For each step of the chain of infection, ask students to provide specific examples of different possible infectious agents, reservoirs, portals of exit, modes of transmission, portals of entry, and susceptible hosts.

3. Review what is entailed in the infectious process. Have students identify positive and negative nursing interventions in response to the infectious process.

4. Review normal body defenses against infection.

5. Describe the inflammatory process and immune response and resultant physiological manifestations. Have students specify client signs and symptoms that indicate that body defenses have been mobilized against an infection.

6. Review the types of immunity and the role of vaccines and immunizations.

7. Discuss nosocomial infections: iatrogenic, endogenous/exogenous. Ask students to determine what may contribute to or reduce the development of these infections in the health care setting.

8. Explain the concept of asepsis in the health care environment, including the differences between medical and surgical aseptic practices. Have students provide situations where each type of asepsis should be applied.

9. Discuss factors that may put the client at a greater risk for infection: age, altered nutrition, stress, heredity, disease processes, medications, and medical treatments.

   Have students specify assessment findings that would indicate that the client might be at greater risk for developing an infection (e.g., infancy, diabetes, and urinary catheterization).

10. Describe local and systemic signs and symptoms of infection (see Resource for Student Activities, p. 170).

11. Discuss the laboratory tests used and the results that are indicative of an infectious process.

12. Guide students in the application of the critical thinking model and the nursing process for a client who is experiencing an infectious process.

13. Discuss nursing interventions that may be implemented to reduce or eliminate the infectious process. Ask students to specify additional strategies to break the chain of infection.

14. Have students discuss what they believe is meant by an "infection control conscience."

15. Identify and/or have students identify supportive measures that may be used to promote the client's defenses against infection.

16. Describe the specific measures that are incorporated in medical asepsis, and the nurse's role in the implementation of this type of asepsis. Have students identify what principles or procedures of medical asepsis should be applied in the following or similar examples:
    a. Disposing of an exudate-filled dressing
    b. Removal of contaminated body fluids
    c. Changing of bed linens
    d. Discarding used equipment — syringes, needles, tubing

17. Explain the different types of isolation measures/barrier precautions, per Centers for Disease Control and Prevention (CDC) guidelines.

18. Discuss the application of and measures included in standard precautions, including the two-tiered approach.

19. Ask students to identify how clients, prior to the CDC guidelines, may have been over-isolated or under-isolated.

20. Stimulate a discussion on how the frequent use of nonsterile gloves may have a negative impact upon the client or how health care providers may "misuse" them.

21. Identify the basic principles of isolation, commonly used equipment (gloves, gowns, masks, protective eyewear), and specific guidelines for selected disease processes (e.g., tuberculosis).

22. Ask students how the psychological effect of isolation may be minimized for the client.

23. Invite a risk manager nurse to speak to the class about his or her role in infection control and promotion of client defenses.

24. Describe the principles and measures that are specific to surgical asepsis, including when objects are considered contaminated. Ask students to provide examples of breaks in sterile technique.

25. Discuss the difference between routine hand washing and a surgical scrub.

26. Have students indicate whether the following nursing interventions require clean or sterile gloves:
    a. Changing a surgical dressing
    b. Taking an oral temperature
    c. Obtaining a venous blood sample
    d. Providing hygienic care
    e. Inserting a urinary catheter
    f. Preparing an intramuscular injection

27. Ask students how aseptic practices may be amended, without being abandoned, in the client's home environment.

INTERACTIVE EXERCISES

1. Working individually or in small groups, have students design a teaching plan on measures to implement to control the spread of infection for a client in the acute or home care environment.

2. Provide students with the following or another similar list of client situations, and ask students to identify what precautions should be implemented in the acute care setting (including transfers within the institution) or home environment:
   a. A child with gastroenteritis
   b. Purulent drainage seeping from a client's surgical wound
   c. Clients with hepatitis A, B, or C
   d. A middle adult client with TB
   e. An adolescent with leukemia

3. Assign students to participate in an affiliating agency's in-service programs on infection control and health care worker responsibilities (as available).

4. Have students investigate and report on resources pertinent to infection control that are available for nurses within an affiliating agency.

5. Organize a role-playing experience with one group of students demonstrating both good and bad aseptic technique, and the other students identifying the positive and negative examples.

CLINICAL SKILLS

1. Have students simulate the preparation of an acute care room for a client who requires second-tier precautions.

2. Explain and demonstrate the procedure for opening a sterile package, and have students practice the technique.

3. Explain and demonstrate (using appropriate supplies and equipment and educational media, as available) the following skills associated with medical or surgical asepsis:
   a. Hand washing
   b. Isolation precautions
   c. Applying a surgical mask
   d. Preparing a sterile field
   e. Performing a surgical scrub
   f. Applying a sterile gown and performing closed gloving
   g. Performing open gloving

4. Have small groups of students practice the skills of medical and surgical asepsis, using the appropriate equipment and supplies.

166   Unit 6: Scientific Basis for Nursing Practice

5. Evaluate the students' ability to implement the skills of medical and surgical asepsis through return demonstration and skill testing before clinical experience.

CLIENT CARE EXPERIENCES

1. Have students present a teaching plan on measures to control the spread of infection to a client or family who is experiencing an infectious process.

2. Assign students to observe and participate in the nursing care of clients experiencing, or at risk for developing, an infectious process within an acute, extended, rehabilitation, and/or home care setting.

   Discuss expectations with the group before the experience, and have students report on their interactions, specific to infection control, after the assignment.

3. Have students complete a care plan/pathway for an assigned client who has an infection present, or who is at risk of developing an infection.

RESOURCE FOR STUDENT ACTIVITIES

Comparison of local and systemic infections—client responses

COMPARISON OF LOCAL AND SYSTEMIC INFECTIONS—CLIENT RESPONSES

Type of Infection	Client Responses
Local	
Systemic	

CRITICAL THINKING EXERCISES

1. Mrs. Jaycock had an indwelling urethral catheter for 1 week. The catheter has now been out for 24 hours. She complains of frequency and pain on urination. Mrs. Jaycock suggests reinsertion of the catheter because of the need to get up frequently. What can frequency or pain on urination be an indication of? Should the catheter be reinserted? Why or why not? Describe at least two independent clinical actions for Mrs. Jaycock.

2. You are caring for Mr. Huang, who has a large, open, and draining abdominal wound. You notice another health care worker changing Mr. Huang's dressing without wearing gloves or using sterile supplies or sterile technique. When you question the health care worker regarding his or her practice, this person says, "Don't worry, the wound is already infected, and the antibiotics and draining will take care of any contaminants." How would you respond to this comment? What would your next steps be in following up on this incident?

3. Ms. Long became ill suddenly with fever, conjunctivitis, and a rash. Her doctor diagnosed measles. Describe the phase of the immune response in which the viral cells are attacked by the body. What class of immunoglobulins would be measured at this time?

4. Mrs. Niles is 83 years of age and lives alone. She has difficulty walking and relies on a church volunteer group to deliver lunches during the week. Her fixed income limits her ability to buy food. Last week, Mrs. Niles's 79-year-old sister died. The two sisters had been very close. As a home health care nurse, explain the factors that might increase Mrs. Niles's risk for infection.

ANSWERS TO CRITICAL THINKING EXERCISES

1. Frequency or pain on urination can be an indication of a urinary tract infection. No—reinsertion of the catheter could complicate the urinary tract infection and would not help in curing the problem.

   Clinical actions: increase fluid intake, encourage frequent voiding, teach client to wipe from front to back after having a bowel movement

2. It is important not to further contaminate the wound. In addition, you do not want to contaminate yourself. It is important to be consistent in the care provided to Mr. Huang. The next steps would be to approach the worker on the issue and report it to management if it is not resolved.

3. Through the process of phagocytosis, specialized WBCs, called neutrophils and monocytes, ingest and destroy microorganisms or other small particles. IgM would be measured at this time.

4. Factors that may increase the risk for infection include age, stress, and nutritional status.

Medication Administration

Chapter 34

CLASSROOM DISCUSSION

1. Discuss terminology related to drugs – names, classifications, and forms.

2. Identify legislation and standards associated with the administration and use of drugs. Ask students to identify how legal guidelines influence the nurse's role in the control and administration of medications.

3. Describe the different drug actions, including the pharmacokinetics: absorption, distribution, metabolism, and excretion of drugs. Have students provide specific examples of how drug actions are influenced by the following factors: type and dosage of drug administered, route of administration, and individual client status (e.g., age, weight, medical condition).

4. Discuss how the following effects of a medication may be differentiated, and the nursing responsibilities associated with each:
   a. Therapeutic effect
   b. Side effect
   c. Toxic effect
   d. Idiosyncratic reaction
   e. Allergic reaction
   f. Drug interaction
   g. Dose response

5. Review factors that influence the actions of drugs: genetics, physiological and psychological variables, environment, and diet. Ask students to provide examples of how the influence may be increased or decreased therapeutically.

6. Identify the different routes by which medications may be administered and the factors involved in the selection of different routes. Ask students to identify the advantages and disadvantages that are associated with each route.

7. Review the metric, apothecary, and household measurement systems and the conversion and calculation of drug dosages. Review the specific calculation for pediatric dosages.

8. Discuss the roles of the physician, pharmacist, and nurse or nurse practitioner in the preparation and administration of medications.

9. Invite a nurse practitioner to speak to the class about his or her preparation for and the responsibilities entailed in the prescription of medications.

10. Guide students in the application of the critical thinking model and the nursing process for clients requiring medications.

11. Ask students what client assessment information is crucial to obtain to safely administer medications.

12. Describe the documentation required after the administration of client medications. Review the legal and safety implications of accurate and timely documentation.

13. Discuss what is incorporated in the nurse's evaluation of the client responses to medications, and the resultant responsibilities based on the evaluation.

14. Discuss the five rights of medication administration. Have students identify how each "right" is determined.

15. Ask students what should be done in the following situations:
    a. Two clients on a unit have the same name
    b. Client has no ID band
    c. Client questions the medication being given
    d. Nurse cannot read the smeared label of a medication bottle
    e. Tablets need to be scored or crushed
    f. Child requires an extremely small liquid dosage
    g. Client is not able to tolerate swallowing pills
    h. An IM site appears hard
    i. A prn pain medication is ordered
    j. A medication to be given is more effective when given on an empty stomach

16. Have students suggest possible reasons for medication errors and how errors might be prevented, and identify the responsibilities of the nurse if an error does occur.

17. Discuss special considerations associated with the administration of medications to infants, children, and older adults. Have students identify particular examples of how the nurse may adapt his or her approach in administering medications for clients in these age groups.

18. Ask students to identify the nurse's responsibility for each of the following client situations:
    a. One of the end-of-shift narcotics counts is incorrect
    b. A needle stick occurs after the injection is given
    c. The client refuses to take the medication that is ordered
    d. Blood is aspirated back into the syringe during an IM injection
    e. The client's vital signs, pulse, respiration, and/or blood pressure have decreased significantly
    f. A rash is noted on the client's upper chest and arms
    g. The client cannot hold the medication cup to swallow the tablets
    h. Another nurse requests that you give the client medications already prepared
    i. The dosage of the medication ordered is double the usual amount for the drug
    j. The client is at physical therapy when the medications are ready to be given
    k. An extremely thin or obese client requires IM injections
    l. An IM medication is extremely irritating to the tissues
    m. A newborn requires an IM injection
    n. A 1-year-old child has an IV infusion to be maintained

INTERACTIVE EXERCISES

1. Provide students with a variety of drug calculations for practise and/or determination of competence in preparation to administer drugs. Use the following and/or similar examples:
   a. Ordered: Demerol 75 mg IM; Available: Demerol 100 mg/cc
   b. Ordered: digoxin 0.25 mg PO; Available: digoxin 0.125-mg tablets
   c. Ordered: Tylenol 40 mg PO; Available: Tylenol 80 mg/2.5 mL

2. Organize a debate on the topic of whether the nurse or another ancillary health care worker (e.g., pharmacy technician) should be responsible for the administration of medications.

3. Arrange for students to visit the pharmacy in an acute care facility to observe the preparation and dispensing of medications. Ask the pharmacist to discuss his or her role in drug preparation and distribution, and coordination with the nursing staff.

4. Working individually or in small groups, have students design a client teaching plan related to self-administration of medications (e.g., home IV therapy, insulin injections).

5. Assign students to investigate the resources available to clients in the affiliating agency or community that will facilitate self- or family administration of medications in the home. Students may report, verbally or in writing, on available referral sources (i.e., home care, visiting nursing services) that have been determined and the criteria for client referrals.

6. Provide examples of forms from different agencies for students to review and practise documentation of medication administration.

7. Have students develop creative strategies to enhance medication compliance that may be implemented for an older adult client who lives alone, and has diminished vision and occasional lapses of memory.

CLINICAL SKILLS

1. Explain and demonstrate (using simulation mannequins/models, appropriate equipment, and educational media) the preparation and administration of medications as follows:
   a. Oral administration
   b. Parenteral administration
      Injections
         Preparation from an ampule or a vial
         Mixing of medications
         Subcutaneous, intramuscular, and intradermal routes/sites
         Z-track and air-lock techniques
         Safe handling and disposal of equipment
      IV infusions
         Large volume
         Bolus (if appropriate for class)
         Volume-controlled
         Piggyback
         Intermittent access

    c. Topical applications
        Skin applications
        Eye, ear, nasal instillations
        Vaginal instillations
        Rectal suppositories
    d. Metered-dose inhalers
    e. Irrigations

2. Have small groups of students practise, with supervision, the preparation and administration of medications via the specified routes, using simulation mannequins/models, grapefruits (or similar "practise" fruits), and/or injection pads. Focus on the selection of the appropriate equipment (e.g., needle length and gauge, syringe, IV setup) for the specific administration route and the accurate calculation of dosage to be administered.

3. Describe the preparation and administration of medications through enteral tubes (nasogastric, jejunostomy, gastrostomy, and feeding tubes). Demonstrate the procedure using available educational media, appropriate equipment, and simulation mannequins/models.

4. Have students practise the preparation and administration of medications through enteral tubes (as available).

5. Evaluate, through return demonstration and skill testing, the students' ability to accurately and safely prepare and administer medications and document the procedure appropriately before clinical experience.

CLIENT CARE EXPERIENCES

1. Have students present a teaching plan on self-medication administration to an adult client or parent.

2. Assign students to observe and participate, with supervision, in the preparation and administration of medications to clients in a health care setting.

3. Discuss expectations with the group before the experience, having students follow through on the "five rights." Have students identify the therapeutic use of the medications for their clients. Review general observations of their medication administration with the group. Have students report back on their experience.

4. Ask students to identify situations that may have been noted in the clinical area that could contribute to medication errors, and have them suggest strategies that may eliminate the problems.

5. Have students complete a care plan/pathway for an assigned client in which the administration of medications is integrated into the approach.

RESOURCES FOR STUDENT ACTIVITIES

Effects of medications chart
Comparison chart of subcutaneous, intramuscular, and intradermal injections
Routes of medication administrationùnursing responsibilities

EFFECTS OF MEDICATIONS CHART

Effects	Nursing Assessment
Therapeutic Action	
Side Effect	
Toxic Effect	
Idiosyncratic Reaction	
Allergic Reaction	
Drug Interaction	
Drug Dose Response	

COMPARISON CHART OF SUBCUTANEOUS, INTRAMUSCULAR, AND INTRADERMAL INJECTIONS

	Subcutaneous	Intramuscular	Intradermal
Needle Gauge/ Length			
Sites Used			
Angle of Injection			
Maximum Amount of Medication			
Specific Medications Given by Route			

ROUTES OF MEDICATION ADMINISTRATION – NURSING RESPONSIBILITIES

Routes	Nursing Responsibilities
Oral	
Parenteral	
Topical	
Inhalation	
Intraocular	

CRITICAL THINKING EXERCISES

1. You are the nurse in charge of a medical unit. A new nurse tells you that there are too many medications to administer to the clients under her care and that she would never be able to administer all of the medications on time. As the charge nurse on this unit, how would you intervene in this situation? What would you tell this new nurse?

2. You are preparing to administer an anticoagulant medication (Coumadin) to a client. When you review the medication with the client, he tells you that the colour of the "blood thinner" (Coumadin) does not look like the one he takes at home. How would you respond to this client?

3. You receive a computerized medical order for a medication with which you are very familiar. However, it does not seem clear to you why this medication was ordered for your client, as she does not have a condition for which this medication is commonly used. How would you proceed in this case?

4. Your client is receiving insulin at home and has run out of syringes. You have some 1-mL tuberculin syringes on hand. The client needs to receive 18 U of NPH and 4 U of regular insulin. How would you draw this up? How many tenths of a millilitre of each insulin would you draw up?

ANSWERS TO CRITICAL THINKING EXERCISES

1. To ensure that the clients under this nurse's care receive all of their medications on time, your most immediate response should be to assist this nurse with medication administration. It is not uncommon for many new nurses to experience this particular situation. Provide coaching to this nurse by informing her that with time and sharpened time-management skills, her medication administration skills will improve.

2. You should tell the client that his "blood thinner" (Coumadin) comes in many different colours (dosage forms) and that you will make sure that this (Coumadin) is the medication that has been ordered for him. You should check the client's medical record for the order that corresponds to the dosage in hand. Check the MAR for proper transcription of the order. If all are correct, the medication dosage was probably changed for a clinical reason or due to a laboratory finding. The nurse should clearly understand the reason for the change, so that it can be explained thoroughly to the client.

3. Medications administered to clients may have more than one intended effect. To adequately monitor a client for the therapeutic response to a medication, it is essential that you understand why a medication is ordered and how it works on the body. It is also possible that this medication has been ordered for this client in error. You should immediately notify the prescriber and clarify the medication order. You should never administer a medication that you feel uncomfortable administering. If this is the case, you should notify the nurse in charge or the nursing supervisor.

4. It is not advisable to use syringes for purposes for which they are not intended. Using tuberculin syringes instead of insulin syringes may confuse the client about the proper procedure for insulin administration. You should call the client's pharmacy or health care provider to obtain a new supply of syringes. In a pinch, one-tenth of a millilitre on a tuberculin syringe is equivalent to ten U on an insulin syringe.

Complementary and Alternative Therapies

Chapter 35

CLASSROOM DISCUSSION

1. Discuss complementary and alternative therapies, their relationship to allopathic medicine, and the difficulties in arriving at a definition of each.

2. Discuss the reasons for Canadians' increased interest in CAM therapies in the past decade.

3. Have students share their personal and family experiences with the use of CAM therapies.

4. Describe biobehaviour therapies and their use with clients experiencing the following:
   a. Dysfunctional grieving
   b. Sleep disorders
   c. Hypertension
   d. Cardiac dysrhythmias
   e. Cerebrovascular or neurological injury
   f. End-stage cancer

5. Describe manual healing therapies and their advantages, limitations, and appropriate use in various clinical situations with which the students are familiar.

6. Discuss the advantages of an integrative medicine approach for both client and health care provider.

7. Discuss factors that have influenced the lack of funding of CAM therapies by Canada's system of universal health care insurance.

8. Discuss how culture and socioeconomic status may influence personal choice in the selection of an allopathic or CAM practitioner or therapist.

9. Outline the role of the nurse with clients who would benefit from CAM therapies. Discuss assessment, client education, and support with specific reference to each of the following:
   a. Traditional and ethnomedicine therapies
   b. Behavioural therapies
   c. Manual healing therapies

Comparison chart of biobehavioural therapies

COMPARISON CHART OF BIOBEHAVIOURAL THERAPIES

	Description/Effects	Clinical Applications	Limitations
Relaxation			
Imagery			
Biofeedback			
Hypnotherapy			
Meditation			

INTERACTIVE EXERCISES

1. Organize a debate: CAM therapies should be funded by Canada's publicly funded health insurance program.

2. Assign students to investigate available community resources for CAM therapies.

3. Ask students to interview a CAM health practitioner or therapist regarding his or her practice. Have the students determine factors such as the cost to the client to access care, the treatments offered, the number of repeat visits required, and a description of clients seeking care (e.g., age range, disease entities). The students should report these findings to the class.

CLINICAL SKILL

1. Require students to practise, and then demonstrate, therapies in a laboratory setting (e.g., relaxation therapy, meditation, qigong, dance and music therapy, or massage — depending on the particular interest and skills of the students).

CLIENT CARE EXPERIENCES

1. Have students in the clinical setting assess their clients to determine whether CAM therapies would be beneficial. Discuss how the client and the primary health care provider may be approached to suggest the use of selected therapies.

2. Require students to incorporate the use of CAM therapies into the nursing care plan or critical pathway for assigned clients.

CRITICAL THINKING EXERCISES

Client profile: Tasha, a 21-year-old college student, was seen in the student health centre for increasing episodes of abdominal fullness and discomfort with alternating diarrhea and constipation. She reports that she was diagnosed with irritable bowel syndrome several years ago and was told to eat more fibre. Nothing has been effective in reducing her abdominal distress. She is taking a heavy course load this semester and has to work twenty hours each week for her work-study contract. She eats mainly fast food and drinks several colas daily.

1. Explain the psychological stressors that may be contributing to Tasha's abdominal discomfort.

2. Describe how Tasha's curent diet may be affecting her, both physiologically and psychologically.

3. What complementary and alternative therapy (or therapies) might be appropriate for Tasha? What information would you discuss with her before implementing any therapy?

4. How would you recommend complementary therapies to Tasha's physican? What important points should you discuss with the physician regarding the therapies you and Tasha feel might be useful?

ANSWERS TO CRITICAL THINKING EXERCISES

Background Information: Irritable bowel syndrome (IBS) is a disorder of gastrointestinal function, characterized by abdominal pain and alteration in bowel habits. In some cases it is also accompanied by extraintestinal symptoms such as urinary frequency, dysuria, headaches, fatigue, dysmenorrhea, and nausea. The etiology is unknown but is thought to be the result of psychological, physiological, and behavioural factors. The symptoms of IBS frequently worsen during stress. Dietary habits also may increase symptoms and may be related to dairy and grain allergies and lactose intolerance.

1. Symptoms of IBS worsen during stress. If Tasha is experiencing stress because of her heavy course and work load, she may well have elevated catecholamine levels (norepinephrine and epinephrine), which increase heart rate and blood pressure and can change mood states in chronic situations.

2. Tasha's diet is less than optimal. She is eating mainly fast food and drinks a lot of cola. She is not getting the recommended increase in fibre. Her diet is likely lacking in vitamins, vegetables, fruit, and calcium and contains higher-than-recommended quantities of fats. Both the lack of fibre and the caffeine-containing colas are irritants that may be contributing to her abdominal discomfort. Caffeine also contributes to the excitatory state caused by high catecholamine levels associated with stress. This information needs to be discussed with Tasha, and she requires assistance in planning some adjustments in her diet.

3. Tasha would probably benefit from relaxation and imagery therapies. Persons who practise relaxation and imagery for 15 to 20 minutes at least once daily (twice is preferred) may have significant decreases in abdominal discomfort. In addition, Tasha should evaluate how she perceives and responds to environmental stressors. Cognitive restructuring allows people to change the way in which they perceive situations, and may result in more positive psychological and physiological responses. It is important to discuss with Tasha her motivation for change – how much time and energy is she willing to commit to make a change in her life. She needs information regarding time commitments, costs, benefits, risks, healing potential, and side effects of these therapies. (If you were to recommend a therapy that might have any contraindications, these should be discussed also.) Tasha needs to be encouraged to inform her physician and other "healers" of any lifestyle changes and therapies in which she is engaging.

4. Presuming that Tasha is under the care of a physician, it is important as a member of the health care team to inform the physician (with Tasha's permission) of changes in lifestyle and any therapies in which Tasha is engaging. You should attempt to discern the physician's attitude toward complementary therapies. It is important to be ready to discuss with the physician and other health care providers research regarding appropriateness and efficacy of the prescribed lifestyle change or therapy recommended with regard to Tasha's condition. In terms of relaxation therapy, there is substantial data indicating the beneficial effects of reduced sympathetic nervous system activity for those with IBS. You also should discuss cognitive restructuring, which would be beneficial in changing the way Tasha responds to stress.

Activity and Exercise

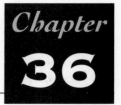

Chapter **36**

CLASSROOM DISCUSSION

1. Discuss body mechanics, exercise, and activity, including the following:
   a. Body alignment
   b. Body balance
   c. Coordinated body movement
   d. Friction
   e. Exercise and activity

2. Review the regulation and coordination of body movement by the musculoskeletal and nervous systems.

3. Discuss the principles of body mechanics and their integration into nursing care.

4. Describe pathological influences on body alignment and mobility, including congenital abnormalities; disorders of the bone, joints, and muscles; CNS damage; and musculoskeletal trauma. Ask students to identify specific pathological problems that may be experienced by clients.

5. Review growth and development across the life span in respect to musculoskeletal and neurological function and mobility. Ask students to identify specific changes that may influence mobility status and place the individual at risk.

6. Discuss the following in relation to an individual's activity and exercise:
   a. Behavioral aspects and lifestyle
   b. Environmental issues—work, school, community
   c. Cultural and ethnic influences
   d. Family and social support

7. Describe the assessment of client mobility in the following areas:
   a. Posture/positioning
   b. Mobility/gait
   c. Activity tolerance

   Ask students about what constitutes expected or abnormal findings in the assessment of mobility.

8. Describe the general effects of exercise on the body systems and the specific benefits of specific types of exercise (e.g., isometric).

9. Guide students in the application of the nursing process for clients who need to maintain or regain their activity and exercise abilities.

Chapter 36: Activity and Exercise   181

10. Discuss joint mobility and range of motion (ROM). Explain the use of the continuous passive range of motion (CPM) machine. Have students identify how ROM exercises may be integrated into other nursing care activities.

11. Ask students to identify possible situations in which additional assistance may be needed to position or ambulate a client.

12. Invite a physical therapist to speak to the class about measures to promote exercise and activity for clients in the community and acute and restorative care agencies.

13. Review the importance of safety and comfort measures when assisting clients with activity and exercise.

14. Ask students to share their own activity and exercise regimens.

INTERACTIVE EXERCISES

1. Have students develop a teaching plan that incorporates basic exercise for an older adult or correct use of an assistive device.

2. Have students identify the activity and exercise needs and the nursing approaches for the following or similar client situations:
   a. An 8 year old with acute asthma
   b. An 86 year old who has had a CVA with resultant left-sided hemiplegia
   c. A 45 year old who is overweight
   d. A 16 year old with a casted fracture of the right tibia and limited weight bearing (crutches required)

CLINICAL SKILLS

1. Explain and demonstrate (using a simulation mannequin/model or volunteer, appropriate equipment, and educational media, as available) specific nursing interventions that may be implemented to promote proper body alignment and mobility, including the following:
   a. Lifting (by the nurse)
   b. Use of assistive devices for ambulation—walking belt, walker, cane, crutches

2. Have small groups of students practice the skills to promote body alignment and mobility, using the appropriate equipment and supplies, and document the procedure and status of the client accordingly. Supervise activities such as lifting and crutch walking.

3. Evaluate the students' ability to implement and document selected skills through return demonstration and skill testing before clinical experience.

CLIENT CARE EXPERIENCES

1. Assign students to observe and participate in the nursing care of clients in acute, restorative, or home care settings, with focus placed on the promotion of body alignment and mobility. Discuss expectations of students before the experience, specifically emphasizing client safety and requesting assistance in moving clients. Review the students' assessments, strategies employed, and evaluation of clients' mobility status after the experience.

2. Have students complete care plans/pathways for their assigned clients, incorporating interventions designed to promote activity and exercise.

RESOURCES FOR STUDENT ACTIVITIES

Musculoskeletal development across the life span chart
Benefits of exercise

MUSCULOSKELETAL DEVELOPMENT ACROSS THE LIFE SPAN CHART

Age-Group	Musculoskeletal Changes
Infants	
Toddlers	
Preschool Children to Adolescents	
Young to Middle Adults	
Older Adult	

BENEFITS OF EXERCISE

Target Individual	Benefits of Exercise
Client with coronary heart disease	
Client with hypertension	
Client with chronic pulmonary disease	
Client with diabetes mellitus	
Older adult client	
Immobile client	
Client with multiple sclerosis	

CRITICAL THINKING EXERCISES

1. Mr. Schmidt is a 65-year-old man who has enrolled in a cardiac rehabilitation program following a coronary artery bypass graft (CABG). What factors do you consider in developing an exercise program for Mr. Schmidt? What interventions could be incorporated to help motivate this client to exercise on a daily basis?

2. You are caring for an 81-year-old woman in her home. She sustained a fracture of the left femur and must use crutches for 1 week until her follow-up visit at the orthopedic clinic. You notice that she has not bathed or combed her hair. When you ask her if she needs assistance in bathing, she replies, "My shower is on the second floor, and I'm afraid to go up and down the stairs." What is a priority nursing intervention at this time?

3. A 30-year-old woman has sustained a spinal cord injury. The client is to be maintained on bed rest. She is becoming increasingly depressed and withdrawn. What actions are important at this point in the client's care?

4. You have been asked to develop an exercise program for a support group for clients with type I diabetes. List some of the precautions and guidelines when developing an exercise prescription specific for persons with type I diabetes. What are some of the factors to consider when planning this program?

ANSWERS TO CRITICAL THINKING EXERCISES

1. First, contact Mr. Schmidt's primary care provider to determine any contraindications in type, frequency, and duration of exercise. Obtain baseline blood pressure, weight, height, pulse, and respiratory rate. Discuss with Mr. Schmidt his preferences for types of exercise and whether these exercises can be carried out after the cardiac rehabilitation has ended. For example, you may question Mr. Schmidt to determine whether there is a safe walking track near his home. Once an exercise program has been developed by the nurse in collaboration with Mr. Schmidt, allow him to perform one session while being monitored at the clinic. Instruct Mr. Schmidt carefully on performing the same exercise program 3 times during the next week until the next rehabilitation session. To potentially increase motivation, give him an exercise log and instruct him on its use.

2. A priority nursing intervention at this time is to instruct the client on crutch walking on stairs. When ascending stairs on crutches, the client usually uses a modified three-point gait. The client stands at the bottom of the stairs and transfers body weight to the crutches. The unaffected leg is advanced between the crutches to the stairs. The client then shifts weight from the crutches to the unaffected leg. Finally, the client aligns both crutches on the stairs. To descend the stairs, a three-phase sequence is also used. The client transfers body weight to the unaffected leg. The crutches are placed on the stair, and the client begins to transfer body weight to the crutches, moving the affected leg forward. Finally, the unaffected leg is moved to the stairs with the crutches. Allow the client to try these skills in your presence while reinforcing the instructions.

3. Maintenance of body image (e.g., clean hair and makeup) and development of an isometric exercise program, particularly tailored to the large muscle groups used for walking, are important. Exercise and activity can enhance a feeling of well-being in the client. Include the client's family in the exercise program to increase socialization and contact with her family.

4. Exercise is an important component in the care of clients with diabetes mellitus, along with diet, glucose monitoring, and medication. Individuals with diabetes mellitus type 1 are encouraged to exercise to improve cardiovascular fitness and psychological well-being. You should instruct the client with type 1 diabetes about certain risks and precautions regarding exercise, such as the following: (a) monitoring blood glucose before and after exercise, (b) avoiding injecting insulin into muscles that will be active during exercise, (c) performing low-intensity to moderate-intensity exercises, (d) carrying a concentrated form of carbohydrates (sugar packets, hard candy), and (e) wearing a diabetes identification bracelet.

Safety

CLASSROOM DISCUSSION

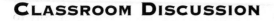

1. Discuss the concept of a "safe environment" in respect to health care and community settings.

2. Review the basic needs that should be met in a safe environment: oxygen, humidity, nutrition, and temperature. Ask students to provide specific examples of how those needs may be met by the client and/or nurse in diverse health care settings.

3. Discuss the major causes of accidents and accidental deaths in the home and health care environment. Ask students to contribute the possible underlying causes of these accidents.

4. Identify physical hazards and how they may be reduced in the home and health care setting. Have students indicate specific measures that may be implemented to reduce hazards. Ask students to share personal experiences of safety hazards that have been identified and/or eliminated in their home or occupational setting.

5. Review concepts of growth and development that have an impact upon safety throughout the life span.

6. Review how reducing the transmission of pathogens contributes to overall client safety and well-being. Have students specify nursing interventions and client instructions that may be implemented to reduce pathogens in the home and health care setting.

7. Given the following or similar situations, have students determine possible safety hazards and preventive measures:
   a. New parents going home with their first child
   b. An older adult living alone in a third floor apartment that has wooden floors, throw rugs, cluttered areas, and dark hallways and stairwells
   c. A single-parent family living in an inner city area where crime and drug abuse are prevalent
   d. New homes built on and around an old chemical plant site
   e. A client with TB going home to live with his large family
   f. An individual whose sexual partner is a known drug user

8. Discuss the types of pollution present today and their effects on people and the environment. Ask students what the role of the nurse should be in reducing or eliminating environmental pollution.

9. Guide students in the application of the nursing process for clients who are at risk of injury.

10. Describe the components of a home safety assessment.

11. Review specific safety concerns of different age-groups from infancy to older adulthood. Ask students to identify target areas for prevention of age-related injuries (e.g., helmets for bicycle riding).

12. Identify and/or ask students to identify risk factors that contribute to safety hazards, including lifestyle behaviors, mobility, sensory impairment, and overall awareness.

13. Discuss safety risks (e.g., falls, accidents) that are specific to the health care setting, including client-inherent, procedure-related, and equipment-related situations. Ask students to identify potential risks and preventive measures in acute, extended, rehabilitative, and home care settings. Stimulate a discussion on similarities and differences in these different settings with respect to safety hazards and prevention of accidents.

14. Explain the nursing responsibilities associated with the following interventions:
    a. Seizure precautions
    b. Use of restraints
    c. Intervening in poisoning
    d. Fire, electrical, and radiation safety

    Ask students to provide examples of situations in which these interventions may be implemented and the decision making that is required of the nurse.

15. Ask students to identify hazard prevention resources that are readily available to consumers, such as carbon monoxide and fire/smoke detectors, bicycle helmets, and childproof locks.

16. Review overall measures to promote and maintain client safety in the home, community, and health care setting.

17. Invite a nurse risk manager to speak to the class about his or her role in reducing or eliminating safety hazards in the health care environment.

18. Invite a representative from a local fire department to speak to the class about home and health care agency fire safety measures and the nurse's responsibility for fire control and evacuation.

19. Using the following or similar situations, have students identify the health and safety risks for clients and families and specify possible measures to alleviate or prevent them:
    a. A living environment with flaking paint, crowding, poor lighting, and poor ventilation
    b. An adolescent having unprotected sex
    c. An older adult with diminished eyesight and peripheral sensation

INTERACTIVE EXERCISES

1. Have students investigate the types of pollution that may be evident in their own neighborhood and/or work environment.

2. Assign students to complete the Home Hazard Assessment (see Resources for Student Activities, p. 193) and report, verbally and/or in writing, on their findings.

3. Assign students to investigate and report on media examples, such as Public Service Announcements, that focus on safety issues.

188   Unit 7: Basic Human Needs

4. Have students investigate where hazard prevention resources (e.g., smoke detectors) may be obtained if the client and family does not have sufficient finances.

5. Arrange for students to attend, if possible, a mandatory employee safety program in an acute care facility.

6. Assign students to investigate and report on safety statistics (e.g., patient falls) within an affiliating health care agency and the agency's plans to reduce the overall incidence of accidents and injuries.

7. Have students contact the local poison control center and ask about common poisoning situations and treatments.

CLINICAL SKILLS

1. Explain and demonstrate the following skills, using simulation mannequins or models, appropriate equipment, and available educational media:
   a. Applying restraints
   b. Seizure precautions

2. Have small groups of students practice the above skills using the appropriate equipment and supplies and document the procedure.

3. Evaluate the students' ability to implement and document the hazard prevention skills through return demonstration and skill testing before clinical experience.

CLIENT CARE EXPERIENCES

1. Have students identify and implement a hazard prevention plan for a specific target group or community, such as home childproofing, sport injury prevention, adolescent suicide, or fire and burn safety for older individuals.

2. Assign students to observe and participate in the nursing care of clients within an acute, restorative, community, and/or home care environment, focusing on the promotion of safety and reduction of hazards. Discuss expectations with the group before the experience, identifying the parameters for assessment of client risk and the implementation and evaluation of preventive strategies.

3. Have students report back on their clients' teaching and learning needs, interactions, and other identified risks for injury.

4. Have students complete a care plan/pathway for an assigned client who is at risk for injury.

RESOURCES FOR STUDENT ACTIVITIES

Home hazard assessment
Safety concerns across the life span chart
RISK assessment tool for fall prevention

HOME HAZARD ASSESSMENT

HOME EXTERIOR

Are sidewalks uneven?

Are steps in good repair?

Do steps have securely fastened handrails?

Is there adequate lighting?

Is outdoor furniture sturdy?

HOME INTERIOR

Do all rooms, stairways, and halls have adequate, nonglare lighting?

Are night-lights available?

Are area rugs secured?

Are wooden floors nonslippery?

Is furniture placed appropriately to permit mobility?

Is furniture sturdy enough to provide support for getting up and down?

Are temperature and humidity within normal range?

Are there any steps or thresholds that may pose a hazard?

Are step edges clearly marked with colored tape?

Are handrails available and secure?

In homes with young children, are window guards installed?

Can all doors and windows with security gates and locks be opened from the inside without a key?

KITCHEN

Are hand-washing facilities available?

Is the pilot light on for the gas stove?

Are the stove top and oven clean?

Are the dials on the stove readable?

Are storage areas within easy reach?

Are fluids such as cleaners and bleach in original containers and stored properly?

Is the water temperature within normal range?

Are there clean areas for food storage and preparation?

Is refrigeration adequate? Are the refrigerator and freezer temperatures correct?

BATHROOM

Are hand-washing facilities available?

Are there skidproof strips or surfaces in the tub or shower?

Are bath mats secured?

Does the client need grab bars near the bathtub and toilet?

Does the client need an elevated toilet seat?

Is the medicine cabinet well lighted?

Are medications in their original containers?

Are medication containers child resistant if children live in the home or visit?

Have outdated medications been discarded?

BEDROOM

Are beds of adequate height to allow getting on and off easily?

Is day and night lighting adequate?

Are floor coverings nonskid?

Does the client have a telephone nearby?

Are emergency numbers visible near the telephone?

ELECTRICAL AND FIRE HAZARDS

Are smoke and carbon monoxide detectors installed?

Are the batteries for all detectors tested every month and changed twice a year?

Have furnaces, chimneys, and stoves been checked for proper ventilation?

Are extension cords in good condition and used appropriately?

Are appliances in good working order?

Are electrical appliances located away from water sources?

Is there a fire extinguisher near the cooking area?

Are combustible items such as oil-based paints, gasoline, and oily rags being stored in a garage and/or basement?

Are flashlights available?

Is there a first aid kit available to the adult members of the household?

Does everyone in the family have easy access to emergency phone numbers?

Data from Tideiksaar R: Home safe home: practical tips for fall-proofing, *Geriatr Nurs* 11(6):280, 1989; Ebersole P, Hess P: *Toward healthy aging*, ed 5, St. Louis, 1998, Mosby; A room by room checklist for fire safety, Fall 1997; and Safety items no home should be without, 1998.

SAFETY CONCERNS ACROSS THE LIFE SPAN CHART

Age-Group	Specific Safety Concerns	Preventive Measures/Teaching
Infant		
Toddler/Pre-school Child		
School-Age Child		
Adolescent		
Adult		
Older Adult		

RISK ASSESSMENT TOOL FOR FALL PREVENTION

TOOL 1: RISK ASSESSMENT TOOL FOR FALLS

Directions: Place a check mark in front of elements that apply to your client. The decision as to whether a client is at risk for falls is based on your nursing judgment.

Guideline: A client with a check next to an item with an asterisk (*) or four or more of the other items would be identified as at risk for falls.

General Data
__ Over 60 years of age
__ History of falls before admission*
__ History of smoking, alcohol, drug use
__ Perioperative status

Physical Condition
__ Vertigo
__ Unsteady gait
__ Problems affecting weight-bearing joints
__ Weakness
__ Paresis/paralysis
__ Seizure disorder
__ Impaired vision
__ Impaired hearing
__ Slow reaction times
__ Diarrhea
__ Urinary frequency, urgency, nocturia

Mental Status
__ Lethargic
__ Confused or disoriented
__ Inability to understand or follow directions

Medications
__ Diuretics
__ Hypotensive or central nervous system depressants (e.g., narcotics, sedatives, psychotropics, hypnotics, tranquilizers, antihypertensives, antidepressants)
__ Medication that increases gastrointestinal motility (e.g., laxatives)
__ Effect of drug interactions

Ambulatory Devices Used
__ Cane
__ Crutches
__ Walker
__ Wheelchair
__ Geriatric (geri) chair
__ Braces

TOOL 2: REASSESSMENT IS SAFE "KARE" (RISK) TOOL

Directions: Place a check mark in front of any element that applies to your client. A client who has a check mark in front of any of the first four elements would be identified as at risk for falls. In addition, when a high-risk client has a check mark in front of the element "use of a wheelchair," the client is considered to be at greater risk for falls.
__ Unsteady gait/dizziness/imbalance
__ Impaired memory or judgment
__ Weakness
__ History of falls
__ Use of a wheelchair

From Brians LK and others: The development of the RISK tool for fall prevention, *Rehabil Nurs* 16(2):67, 1991.

CRITICAL THINKING EXERCISES

1. Mr. Santiago, who is 88 years old, lives alone. Within the past year he has fallen twice at home, once by tripping over a rug and once when he got up to go to the bathroom at night. He has become increasingly afraid of falling again and tends to restrict his activities in the home. He goes out only when accompanied by a son.
   a. What physical assessment findings would be significant?
   b. What aspects of the environment need to be assessed?
   c. Design specific interventions to ensure the client's safety in his home.
   d. In terms of evaluation, what findings indicate that Mr. Santiago cannot live alone in the house?

2. Mr. Carr, who is 20 years old, comes to the emergency department following a night of drinking and illegal drug use. He is extremely combative with the staff.
   a. Describe in detail the steps the nurse should take to protect Mr. Carr, staff, and other clients.

3. A nurse does health teaching in a senior center. The nurse believes that the clients, who are all ambulatory and in good health, would benefit from exercises to increase their strength, balance, and flexibility.
   a. How should the nurse validate these beliefs?
   b. What benefits would the clients gain from increased strength, balance, and flexibility?
   c. What steps should the nurse take to initiate a program for these clients?

ANSWERS TO CRITICAL THINKING EXERCISES

1. a. Significant physical assessment findings include changes in blood pressure (hypotension or hypertension), decreased vision and/or hearing, altered gait, poor balance and coordination, decreased muscle strength, and increased nocturia.
   b. A complete home assessment is indicated.
   c. Hazards to safety, such as loose throw rugs and lack of lighting at night in bedrooms, halls, and bathrooms, need to be corrected. Abnormal physical assessment findings need to be investigated and corrected when possible.
   d. Increasing memory loss or cognitive changes, severe fear of falling, or increased weakness may indicate that the client is in danger by living alone. The client and family need to consider options such as a live-in aide, moving in with an adult child, and long-term care.

2. The nurse must use critical thinking elements and quickly respond to a potentially dangerous situation. The nurse must be familiar with the agency's policies regarding emergency situations.
   a. Obtaining sufficient staff to assist, the nurse must determine which restraints to apply, restrain correctly, and constantly assess the client for airway, breathing, and circulation, as well as continued need for the restraint. The nurse must document assessment and interventions employed, and obtain an order for the restraint.

3. a. The nurse should consult with the clients at the center and see whether they think the belief is true.
   b. Increased strength, balance, and flexibility could decrease the risk of falling, and the clients would most likely feel better.
   c. The nurse should consult with a physical therapist to set up classes at the center, stressing simple exercises that clients can continue to do at home.

Hygiene

Chapter
38

CLASSROOM DISCUSSION

1. Discuss the measures that constitute personal hygiene and the usual hygienic care that is provided in the acute and extended care health setting.

2. Discuss factors that may influence hygienic care practices. Have students identify how these factors may alter the nurse's approach to the client.

3. Review the anatomy and physiology of the integumentary system.

4. Review the physical assessment of the skin, hair, nails, mouth, teeth, and feet (refer to Chapter 32 of *Canadian Fundamentals of Nursing*, Second Edition). Use photos, illustrations, models, and videos, as available. Ask students to identify how the physical assessment may be integrated into hygienic care and to specify expected and unexpected findings of the assessment.

5. Review developmental changes that occur in the skin, hair, nails, and teeth throughout the life span.

6. Ask students to identify the information about the client's self-care abilities and personal hygienic practices that determines the type of hygienic care and amount of assistance provided by the nurse.

7. Review possible risks for skin impairment. Have students provide additional situations in which preventive measures may be indicated for the client.

8. Explain the multiple purposes of hygienic care, including cleanliness, exercise, relaxation, improved self-image, and stimulation of circulation and respiration. Ask students how the hygienic care routine may provide an opportunity for communication with the client.

9. Review the guidelines for bathing a client: privacy, safety, warmth, and independence. Have students provide specific examples of how the nurse achieves these guidelines.

10. Discuss the principles of perineal care for male and female clients.

11. Ask students how the bath of a newborn/infant and young child differs from that of an adult.

12. Discuss general foot care and appropriate footwear. Describe and demonstrate special foot care that is provided for clients with reduced peripheral circulation (e.g., clients with diabetes).

13. Identify and/or ask students to identify risk factors that may contribute to oral hygiene problems. Describe common oral problems that the nurse may encounter (use photographs and illustrations).

14. Discuss general guidelines for oral hygiene. Ask students to identify the special considerations that would be indicated for clients who are unconscious, prone to stomatitis, diabetic, or experiencing an oral infection.

15. Identify common hair and scalp problems.

16. Describe general measures that may be implemented to assist the client with hair care, including brushing, combing, shampooing, and shaving. Ask students to identify specific precautions that may need to be taken to avoid client injury.

17. Review the physical assessment of the eyes, ears, and nose (refer to Chapter 32 of *Canadian Fundamentals of Nursing*, Second Edition). Discuss the expected and unexpected findings that may be assessed by the nurse.

18. Describe general measures that are incorporated into the hygienic care of the eyes, ears, and nose and the maintenance of sensory aids (e.g., glasses, contact lenses, artificial eyes, and hearing aids).

19. Ask students how the client's environment, in the home or health care setting, may be modified to increase comfort, cleanliness, and a feeling of security.

20. Discuss general principles of bed making, including the situations that warrant making unoccupied or occupied beds.

21. Have students discuss how sociocultural practices may influence a client's hygienic care.

22. For the following situations, have students identify how hygienic care measures may be adapted by the nurse to meet the client's needs:
    a. A client with right-sided weakness after a CVA
    b. An obese client with shortness of breath, residing at home, who only has access to a bathtub
    c. An older client with some difficulty in balance
    d. A newborn, 2 year old, or 8 year old
    e. A client with casts on both arms and/or legs
    f. An unconscious client
    g. A severely depressed client

INTERACTIVE EXERCISES

1. Assign students to design a teaching plan for the following or similar client situations, with respect to hygienic care practices:
   a. New parents with a 3-day-old newborn
   b. A client with diabetes
   c. An older client with dry skin
   d. A client on anticoagulant medication

2. Ask students to determine what resources may be available and what adaptations may be indicated for implementation of hygienic care in the client's home environment (e.g., availability of hot water).

CLINICAL SKILLS

1. Demonstrate the proper technique for bathing a newborn/infant using a simulation mannequin or doll. Have students return demonstrate the procedure.

2. Have students modify a simulated acute or restorative care client environment to increase client comfort and privacy by manipulating available equipment and furniture.

3. Explain and demonstrate (using a simulation mannequin/model or volunteer, appropriate equipment/supplies, and educational media, as available) the following selected nursing interventions for promotion of client hygiene:
   a. Bathing, perineal care, back rub, "bag bath"
   b. Nail and foot care
   c. Mouth care, denture cleansing
   d. Hair and scalp care
   e. Care of sensory aids—contact lenses and hearing aids
   f. Unoccupied and occupied bed making

4. Have small groups or pairs of students practice the performance and documentation of the skills, using the appropriate equipment and supplies.

5. Evaluate the students' ability to implement and document the selected hygienic care interventions through return demonstration and skill testing before clinical experience.

CLIENT CARE EXPERIENCES

1. Assign students to participate in the nursing care of clients in a variety of health care settings, specifically focusing on the implementation of hygienic care measures. Discuss with the group, before the experience, the decision making involved in determining the client's hygienic care needs.

2. Have students complete a care plan/pathway for an assigned client in which a self-care limitation exists that influences the achievement of hygienic care.

RESOURCE FOR STUDENT ACTIVITIES

Specific hygienic care measures across the life span chart

SPECIFIC HYGIENIC CARE MEASURES
ACROSS THE LIFE SPAN CHART

Age-Group	Specific Hygienic Care
Newborn	
Infant	
Toddler/Preschooler	
School-Age Child	
Adolescent	
Adult	
Older Adult	

CRITICAL THINKING EXERCISES

1. Mrs. Truman is a 62-year-old female being seen in the internal medicine clinic during her follow-up appointment for management of her diabetes mellitus. During the nurse's conversation with Mrs. Truman, the client says, "You know, last week I found a sore on my left foot; I didn't even know it was there." What type of assessment should the nurse conduct for Mrs. Truman, and what might be the implications of her findings?

2. Mr. Wilkes is a 54-year-old client with advanced stages of lung cancer. The tumor has spread to the bone, causing Mr. Wilkes considerable pain and predisposing him to pathologic fractures (fractures that result when bone is weakened by tumor growth). The client has been experiencing a high fever almost on a daily basis. What considerations might you give in anticipating Mr. Wilkes's hygiene needs?

3. Peter Nixon is an 18-year-old admitted to the neurosurgical intensive care unit following a head injury. Peter is currently unconscious, responsive only to painful stimulus. What assessment is critical for the nurse to perform prior to providing oral hygiene?

ANSWERS TO CRITICAL THINKING EXERCISES

1. The nurse should perform a complete assessment of Mrs. Truman's feet. Having diabetes, Mrs. Truman is at risk for the development of foot ulcers because of reduced peripheral circulation. The fact that Mrs. Truman did not know that a sore was on her foot suggests that she has reduced sensation from the peripheral neuropathy that develops with diabetes mellitus. The nurse will inspect all surfaces of both feet, carefully examine the condition of the existing ulcer, and conduct necessary assessment of circulation and sensation. The nurse will also review with Mrs. Truman the client's understanding of regular daily foot care. It would help if the nurse would ask Mrs. Truman to demonstrate a self-assessment of the feet. The client may require instruction on hygiene practices and selection of footwear.

2. The advanced stages of cancer, coupled with Mr. Wilkes's severe pain and risk for bone fracture, make him a likely candidate to be confined to bed. If that is the case, you will need to plan an approach to provide the client a complete bed bath and to make an occupied bed. You will need to consider ways to make the client as comfortable as possible while the bath is administered. This may require administering analgesics before the bath. In addition, good body mechanics used in moving and positioning the client will help to minimize stress on the client's extremities. Since Mr. Wilkes has had a fever, the associated diaphoresis can increase the risk for skin breakdown. You must monitor the client's skin regularly and be sure that bed linens remain dry throughout the day. Mr. Wilkes's level of pain and the extent to which it limits range of motion, in addition to the client's overall level of physical energy, will influence the extent to which assistance will be needed with other hygiene activities.

3. Clients who have had serious neurological injury involving the brain must be assessed for the presence of a gag reflex. Absence of a gag reflex will make the client more prone to aspiration during cleansing of the oral cavity.

Oxygenation

Chapter 39

CLASSROOM DISCUSSION

1. Review normal anatomy and physiology and common pathophysiological changes in the cardiac and respiratory systems.

2. Discuss factors that affect oxygenation, including physiological, developmental, lifestyle, stress or anxiety, and environmental. Ask students to identify specific examples of how and why these factors affect oxygenation.

3. Describe the following alterations in cardiac function that influence oxygenation and the signs and symptoms associated with each: conduction disturbances, altered cardiac output, impaired valvular function, and myocardial ischemia.

4. Describe the following alterations in respiratory function and the signs and symptoms associated with each: hyperventilation, hypoventilation, and hypoxia.

5. Describe the assessment of the client's oxygenation status, including the history, physical examination, and diagnostic and laboratory tests.

6. Identify components of the nursing history relevant to the client's oxygenation status, such as fatigue, dyspnea, coughing, wheezing, pain, possible exposure, infections, risk factors, and medication administration.

7. Review the physical assessment techniques and components that are specific to determining a client's oxygenation status.

8. Identify and describe diagnostic and laboratory tests that are used to determine the client's cardiopulmonary function and oxygenation status (see Resources for Student Activities, p. 206). Have students identify the client preparation and education that is necessary before these diagnostic and laboratory tests are performed.

9. Identify and/or have students identify nursing interventions that may be implemented for the promotion and maintenance of a client's oxygenation. Incorporate how the interventions may be adapted according to the client's developmental status.

10. Discuss the use of influenza and pneumococcal vaccines, including their indications and contraindications for use.

11. Discuss which clients are at a greater risk for reduced oxygenation because of occupational or geographic exposure.

12. Describe secondary and tertiary care for clients with alterations in oxygenation:
    a. Dyspnea management
    b. Maintenance of patent airway
    c. Mobilization of pulmonary secretions
    d. Suctioning

13. Ask students to identify the rationale for nursing interventions that promote oxygenation.

14. Describe the placement and suctioning of artifical airways, using photos/illustrations and/or videos, as available.

15. Discuss oxygen therapy and the nurse's responsibilities associated with its use in the health care and home environment. Have students identify the specific safety measures that must be implemented in the presence of oxygen therapy.

16. Invite a respiratory therapist to speak to the class about client oxygenation needs. Ask the therapist to demonstrate different types of equipment, their uses, and monitoring requirements.

17. Discuss the purpose, insertion, and maintenance of chest tubes.

18. Discuss the maintenance and promotion of oxygenation in the restorative and home care environments and the role of the nurse in client education and monitoring.

19. Guide students in the application of the critical thinking model and the nursing process for clients experiencing alterations in oxygenation.

INTERACTIVE EXERCISES

1. Have students investigate and report on environmental pollutants that are present in their community, what their influence may be on the health status of that community, and what measures may be taken to eliminate or reduce the level of pollutants.

2. Provide photos/illustrations of different types of oxygen equipment, and have students identify the use, flow rate, and client considerations for each one.

CLINICAL SKILLS

1. Demonstrate select cardiovascular and pulmonary assessment techniques to reinforce the information.

2. Demonstrate coughing, deep breathing, use of the incentive spirometer, positioning, chest physiotherapy, and postural drainage to the class. Have students practice the techniques individually and/or with a partner.

3. Explain and demonstrate (using a simulation mannequin/model, appropriate equipment/supplies, and educational media) the following nursing interventions for the promotion and evaluation of client oxygenation:
   a. Pulse oximetry (refer to Chapter 31 of *Canadian Fundamentals of Nursing,* Second Edition)
   b. Suctioning
   c. Care of chest tubes
   d. Application of a nasal cannula and oxygen mask
   e. Use of home oxygen equipment (as available)

4. Have pairs or small groups of students practice the implementation and documentation of the specified nursing interventions for promotion of oxygenation.

5. Evaluate the students' ability to implement and document the interventions to promote client oxygenation through return demonstration and skill testing before clinical experience.

6. Discuss and demonstrate cardiopulmonary resuscitation (CPR).

7. Assign students to complete a CPR class (preferably health care provider level) through an approved provider, and verify with possession of certification card.

CLIENT CARE EXPERIENCES

1. Assign students to observe and participate in the nursing care of clients with actual or potential alterations in oxygenation in a variety of health care settings. Focus on the assessment of the client's oxygenation status and the implementation of measures to support and/or improve cardiopulmonary function (e.g., positioning, coughing, or deep breathing).

2. Supervise the administration of appropriate medications and oxygen therapy.

3. Evaluate the students' ability to implement and document nursing interventions for the promotion of oxygenation.

4. Have students design and implement a teaching plan for an assigned client who has an oxygenation deficit and requires oxygen therapy in the home.

5. Have students complete a care plan/pathway for a client experiencing alterations in oxygenation and requiring strategies for the promotion of cardiopulmonary function.

RESOURCES FOR STUDENT ACTIVITIES

Select factors and their affect on oxygenation chart
Diagnostic tests for oxygenation status—client preparation and data obtained

Factors	Affect on Oxygenation Status
Hypovolemia	
Pregnancy	
Obesity	
Kyphosis	
Exercise	
Smoking	
Substance Abuse	
Anxiety	
Premature Birth	

DIAGNOSTIC TESTS FOR OXYGENATION STATUS—CLIENT PREPARATION AND DATA OBTAINED

Focus	Diagnostic Tests	Client Preparation	Data Obtained
Cardiac Conduction			
Cardiac Contraction/ Blood Flow			
Ventilation/ Oxygenation			
Blood Studies			
Visualization of Structures			
Determination of Infection			

CRITICAL THINKING EXERCISES

1. Ms. Wanda Johnson is a 56-year-old postmenopausal woman with a history of hypertension. What would you include in the teaching portion of her plan of care?

2. Mr. Jose Martinez has recently immigrated to the United States from his homeland of Cuba to join his family. He comes to the primary care office to establish a health care provider and because he has been increasingly fatigued, has had a persistent cough, and has been losing weight. What questions would be important to ask when completing the health history interview?

3. Mrs. Amanda Miller, age 45, has been admitted to the hospital with community-acquired pneumonia. She has a productive cough, fever, chills, crackles and wheezes on auscultation of her chest, and a heart rate of 104 beats per minute. What nursing diagnosis would you consider for this client?

4. Mr. Chen Lee, age 72, has been having chest pain, shortness of breath, and pain down his left arm for about 2 hours. He comes to the emergency department for care. What nursing diagnosis would be appropriate for this client?

ANSWERS TO CRITICAL THINKING EXERCISES

1. Ms. Johnson should be taught about risk factors for the development of coronary artery disease. These include estrogen replacement therapy for postmenopausal women, hypertension, inappropriate diet and exercise, and excess body weight. She should also be taught about the signs and symptoms of coronary artery disease in women and prevention measures, such as a diet and exercise plan.

2. When completing Mr. Martinez's health history, the nurse would include questions about sputum production, the presence of blood in the sputum, night sweats, length of time he has had the cough, how quickly he has lost the weight, and if anyone else in his family, either here or in Cuba, has the same symptoms. Given the history, the nurse should suspect the client might have tuberculosis.

3. With the presenting symptoms, you should consider ineffective airway clearance related to retained secretions, pain related to frequent coughing, impaired gas exchange related to alveolar hypoventilation, and hyperthermia related to infectious process. The priority diagnoses for this client include ineffective airway clearance and impaired gas exchange.

4. Nursing diagnoses for Mr. Chen might include pain related to myocardial ischemia, knowledge deficit (coronary artery disease, emergency department procedures), and decreased cardiac output related to chest pain. The priority for Mr. Chen would be to reduce his pain and provide him with some information about what is happening to him to help reduce his stress and anxiety. His family should be included in the plan of care.

Fluid, Electrolyte, and Acid-Base Balances

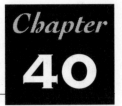

Chapter

40

CLASSROOM DISCUSSION

1. Using educational media (e.g., illustrations, overhead transparencies), review the distribution, movement, and regulation of body fluids, including the following:
    a. ECF and ICF compartments
    b. Examples of body movement
    c. Fluid intake
    d. Fluid output
    e. Hormonal regulation

    Provide examples of different types of IV solutions, and ask students how they will influence fluid movement within the body.

2. Review the major cations and anions, their functions, regulatory mechanisms, sources, and normal blood values. Ask students to provide examples of food sources for each electrolyte.

3. Discuss acid-base balance and the chemical, biological, and physiological mechanisms of regulation within the body.

4. Discuss disturbances in fluid, electrolyte, and acid-base balance, including possible etiology, signs and symptoms, and clients with a greater risk of developing the imbalances. Ask students to give the rationale for the physiological manifestations and the reasons why particular clients are at risk to develop these imbalances.

5. Identify variables that affect fluid, electrolyte, and acid-base balance, including age, illness, environment, diet, lifestyle, and medication. Have students provide specific examples of the affects of these variables on different clients (e.g., why an infant is more susceptible to fluid imbalances).

6. Guide students in the application of the critical thinking model and nursing process for clients experiencing an alteration in fluid, electrolyte, and/or acid-base balance.

7. Describe the nursing assessment and physical examination of clients to determine actual or potential fluid, electrolyte, or acid-base disturbances.

8. Discuss common health problems and client situations in which there are greater risks for imbalances, including surgery, burns, cardiovascular disorders, respiratory disorders, renal disorders, cancer, head injuries, and gastrointestinal disturbances. Ask students to identify which imbalances may be present in these situations and how they may be assessed by the nurse.

9. Explain the role of daily weights and intake and output measurements in the determination of fluid balance. Discuss what is included in fluid I&O, and have students practice the calculation and documentation of sample or actual client intake and output measurements for a prescribed period of time.

10. Identify laboratory tests that may be used to determine fluid, electrolyte, and acid-base disturbances.

11. Discuss the following measures that may be implemented to correct fluid, electrolyte, and/or acid-base disturbances and the associated nursing responsibilities for each:
    a. Enteral replacement
    b. Fluid restriction
    c. Parenteral replacement

12. Discuss the initiation, monitoring and maintenance, and discontinuation of IV therapy. Review aseptic technique.

13. Describe potential complications associated with IV therapy, including phlebitis, infiltration, fluid overload, bleeding, and infection.

14. Discuss blood replacement and administration, nursing responsibilities, and precautions. Have students identify the nursing interventions particular to the IV administration of blood products.

15. Discuss medical interventions and associated nursing strategies that may be implemented to correct problems underlying acid-base disturbances.

16. Discuss the assessment of fluid, electrolyte, and acid-base imbalances and how nursing strategies may be altered to monitor and assist clients in extended and community health care settings.

INTERACTIVE EXERCISES

1. Provide students with sample client weights, and have them calculate fluid volume changes (using 5 lb = 2.5 L).

2. Using the following and/or a similar sample situation, have students determine the client's intake and output in cc:
   ½ cup ice cream   urine—480 cc
   1 cup coffee   wound drainage—120 cc
   ⅛ cup cream
   2 cups corn flakes
   ½ cup milk
   2 cups water
   IV began with 950 cc—currently 290 cc left in bag

3. Provide students with sample test results, and have them analyze the values and decide what imbalance the client may be experiencing (see Resources for Student Activities, p. 211).

4. Provide examples and/or show students photos or illustrations of different IV complications, and ask them to identify each problem.

5. Using the following or similar situations, ask students to identify what fluid, electrolyte, and/or acid-base disturbance the client may be experiencing and what nursing interventions may be implemented:
   a. A client in labor who is hyperventilating
   b. An individual working outside in extremely hot weather
   c. A 4 year old with a high fever
   d. An 80 year old living alone, with diminished appetite and thirst
   e. An individual who has cut himself on a lawn mower blade
   f. An infant with gastroenteritis and severe diarrhea
   g. An adult experiencing prolonged episodes of vomiting
   h. A client with bone cancer
   i. A client with known coronary insufficiency
   j. A client who has smoked consistently for years and has emphysema
   k. A child who ingests a large amount of aspirin
   l. An adult suffering from second- and third-degree burns over 30% of her body
   m. A client who develops tachycardia, dyspnea, and chills in the first 5 minutes of a blood transfusion

CLINICAL SKILLS

1. Explain and demonstrate (using a simulation mannequin/model, appropriate equipment, and educational media, as available) the following nursing interventions associated with intravenous therapy:
   a. Initiating a peripheral intravenous infusion
   b. Regulation of IV flow rate
   c. Changing a peripheral IV solution, tubing, and dressing
   d. Administering a blood transfusion

2. Have small groups of students practice, with supervision, the performance and documentation of the specified nursing interventions, using appropriate equipment and supplies.

3. Evaluate the students' ability to implement and document the interventions for IV therapy through return demonstration and skill testing before clinical experience.

4. Explain and demonstrate the procedure for an arterial puncture for blood gas analysis. Have students observe a nurse or skilled technician perform the procedure in an acute care setting.

CLIENT CARE EXPERIENCES

1. Assign students to observe and participate in the nursing care of clients in acute health care settings, focusing on the assessment of fluid, electrolyte, and acid-base disturbances. Discuss physical assessment and analysis of laboratory values with the group.

2. Supervise the initiation (if appropriate) and maintenance of IV therapy.

3. Have students design and implement teaching plans to meet client needs in relation to fluid, electrolyte, and acid-base imbalances. Review client discharge planning and referral with the students.

4. Have students complete a care plan/pathway for an assigned client who is experiencing an alteration in fluid, electrolyte, and/or acid-base balance.

RESOURCES FOR STUDENT ACTIVITIES

Analysis of blood chemistry values
Comparison chart of acid-base imbalances

ANALYSIS OF BLOOD CHEMISTRY VALUES

Client Values	Normal Levels	Analysis
Sodium, 155 mEq/L		
Chloride, 95 mEq/L		
Calcium, 3.5 mEq/L		
Potassium, 3.0 mEq/L		
Magnesium, 3.2 mEq/L		
Phosphate, 5.2 mEq/L		
Urine Specific Gravity, 1.1		

Arterial Blood Gases
   pH, 7.3
   $PaCO_2$, 50 mm Hg
   PaO_2, 82 mm Hg
   Bicarbonate, 19 mEq/L		

COMPARISON CHART OF ACID-BASE IMBALANCES

Body State	Etiology	Signs and Symptoms	Treatment
Metabolic Acidosis			
Metabolic Alkalosis			
Respiratory Acidosis			
Respiratory Alkalosis			

CRITICAL THINKING EXERCISES

1. Mrs. Emanuele is an 81-year-old admitted to the hospital with a 3-day history of vomiting and diarrhea. She has had only ice chips since the first episode of vomiting and is now complaining of malaise, cramping muscles, and a temperature of 101° F. Which laboratory findings would you expect to be abnormal based on her complaints? What interventions would you expect the physician to order?

2. Alexandra is the nurse assigned to Mrs. Emanuele. What nursing measures should she employ to make her comfortable and why? Will Alexandra need to provide for Mrs. Emanuele's safety? If so, how might she do this?

3. Caroline has just received a new client on her unit, who is to receive 1 unit of RBCs within the next hour. What nursing actions are necessary before administering blood? What are the signs and symptoms of a transfusion reaction? Can Caroline delegate the administration of blood to a licensed practical nurse or a nursing assistant on her team?

4. Bob is caring for a 52-year-old man who has been seen in the emergency department after being involved in a motor vehicle accident. He is complaining of difficulty breathing and a respiratory rate of 40 breaths per minute. Bob's client is transferred to the intensive care unit, intubated, and placed on a ventilator. After the client leaves, a nursing student asks Bob to interpret his client's last ABG results: pH, 7.30; PaO_2, 70; $PaCO_2$, 50; HCO_3, 24. What interpretation will Bob give to the student nurse? What is the relationship between the ABG results and the client being intubated and ventilated?

Chapter 40: Fluid, Electrolyte, and Acid-Base Balances   209

5. Jane is the nurse caring for Betty, a 59-year-old who has just had a total knee replacement. The physician has ordered Ancef 1 gm in 50 ml to run over 30 minutes IV piggyback tid. Betty has a continuous infusion of Ringer's lactate at 75 ml/hr in the left forearm. What type of tubing will Jane use to administer the IV piggyback medication? Calculate the drops per minute of the piggyback using both microtubing (60 drops/ml) and macrotubing (15 drops/ml).

ANSWERS TO CRITICAL THINKING EXERCISES

1. Any of the following laboratory values may be low, normal, or below related to the diarrhea and vomiting episodes. Serum potassium low or below normal < 3.5 mEqL, urine specific gravity > 1.025, increased hematocrit > 50%, and an increased BUN level > 25 mg/100 ml (hemoconcentration) all related to fluid volume deficit. You can anticipate that the physician will order IV therapy and blood work. The physician will begin to investigate the etiology of the vomiting and diarrhea and, based on the assessment, may begin to treat the symptoms and underlying cause.

2. Alexandra will initiate comfort measures such as mouth care. Because of Mrs. Emanuele's complaints and her age, her side rails should be up, in case of orthostatic hypotension. Once the vomiting has been treated and ceases, the client may be ordered to resume a liquid diet. Alexandra may need to assist with feeding or delegate this activity if Mrs. Emanuele's activity status has been restricted because of fluid volume deficit.

3. Adminstering a blood transfusion is a professional nurse's responsibility, and Caroline would not be able to delegate this activity. Transfusing blood requires an assessment of the IV site, vital signs, client status, and potential and actual signs and symptoms related to a transfusion reaction, before, during, and after the infusion. Additionally, because a transfusion reaction can be fatal, it is imperative that the unit of blood be checked properly (review blood transfusion procedure, pp. 1242–1243 of *Canadian Fundamentals of Nursing*, Second Edition).

4. The client's increased respiratory rate is a compensatory method to increase oxygenation that has been ineffective. A client who is laboring to breathe runs the risk of extensive systemic and cerebral hypoxia that may lead to irreversible deficits. The blood gases demonstrate the inability of the client's system to compensate; ventilatory assistance is required.

5. Jane can use either microtubing or macrotubing. Some hospitals have a policy regarding the appropriate tubing for 50-cc/hr or less IV rates. If Jane used microtubing 60 gtts/ml, she will calculate the IV rate at 100 gtts/min. If she uses macrotubing 15 gtts/ml, she will calculate the IV rate at 25 gtts/min.

Sleep

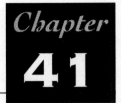

Chapter 41

CLASSROOM DISCUSSION

1. Review the physiology of sleep, including the sleep-wake cycle, circadian rhythm, regulation of sleep, and stages of sleep. Discuss how the physiological mechanisms are determined through the use of selected instruments (e.g., EEG, EMG, and EOG).

2. Stimulate a discussion on how the physiology of sleep may be disrupted in the home and health care environment.

3. Describe the difference between rest and sleep, and discuss how the nurse may promote rest. Have students share what makes them feel "rested."

4. Describe the functions of sleep in restoration and healing, and the importance of dreams.

5. Identify the average sleep requirements and specific concerns for individuals across the life span. Ask students to provide examples of how sleep patterns change with growth and development.

6. Identify factors that may affect sleep patterns, including the following:
   a. Physical illness
   b. Drugs and illegal substances
   c. Lifestyle
   d. Usual sleep patterns and excessive sleepiness
   e. Emotional stress
   f. Environment
   g. Exercise and fatigue
   h. Food and caloric intake

   Ask students to provide specific examples of how and why each factor may affect normal sleep patterns.

7. Have students discuss how the acute care environment specifically may interfere with sleep patterns and how the nurse may eliminate or reduce this interference.

8. Describe common sleep disorders, including insomnia, sleep apnea, narcolepsy, sleep deprivation, and parasomnias.

9. Discuss the assessment of sleep patterns/habits, the possible sources of data that the nurse may utilize to elicit information (e.g., parents, spouse, sleep partner), and questions that may be asked to determine the client's routines.

10. Review the components of a sleep history.

11. Discuss how the sleep history may be correlated with the client's medical history, life events, emotional and mental status, and/or alteration in bedtime routine or environment.

12. Identify behaviors that may be associated with sleep deprivation.

13. Using the following or similar situations, have students identify how the individual's sleep patterns may be disturbed and what interventions the nurse may implement to promote adequate sleep and rest:
    a. An employee who rotates to the night shift (12 AM till 8 AM) every 3 weeks
    b. A 3-year-old child who is admitted to the acute care environment with a respiratory condition
    c. A middle adult who is fearful of losing his or her job
    d. An older adult with chronic arthritic pain
    e. A young adult preparing for her upcoming wedding
    f. A student who is working, caring for a family, and preparing for college examinations
    g. An individual with a bed partner who is restless and snores

14. Guide students in the application of the critical thinking model and the nursing process for clients with a sleep pattern disturbance.

15. Identify interventions that may be implemented to promote a client's sleep and rest. Ask students to specify measures to achieve the following for clients:
    a. A restful and safe environment
    b. Promotion of bedtime routine (as close as possible)
    c. "Sleep friendly" scheduling of treatments
    d. Stress reduction
    e. Physical comfort
    f. Pharmacological management

16. Invite a counselor/therapist who specializes in sleep pattern disturbances to speak to the class about measures to promote relaxation and rest, and the recognition of sleep deprivation behaviors.

INTERACTIVE EXERCISES

1. Have students complete a sleep questionnaire with a peer, family member, or client (see Resources for Student Activities, p. 219).

2. Have students determine what resources are available in the health care setting and community for clients who are experiencing sleep pattern alterations.

CLIENT CARE EXPERIENCES

1. Assign students to observe and participate in the nursing care of clients in a variety of health care settings, focusing on the following:
   a. Assessment of actual and potential sleep pattern disturbances
   b. Promotion of physical and emotional comfort, and relaxation
   c. Administration, with supervision, of prescribed medications for promotion of comfort and rest
   d. Evaluation and documentation of client responses to sleep and rest promotion interventions

2. Have students determine client teaching and learning needs and design a teaching plan specific to the attainment of rest and sleep.

3. Have students complete a care plan/pathway specific to, or incorporating, the client's needs for rest and sleep.

RESOURCES FOR STUDENT ACTIVITIES

Comparison chart for sleep patterns across the life span
Factors affecting sleep patterns
Questions to ask to assess for sleep disorders

COMPARISON CHART FOR SLEEP PATTERNS
ACROSS THE LIFE SPAN

Age-Group	Sleep Pattern/Needs
Neonate/Infant	
Toddler	
Preschooler	
School-Age Child	
Adolescent	
Young Adult	
Middle Adult	
Older Adult	

FACTORS AFFECTING SLEEP PATTERNS

Factors	Sleep Pattern Alterations
Physical Illness	
Drugs/Controlled Substances	
Lifestyle	
Usual Sleep Patterns	
Emotional Stress	
Environment	
Exercise and Fatigue	
Food/Calorie Intake	

QUESTIONS TO ASK TO ASSESS FOR SLEEP DISORDERS

ASSESSMENT QUESTIONS	RATIONALE
Insomnia	Determine nature and severity of insomnia.
How easily do you fall asleep?	Help in selection of sleep therapies.
Do you fall asleep and have difficulty staying asleep? How many times do you awaken?	
Do you awaken early from sleep?	
What time do you awaken for good? What causes you to awaken early?	
What do you do to prepare for sleep? To improve your sleep?	
What do you think about as you try to fall asleep?	
How often do you have trouble sleeping?	
Sleep Apnea	Reveal presence of sleep apnea and severity of condition.
Do you snore loudly?	
Has anyone ever told you that you often stop breathing for short periods during sleep? (Spouse or bed partner/roommate may report this.)	
Do you experience headaches after awakening?	
Do you have difficulty staying awake during the day?	
Does anyone else in your family snore loudly or stop breathing during sleep?	
Narcolepsy	Help diagnose narcolepsy and influence on daily activities.
Are you tired during the day?	
Do you fall asleep at inopportune times? (Friends or relatives may report this.)	
Do you have episodes of losing muscle control or falling to the floor?	
Have you ever had the feeling of being unable to move or talk just before falling asleep?	
Do you have vivid lifelike dreams when going to sleep or waking up?	

CRITICAL THINKING EXERCISES

1. Mrs. Davis, age 66, visits the community clinic for her annual checkup. She tells you as the nurse that she is having trouble sleeping at night because her husband is restless and snores. What assessment data is appropriate to gather regarding this situation?

2. As a nurse you are asked to help develop a health promotion brochure for senior citizens that includes information on how to promote sleep. The brochure will be available in clinics and senior centers. What general information should be included in the brochure for sleep enhancement in this group?

3. Mr. Walker, age 55, is recovering on your unit from heart surgery. You find him awake at 2 AM as you make rounds, and he tells you he has been having trouble sleeping since surgery 3 days ago. Develop a plan of care for Mr. Walker to promote sleep for him while he is in the hospital.

ANSWERS TO CRITICAL THINKING EXERCISES

1. Data should be gathered from both Mrs. Davis (as the spouse) and Mr. Davis, who may have a sleeping disorder. You are interested in gathering information in the following areas:
   What is the main problem with Mr. Davis's sleep, and why does his wife think it is a problem?
   Does Mr. Davis think he has a sleeping problem? If so, how does he describe it?
   How long has the problem existed? How does Mr. Davis rate the quantity and quality of his sleep?
   How frequently does the problem occur?
   How does this problem interfere with their usual activities?
   What has Mr. or Mrs. Davis done to try to remedy the situation?
   Ask for a description of Mr. Davis's sleep-wake pattern and usual bedtime routine.
   Ask about ingestion of caffeine, alcohol, nicotine use, and food intake before bedtime.
   Obtain a complete health history of all systems.
   Obtain a complete medication history of prescription and over-the-counter medications.
   Ask about family history of sleeping problems, especially insomnia, obstructive sleep apnea, narcolepsy, or restless leg syndrome.

   (Reference: Rogers AE: Nursing management of sleep disorders. I. Assessment. *ANNA J* 24(6): 666, 1997a.)

2. The following information should be included in the brochure for senior citizens:
   Keep a regular wake-up and bedtime schedule.
   Get up and do a quiet activity if you cannot fall asleep within 30 minutes of going to bed.
   Avoid daytime naps, if possible; if not, limit naps to 30 minutes or less.
   Avoid alcohol, caffeine, and nicotine late in the afternoon and before bedtime.
   Limit liquids before bedtime so that you do not have to make frequent trips to the bathroom.
   Exercise regularly during the daytime, preferably outdoors.
   Control the room temperature so that it is comfortable; use blankets as needed.

Use relaxation techniques to promote sleep.

Soft music may mask noise and help induce sleep.

(References: Beck-Little R, Weinrich SP: Assessment and management of sleep disorders in the elderly, *J Gerontol Nurs* 24(4):14, 1998; Rogers AE: Nursing management of sleep disorders. II. Behavioral interventions, *ANNA J* 24(6):672, 1997b.)

3. The plan of care should focus on interventions to promote sleep in a hospital setting:

    Administer analgesics as needed to promote comfort.

    Close the door to Mr. Walker's room to reduce noise.

    Pull the curtains between beds in Mr. Walker's room.

    Give a backrub or perform other hygiene measures to promote comfort and relaxation.

    Spend some time talking to Mr. Walker to answer questions and relieve anxiety.

    Try to reduce unnecessary noise (e.g., call lights unanswered, talking in the hallways or at the nurse's station).

    Play soft music in his room if desired.

    Do all procedures, assessments, and vital signs early in the night to allow for uninterrupted periods of sleep.

(References: Appling SE: Sleep: linking research to improved outcomes, *Medsurg Nurs* 6(3):159, 1997; Richards KC: Sleep promotion, *Crit Care Nurs Clin North Am* 8(1):39, 1996.)

Comfort

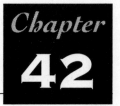

CLASSROOM DISCUSSION

1. Discuss the concept of comfort and the holistic approach that the nurse may use in assisting clients to achieve comfort.

2. Discuss the nature of pain, including the objective and subjective aspects of the experience, sources of pain, and its protective mechanism.

3. Ask students to contribute their ideas about the prejudices and misconceptions that may be associated with the pain experience and how nursing care may be influenced or altered.

4. Explain the neurophysiology of pain. Ask students how alterations in the central nervous system may influence the physiological pain mechanism.

5. Identify physiological and behavioral responses to pain. Ask students to share personal or clinical experiences in which responses to pain have been manifested.

6. Explain the different classifications of pain—acute, chronic, and cancer-related, or nociceptive and neuropathic. Ask students how the client's activities of daily living may be influenced by each type of pain.

7. Discuss factors that influence the pain experience:
   a. Age
   b. Gender
   c. Culture
   d. Meaning of pain
   e. Attention
   f. Anxiety
   g. Fatigue
   h. Prior experience
   i. Coping style

   Ask students to provide specific examples of how and why each factor may influence an individual's pain experience.

8. Describe the assessment guidelines for clients experiencing pain, including the following:
   a. Expression of pain
   b. Classification of pain
   c. Characteristics of pain
   d. Physiological and behavioral effects of pain
   e. Neurological status

9. Have students indicate how the client may express pain verbally and nonverbally and therapeutic measures that may be used to promote nurse-client communication.

10. Discuss the importance of pretreatment or procedure explanation in reducing a client's discomfort.

11. Identify and describe specific pain relief measures that the nurse may implement. Ask students to provide additional examples of possible interventions for different health care settings.

12. Review nonpharmacological pain relief measures, including indications for their use, precautions and contraindications, and nursing responsibilities associated with their implementation.

13. Discuss pharmacological pain therapy, including indications, precautions and contraindications, and nursing responsibilities associated with the following:
   a. Analgesics
   b. Patient-controlled analgesia
   c. Local and regional anesthetics
   d. Epidural analgesia

14. Stimulate a discussion on the advantages of nonpharmacological and pharmacological pain relief measures, and situations in which they may be used most effectively.

15. Identify surgical interventions that may be used to treat a client's pain.

16. Explain the treatment protocol for clients with intractable pain, including the goal of therapy, types of administration routes, and most effective pharmacological agents.

17. Review the evaluation and documentation of the client's responses to pain relief measures.

18. Invite a nurse working in a hospice or on an oncology unit to speak to the class about client assessment, pain relief measures, and nursing accountability.

19. Guide students in the application of the critical thinking model and nursing process for clients experiencing pain.

INTERACTIVE EXERCISES

1. Provide examples of different client situations, and ask students to identify whether the client may experience acute or chronic pain (e.g., a client with a ruptured appendix).

2. Have students investigate and report on different cultural responses to the pain experience.

3. Have students complete an assessment with another student or family member who is currently experiencing or has previously experienced pain.

4. Organize a role-playing situation (e.g., a lumbar puncture) with students explaining a procedure or treatment and the sensations that the client may expect.

5. Have students design a teaching plan for a client using a PCA (patient-controlled analgesia) pump in the home.

6. Have students investigate and report on available resources in the health care setting or community for reduction or relief of pain (e.g., a headache clinic).

7. Assign students to attend a nursing staff conference, if available, on pain relief strategies.

8. Working in small groups, have students plan how they may approach pain relief for the following clients:
   a. An older adult with arthritis
   b. A middle adult who has just had abdominal surgery
   c. A young adult with severe pain from advanced bone cancer
   d. A school-age child after a fracture or severe burn
   e. A toddler who is to have a lumbar puncture
   f. An adolescent with migraine headaches

CLINICAL SKILL

1. Demonstrate selected nonpharmacological pain relief measures to the class, such as relaxation, guided imagery, biofeedback, distraction, and cutaneous stimulation (application of hot/cold, TENS, acupressure, and/or massage).

CLIENT CARE EXPERIENCES

1. Assign students to observe and/or participate in the nursing care of clients experiencing pain in one or more of the following or similar health care settings:
   a. Labor and delivery
   b. Oncology unit
   c. Postoperative/postanesthesia care unit
   d. Hospice care center or home care agency

2. Have students assess the presence and characteristics of a client's pain and the client's responses to the experience. Supervise the students' implementation and documentation of appropriate pain relief measures in the clinical setting.

3. Have students complete a care plan/pathway for clients experiencing pain, and then identify how they individualized interventions to meet the specific clients' needs.

Factors influencing the pain experience
Acute and chronic pain: client responses

FACTORS INFLUENCING THE PAIN EXPERIENCE

Factors	Influence and Response of the Individual in Pain
Age	
Gender	
Culture	
Meaning of Pain	
Level of Attention	
Anxiety	
Fatigue	
Previous Pain Experience	
Coping Style	
Family/Social Support	

Acute Pain		Chronic Pain	
Physiological Responses	Behavioral Responses	Physiological Responses	Behavioral Responses

CRITICAL THINKING EXERCISES

1. John is a 32-year-old construction worker who sustained an injury to the lumbar region of his back during a fall approximately 8 months ago. John is 6 feet tall and weighs 280 pounds. He continues to report pain intensity as a 5 (on a scale of 0 to 10), increasing with activity; he has limited flexibility and is unable to return to work. He has recently been admitted for treatment at a comprehensive pain clinic. What interventions might the health care team employ?

2. Alexis is a 3 year old admitted to the pediatric unit for a third-degree burn to her right lower extremity. What tools might be useful when assessing this child's pain?

3. You are caring for an unconscious client who was involved in an automobile accident and sustained multiple injuries. The client has several lacerations, wounds, and surgical incisions, as well as multiple lines and tubes. What measures might you take to promote the client's comfort?

4. Mary Beth Jones, a 55-year-old woman with metastatic breast cancer to the bone, has been receiving IV morphine sulfate (MSO_4) for a week for severe back and leg pain. Her frequently increased infusion of MSO_4 is not reducing her pain to an acceptable level, and she is becoming increasingly sedated. What other pharmacological interventions might be considered?

ANSWERS TO CRITICAL THINKING EXERCISES

1. After conducting an extensive pain history and assessment, the team may recommend a variety of interventions. Pharmacological interventions may need to be implemented, but additional interventions would be helpful when dealing with chronic pain. The team may consider physical therapy, including activity and exercise, diet control, if necessary, and nonpharmacological interventions such as heat and cold application, biofeedback, distraction, and relaxation. A social worker might assist with any ramifications that his chronic pain has had on his financial status (e.g., unemployment).

2. The Oucher face scale is a very useful tool when assessing pain in toddlers. It is also important to involve the parent in the pain assessment.

3. Because of the extent of the client's injuries and altered level of consciousness, it will be necessary to assess for nonverbal cues of pain (e.g., grimacing). Pharmacological interventions would most likely be used. It would be your responsibility as the RN to assess the client routinely and consider around-the-clock dosing. Nonpharmacological interventions such as massage, range of motion, and positioning might be beneficial.

4. It might be helpful to start the client on a nonsteroidal antiinflammatory drug (NSAID) around the clock as an adjuvant to the morphine sulfate. If this is not effective, the client may benefit from an epidural analgesic with or without a local anesthetic. A test dose may be given to determine effectiveness, and an implantable catheter might be considered.

Nutrition

Chapter 43

CLASSROOM DISCUSSION

1. Review the principles of nutrition, including basal metabolic rate, energy expenditure, nutrients, and nutrient density.

2. Identify the six categories of nutrients, the role and storage of each in the body, and current recommendations for daily intake:
   a. Carbohydrates
   b. Proteins
   c. Lipids
   d. Water
   e. Vitamins — fat soluble and water soluble
   f. Minerals

   Have students identify food sources for each nutrient.

3. Discuss the role of carbohydrates, lipids, and proteins in energy provision.

4. Review the processes of digestion, absorption, and elimination. Define *metabolism;* review anabolism and catabolism, and present situations in which the body performs these activities.

5. Discuss the current dietary guidelines. Using transparencies, photos, illustrations, and/or models, explain *Canada's Food Guide to Healthy Eating.*

6. Discuss how the promotion of nutrition follows the *Nutrition for Health* objectives with guidelines for reducing saturated fat and sodium intake and increasing the intake of fruits and vegetables.

7. Review developmental variables and nutritional needs across the life span. Have students provide specific examples of how growth and development alters nutritional needs (see Resources for Student Activities, p. 231).

8. Explain the potential for nutrient–drug interactions. Ask students for additional examples of possible interactions.

9. Discuss alternative food patterns (e.g., vegetarianism) and the advantages and disadvantages in nutrient intake. Ask students to share personal or clinical experiences with alternative food pattern intake.

10. Identify and explain the aspects of a nutritional assessment and the information that is elicited through the following:
    a. Physical measurements — height, weight, body mass index (BMI), anthropometry, bioelectrical impedance analysis (BIA)
    b. Laboratory tests
    c. Dietary and health history — food records
    d. Clinical observation

11. Identify clients who may be at risk for nutritional problems. Use the following or similar situations, and ask students to provide the rationale for why nutritional problems may develop and how the nurse could determine the presence of the problem(s):
    a. A postoperative client
    b. An immobilized client
    c. An older adult living alone
    d. A preschool child living within a poor socioeconomic setting

12. Guide students in the application of the critical thinking model and the nursing process for clients with an altered nutritional status.

13. Identify measures that may be implemented to promote nutrition for clients in a variety of health care settings. Have students provide additional specific nursing interventions for stimulating a client's appetite, meeting nutritional guidelines for disease-related treatment, and client and family counselling and teaching.

14. Stimulate a discussion on client situations in which referrals for nutritional needs (e.g., Meals-on-Wheels) may be indicated.

15. Discuss nutritional concerns for clients of diverse cultural and spiritual backgrounds (e.g., kosher and Hindu requirements).

16. Invite a nutritionist or a dietitian to speak to the class about dietary health promotion for clients in the acute, restorative, and/or home care setting.

17. Discuss enteral nutrition, including its purpose, uses, complications, and associated nursing responsibilities. Have students identify client situations in which enteral nutrition and tube feedings may be used to promote nutrition.

18. Discuss parenteral nutrition, including its purpose, use, specific solutions, contraindications, complications, and the associated nursing responsibilities of assisting with central venous insertion and maintaining the infusion. Have students identify situations in which parenteral nutrition may be indicated for a client.

INTERACTIVE EXERCISES

1. Have students complete a food intake record (24 h per day for up to 3 days) on themselves, a peer, or a family member, and analyze the total nutrient intake for adequacy. They can use a commercial computer program, if available.

226   Unit 7: Basic Human Needs

2. Have students identify what is available to the consumer regarding nutritional information and guidelines (e.g., food labels, media presentations). Assign students to bring in examples of readily found nutritional information.

3. Provide students with client situations and have them identify, verbally and/or in writing, potential nutritional problems and needs and appropriate nursing interventions. Use examples for clients experiencing one or more of the following: diabetes mellitus; GI, cardiovascular, or renal disease; HIV; or cancer (see Resources for Student Activities, p. 232).

4. Have students design and present a teaching plan on dietary needs for one of the following simulated situations:
   a. Parents with an 8-month-old infant and/or 2-year-old child
   b. An older adult with coronary disease
   c. A family member responsible for care of a client's gastrostomy tube

CLINICAL SKILLS

1. Explain and demonstrate (using a simulation mannequin/model, appropriate equipment, and available educational media) the following nursing interventions for promotion of client nutrition:
   a. Insertion of a small-bore a nasoenteric tube
   b. Initiation of enteral tube feedings via a nasoenteric tube
   c. Administration of enteral feedings via a gastrostomy or a jejunostomy tube

2. Have small groups of students practise the performance and documentation of these interventions, using appropriate equipment (as available).

3. Evaluate the students' ability to implement and document the interventions to promote client nutrition through return demonstration and skill testing before clinical experience.

CLIENT CARE EXPERIENCES

1. Assign students to observe and participate in the nursing care of clients, in a variety of health care settings, focussing on the assessment and promotion of nutritional intake. Have students prepare the environment and assist with oral care to stimulate a client's appetite.

2. Supervise the students' implementation of oral, enteral, or parenteral feedings, as indicated. Review and evaluate their assessment of the client's nutritional status, and discuss possible strategies for improvement, if needed. Have students work with clients in food selection, meal planning, and food preparation according to prescribed diet therapy.

3. Have students complete a care plan/pathway for an assigned client who is experiencing an alteration in nutritional status.

RESOURCES FOR STUDENT ACTIVITIES

Nutritional needs across the life span chart
Disease-related dietary management chart
Nutrition screening tool for older adults

NUTRITIONAL NEEDS ACROSS THE LIFE SPAN CHART

Age Group/ Population	Nutritional Needs
Infant	
Toddler/ Preschooler	
School-Age Child	
Adolescent	
Young and Middle Adult	
Pregnant or Lactating Woman	
Older Adult	

228   Unit 7: Basic Human Needs

Pathophysiology	General Dietary Needs
Gastrointestinal Disease	
Cardiovascular Disease	
Pulmonary Disease	
Diabetes Mellitus	
Renal Disease	
HIV/AIDS	
Cancer	

The Warning Signs of poor nutritional health are often overlooked. Use this checklist to find out if you or someone you know is at nutritional risk.

Read the statements below. Circle the number in the yes column for those that apply. For each yes answer, score the number in the box. Total the nutritional score.

DETERMINE YOUR NUTRITIONAL HEALTH

	YES
I have an illness or condition that made me change the kind and/or amount of food I eat.	2
I eat fewer than 2 meals per day.	3
I eat few fruits or vegetables, or milk products.	2
I have 3 or more drinks of beer, liquor or wine almost every day.	2
I have tooth or mouth problems that make it hard for me to eat.	2
I don't always have enough money to buy the food I need.	4
I eat alone most of the time.	1
I take 3 or more different prescribed or over-the-counter drugs a day.	1
Without wanting to, I have lost or gained 10 pounds in the last 6 months.	2
I am not always physically able to shop, cook and/or feed myself.	2
TOTAL	

Total Your Nutritional Score. If it's –

0–2 **Good!** Recheck your nutritional score in 6 months.

3–5 **You are at moderate nutritional risk.** See what can be done to improve your eating habits and lifestyle. Your office on aging, senior nutrition program, senior citizens center or health department can help. Recheck your nutritional score in 3 months.

6 or more **You are at high nutritional risk.** Bring this checklist the next time you see your doctor, dietitian or other qualified health or social service professional. Talk with them about any problems you may have. Ask for help to improve your nutritional health.

These materials developed and distributed by the Nutritional Screening Initiative, a project of:

AMERICAN ACADEMY OF FAMILY PHYSICIANS

THE AMERICAN DIETETIC ASSOCIATION

NATIONAL COUNCIL ON THE AGING

Remember that warning signs suggest risk, but do not represent diagnosis of any condition.

From the Nutrition Screening Initiative (1998), a project of the American Academy of Family Physicians, the American Dietetic Association, and the National Council of the Aging, Inc. and funded in part by a grant from Ross Products Division, Abbott Laboratories.

CRITICAL THINKING EXERCISES

1. Jean, age 35, has just had surgery for a bowel obstruction. Her medical history includes Crohn's disease. Before this exacerbation, three months ago, Jean's weight was 55.8 kg. Admission weight was 52.2 kg; three days after surgery, she now weighs 49.0 kg. Her height is 165 cm. Reported laboratory values are white blood cell count, 8.3×10^9/L percentage lymphocytes, 13; albumin, 23 gL. What is Jean's BMI? What is her percent weight loss? What is her total lymphocyte count? Jean remains NPO with nasogastric suction; what intervention(s) would you discuss with her physician?

   *(For further information refer to McMorrow ME, Malarkey L: *Laboratory and diagnostic tests: A pocket guide*, Toronto, 1998, W.B. Saunders.)

2. During a well-child check-up, Mrs. Grosboll asks if she should be concerned about John, her 20-month-old son. She complains that his appetite was good until a few months ago, when he became a picky eater. She worries that he is not getting adequate nutrition. What is your response?

3. Roberta is being treated for breast cancer with chemotherapy as adjunct to a lumpectomy. She has maintained a positive attitude as well as possible but is concerned about the side effects of the medication. Roberta has bleeding gums, stomatitis, nausea, and diarrhea. As a result, she has no desire to eat. She is 85 percent of her UBW at present. How could you assist Roberta to improve her nutritional status?

4. Mrs. Caine is 85 years old. She has been hospitalized for a fractured left hip and is now ready for discharge. She has always been active, living alone. She has no family nearby, but a few close friends. What arrangements would you make to continue her nutritional intake at home while she recovers?

ANSWERS TO CRITICAL THINKING EXERCISES

1. a. Jean's body mass index is calculated using the formula kg ÷ metres (ht) squared. Thus, Jean presently weighs 49.0 kg and is 1.65 m in height, which, squared, equals 2.7; her BMI is 18.1. A BMI of 18.1 places Jean within a high-risk category, in need of nutritional intervention.
   b. Jean's percent weight loss is calculated with the formula: usual body weight [UBW] – current body weight [CBW] ÷ UBW × 100; (55.8 kg – 49.0 kg) ÷ 55.8 × 100 = 12. Jean's weight loss within a 3-month time period, is significant. A loss of greater than 7.5 percent over 3 months or of 10 percent over 6 months places clients at high risk.
   c. Jean's total lymphocyte count (TLC) is calculated by percentage lymph × WBC count ÷ 100. A WBC of 8.3×10^9/L is equivalent to 8,300/mm^3; 13 × 8,300 divided by 100 equals 1,079. A TLC of less than 1,500 cells/mm^3 is associated with increased morbidity and mortality.
   d. Jean is a good candidate for parenteral nutrition (PN). When nasogastric suctioning is discontinued, and Jean has bowel sounds in all four quadrants, she should be transitioned to oral intake with calorie counts. PN is decreased as oral intake increases to full dietary requirements.

2. Toddlers are usually "picky eaters" and consume slightly less food. They tend to focus more on developing verbal and motor skills and becoming acquainted with their environment. Always begin with a physical nutritional assessment. This data should guide your advice to Mrs. Grosboll. If assessment results warrant concern, have John's mother keep a food diary for three days and mail it to the office. Offer dietary counselling regarding required servings for John's age from the food groups, using *Canada's Food Guide to Healthy Eating*. Suggest small, frequent, nutrient-dense snacks in place of larger meals.

3. Perform a complete physical assessment. Focus on medications, food preferences, cues that induce nausea and what she does to cope, and frequency and amount of diarrhea. Establish Roberta's energy requirements, and estimate her usual intake. What is her illness/activity factor? Encourage exercise as tolerated. Treat Roberta's symptoms as follows:
   a. Bleeding gums: Have Roberta use an extra-soft bristle, child-size toothbrush.
   b. Stomatitis: Have Roberta eat cool or room temperature foods, increase fluids, avoid course-textured, highly seasoned or acidic foods, tobacco, alcohol, and commercial mouthwashes. Consult with her physician about use of an analgesic mouthrinse. Supplement foods with protein powder or a carbohydrate liquid supplement.
   c. Nausea: Suggest frequent, small, nutrient-dense meals. Roberta should include high-protein/kcal supplements, avoid excess fat, eat slowly, limit fluid intake with meals, rest after meals with her head elevated, and consult with her physician regarding antiemetic medication use.
   d. Diarrhea: Suggest frequent, small meals. Roberta should avoid excess fat and gas-forming foods, drink fluids between meals, and consult with her physician about antidiarrheal medication use.

4. Consult with social services regarding identified nutritional needs after discharge. A referral for Mrs. Caine to receive Meals on Wheels would be helpful, as well as information regarding community grocery stores with delivery services.

Urinary Elimination

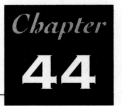

Chapter

44

CLASSROOM DISCUSSION

1. Review the anatomy and physiology of the urinary tract—kidneys, ureters, bladder, urethra, and process of urination.

2. Discuss factors that influence urinary elimination:
   a. Pathophysiology
   b. Growth and development
   c. Sociocultural
   d. Psychological
   e. Muscle tone
   f. Fluid balance
   g. Surgical procedures
   h. Medications
   i. Diagnostic examination

   Have students identify specific examples of how each factor may influence an individual's urinary elimination (see Resource for Student Activities, p. 239).

3. Identify and describe the following alterations in urinary elimination, including possible etiology and client signs and symptoms:
   a. Urinary retention
   b. Lower urinary tract infections
   c. Urinary incontinence

4. Discuss the indications for, surgical treatment of, and resultant client alterations in elimination that are associated with urinary diversions.

5. Discuss the components of the nursing history that will elicit information on a client's urinary function, including patterns of urination, symptoms, and other related factors. Have students determine what initial and follow-up questions may elicit the most accurate information from the client.

6. Discuss the importance of hygiene and asepsis in the control of urinary infections. Ask students how the age, developmental level, and sociocultural practices of the client may have an impact upon urinary hygiene.

7. Review the physical assessment of the client with respect to urinary elimination. Ask students to identify expected and unexpected findings from the assessment (e.g., distended bladder and inflamed mucosa).

8. Describe the nursing assessment of urinary output, including analysis of intake and output and characteristics of urine.

9. Identify and describe common laboratory and diagnostic tests used to evaluate urinary function. Discuss client preparation and nursing responsibilities associated with the testing. Review normal results and the meaning of abnormal findings from urinary diagnostic testing.

10. Discuss the psychological and emotional factors involved in urinary elimination. Ask students to identify how the nurse may promote client dignity and alleviate anxiety in the health care setting.

11. Using the following or similar situations, ask students to specify how urinary elimination may be affected:
    a. A paraplegic client
    b. An older adult with rheumatoid arthritis
    c. A hospitalized 3-year-old child
    d. An adult female with recurrent urinary tract infections
    e. A client diagnosed with bladder cancer

12. Identify nursing interventions that may be implemented to promote urinary function, including the following: client education, stimulation of function, bladder emptying, and prevention of infection. Have students provide additional specific examples of nursing interventions and the rationale for their implementation.

13. Discuss how nursing approaches and procedures to promote urinary elimination may be altered from the acute care setting to the restorative setting to the home care setting.

14. Discuss the types, purposes, complications, nursing responsibilities, and documentation associated with urinary catheterization. Have students identify measures that may be implemented to reduce the incidence of infection associated with catheterization.

15. Describe restorative nursing care measures for promotion of urinary elimination, such as teaching the client Kegel exercises or self-catheterization, maintaining skin integrity and comfort, and bladder retraining. Stimulate a discussion on how the nurse may be creative in implementing these measures with the client, especially in the home environment.

16. Invite a nurse who specializes in dialysis and renal care to speak to the class about specific client needs, assessment, and nursing responsibility for promoting and evaluating urinary function.

17. Guide students in the application of the critical thinking model and the nursing process for clients experiencing alterations in urinary elimination.

INTERACTIVE EXERCISES

1. Assign students to investigate and report on the resources available in an affiliating health care setting or community for clients requiring dialysis, urinary diversion support groups, and/or special ostomy equipment (type available and cost).

2. Provide students with the results of a sample urinalysis, and have them determine the normal and abnormal findings.

3. Provide small groups of students with the name of a urinary diagnostic test, and have them design a teaching plan for and/or role play the preparation of a client for that procedure.

4. Have students design and implement a teaching plan for an adolescent or adult female client in the community on the prevention of urinary tract infections.

CLINICAL SKILLS

1. Explain and demonstrate the procedure for collection of a midstream (clean-voided) specimen. Ask students how the procedure may be altered for clients of different ages and self-care abilities.

2. Demonstrate measures to stimulate urinary elimination by having students place their hands in warm water or hear the sound of running water (if a bathroom is available nearby).

3. Explain and demonstrate (using a simulation mannequin/model, appropriate equipment and supplies, and available educational media) the following nursing interventions to promote urinary elimination:
   a. Insertion of a straight or indwelling catheter
   b. Provision of indwelling catheter care
   c. Closed and open catheter irrigation
   d. Application of a condom catheter

4. Have small groups of students practice, with supervision, the performance and documentation of the specified interventions, using appropriate equipment.

5. Evaluate the students' ability to implement and document the interventions to promote urinary elimination through return demonstration and skill testing before clinical experience.

CLIENT CARE EXPERIENCES

1. Assign students to accompany clients (as possible) and observe urinary diagnostic procedures (e.g., cystoscopy). Have students share their observations after the experience.

2. Assign students to observe and participate in the nursing care of clients in diverse health care settings, who may be experiencing alterations in urinary elimination. Discuss the assessment of urinary function with the group. Review laboratory and diagnostic test results and client manifestations that may indicate altered urinary function.

3. Discuss measures to be implemented to promote urinary elimination, focusing on the maintenance of client dignity, privacy, and control (as possible).

4. Identify actual and potential client educational needs regarding urinary elimination.

5. Have students complete a care plan/pathway for an assigned client who is experiencing an alteration in urinary elimination.

RESOURCE FOR STUDENT ACTIVITIES

Factors influencing urinary elimination

FACTORS INFLUENCING URINARY ELIMINATION

Factors	Influence on Urinary Elimination
Disease Conditions	
Growth and Development	
Sociocultural	
Psychological	
Muscle Tone	
Fluid Balance	
Surgical Procedures	
Medications	
Diagnostic Examinations	

CRITICAL THINKING EXERCISES

1. Mr. Miller is a 75-year-old widower who has had prostate surgery for benign prostatic hypertrophy. He thought his problems would be over, but now he is experiencing continual dribbling of urine. He has been attempting to deal with the problem by using an absorbant pad in his underwear, but he feels as though everyone knows his problem. The embarrassment of having an odor keeps him at home. He has given up attending his senior citizen center.
   a. How can the nurse help him regain control of his urinary elimination?
   b. What are the actual nursing diagnoses that apply to Mr. Miller?
   c. For one diagnosis give one goal/outcome and two nursing interventions.

2. Mrs. Luis is a 37-year-old woman who has been admitted with hematuria. She has noticed blood in her urine for a week, but she was hoping it would go away. She is to undergo a cystoscopy in 4 hours.
   a. What is the purpose of a cystoscopy?
   b. What nursing care is needed before she goes to the operating room?
   c. Give at least two nursing responsibilities for care of the client after undergoing a cystectomy.

3. Mrs. Joseph is a 70-year-old woman with cognitive changes associated with Alzheimer's disease. Her daughter, with whom she lives, has brought her to her family practitioner's office. You are the family nurse practitioner in the practice. As you assess Mrs. Joseph, you ask her daughter how she is coping with her mother. The daughter replies that her mother does not seem to remember how to go to the bathroom. Mrs. Joseph will go into the bathroom but forget to pull down her underwear before going to the bathroom. After the incident her mother becomes upset and blames the daughter for her wetness. She asks you for suggestions on how to manage, as she noticed that her mother's perineal skin is reddened and sore. What assessments does the nurse need to complete before planning interventions for Mrs. Joseph's care?

ANSWERS TO CRITICAL THINKING EXERCISES

1. a. Mr. Miller is suffering from a condition that is a source of embarrassment and shame for him. The nurse, in assessing the situation, knows that in order to make a difference, the urine dribbling must be controlled. With increased muscle control, Mr. Miller can enhance the ability of the external urinary sphincter to control the dribbling. For long-term control, a regimen of pelvic floor exercises will accomplish that goal. For the immediate problem, the nurse needs to help him choose an absorbent pad product that will contain the urine, prevent odor, and be undetectable under his clothes.
   b. Some possible nursing diagnoses for Mr. Miller include the following:
      Total urinary incontinence related to internal urinary sphincter damage as evidenced by continuous urinary dribbling
      Situational low self-esteem related to reduced self-care ability as evidenced by shame and embarrassment
      Social isolation related to perceived urinary odor as evidenced by self-imposed limited social interaction

c. Situational low self-esteem related to reduced self-care ability as evidenced by shame and embarrassment:

Goal/outcome: Client will be able to relate effect of life events (incontinence) on feelings about self.

Interventions: Actively listen to and demonstrate acceptance of client. Provide information about pelvic floor exercises to help him regain urinary control.

2. a. Mrs. Luis has been admitted with hematuria and will undergo a cystoscopy. The purpose of the cystoscopy is to determine, if possible, the source of the bleeding. Hematuria may be an early sign of either bladder cancer or renal cancer. Early detection will greatly improve the success of medical treatment.

b. Before sending Mrs. Luis to the operating room, it is important to assess her level of anxiety concerning both the procedure and the outcome of the surgery. Since she was admitted before going to the operating room, preoperative teaching about what to expect is indicated. Many times the procedure will be done under general anesthesia so that muscle relaxation will be maximized. This will minimize the possibility of urethral or bladder injury during the procedure. Mrs. Luis needs to know that she may return to her room with an indwelling catheter and will probably have an intravenous line in place for fluids until she can tolerate liquids by mouth. She also needs to know that her urine drainage may still be bloody or pink-tinged after the procedure.

c. When Mrs. Luis returns to her room, it is important for the nurse to (1) encourage fluids by mouth and monitor urine output and (2) administer medications to alleviate bladder spasms and/or lower back discomfort.

3. In planning care for Mrs. Joseph, it is important and necessary to include assessment of her caregiver and her environment in order to have a complete picture of the situation.

a. Client assessment—What is her cognitive level? Does she "forget" how to use the toilet all the time, or just sometimes? What is the pattern of incontinence? Are there any specific behavioral changes before an accident (e.g., pacing or fidgeting)? What is the current condition of her perineal skin?

b. Caregiver assessment—Is the daughter working outside the home? From home? Primary responsibilities in the home? Other constraints on the daughter's time and energy (children at home)?

c. Environmental assessment—How long has Mrs. Joseph been in her current living condition? Are there any physical barriers, such as the only bathroom being located on the second floor?

Bowel Elimination

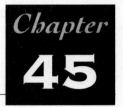

CLASSROOM DISCUSSION

1. Review the anatomy and physiology of digestion and bowel elimination.

2. Identify factors that affect bowel elimination. Have students provide specific examples of how bowel elimination may be affected with each factor.

3. Describe common bowel elimination problems, including their etiology, potential complications, and client signs and symptoms:
   a. Constipation
   b. Fecal impaction
   c. Diarrhea
   d. Incontinence
   e. Flatulence
   f. Hemorrhoids

4. Discuss psychological and emotional factors associated with bowel elimination. Ask students how the nurse may recognize and minimize disturbances in bowel elimination that may be related to the health care environment (e.g., lack of privacy, positioning).

5. Discuss the indications for, surgical treatment of, and resultant client alterations in elimination that are associated with bowel diversions—ileostomies and colostomies. Using educational media (photos/illustrations, videos, models), demonstrate how the incontinent and continent ostomies differ in location, drainage, and nursing and client care management.

6. Stimulate a discussion on the potential affect on a client's self-concept and body image after the creation of an ostomy.

7. Invite an enterostomal therapy nurse to speak to the class about specific physical and psychological needs of the client with an ostomy and measures that the nurse may implement to support the client.

8. Describe the aspects of the nursing history that will elicit information about the client's bowel elimination status.

9. Review the physical assessment of the client in relation to digestion and bowel elimination. Ask students to identify unexpected findings from the physical assessment that may indicate a problem with digestion and/or bowel elimination.

10. Discuss the nurse's analysis of fecal characteristics for determination of abnormalities.

11. Identify and describe laboratory and diagnostic tests that may be used to determine problems with digestion and bowel elimination. Discuss client preparation and the nursing responsibilities associated with the testing. Review normal results and the meaning of abnormal findings from digestive and bowel elimination testing.

12. Explain the procedure for collection of a fecal sample for the measurement of occult blood. Ask students what information is necessary to provide to clients who will use the test at home.

13. Identify specific nursing measures that may be implemented to promote bowel elimination and support the client's self-concept, including bowel training, fluid and dietary intake, exercise, privacy, and proper positioning. Have students specify additional measures that may be used by the nurse, particularly in the acute and extended care setting, to establish client comfort and routine.

14. Discuss the use of medications (laxatives, cathartics, stool softeners, antidiarrheals) to promote or restore normal bowel elimination. Ask students how these medications may also create bowel elimination problems.

15. Discuss the types, purposes, and administration of enemas.

16. Review the indications and the procedure for the digital removal of stool.

17. Discuss the nursing care and client and family educational needs associated with ileostomies and colostomies. Ask students to provide specific concerns related to skin care, diet therapy, and body image.

18. Have students identify how bowel elimination may be affected and the nursing measures that may be implemented for the following client situations:
    a. A client with a cardiac condition
    b. A client with a new ileostomy or colostomy
    c. A salesman who is on the road for long periods of time and is under a great deal of occupational stress
    d. An immobilized client with a head trauma
    e. An adult client with multiple sclerosis
    f. A 3 year old hospitalized for a minor surgical procedure
    g. A client after abdominal surgery
    h. An individual taking narcotic analgesics
    i. An older adult with osteoarthritis

19. Guide students in the application of the critical thinking model and the nursing process for clients experiencing alterations in bowel elimination.

INTERACTIVE EXERCISES

1. Assign students to investigate resources that are available within the affiliating agency and community for clients with an ileostomy or colostomy. Have students identify the types and costs of equipment that the client may need to purchase and whether medical insurance will cover the expenses.

2. Have students practice completing the bowel elimination component of the health history with a peer to better experience the embarrassment that may be felt by the client in response to these questions.

3. Have students design and present a teaching plan based on one of the following:
   a. Client or family member care of an ileostomy or sigmoid colostomy
   b. Maintenance of regular bowel elimination patterns during pregnancy
   c. Bowel retraining
   d. Hazards of overuse of laxatives, cathartics, and enemas
   e. Client scheduled to have an upper or lower GI series

CLINICAL SKILLS

1. Demonstrate the procedure for collection of a fecal sample for the measurement of occult blood.

2. Explain and demonstrate (using a simulation mannequin/model, appropriate equipment and supplies, and available educational media) the following nursing interventions to promote bowel elimination:
   a. Administration of a cleansing enema
   b. Pouching of a colostomy or ileostomy
   c. Irrigation of a colostomy
   d. Insertion and maintenance of a nasogastric tube

3. Have small groups of students practice the performance and documentation of the specified interventions, using appropriate equipment and supplies.

4. Evaluate the students' ability to implement and document the interventions for promotion of bowel elimination through return demonstration and skill testing before clinical experience.

CLIENT CARE EXPERIENCES

1. Assign students to accompany clients (as possible) and observe diagnostic testing for digestive or bowel elimination disorders. Have students share their observations after the experience.

2. Assign students to observe and participate in the nursing care of clients in a variety of health care settings, with the focus on the assessment and promotion of bowel elimination. Discuss client manifestations and laboratory and diagnostic test results that may indicate a problem with bowel elimination.

3. Have the students collaborate with the nursing staff and clients to promote food and fluid intake, provide exercise and comfort, maintain skin integrity, and support client self-concept.

4. Evaluate the students' implementation of nursing measures, being alert to the maintenance of client dignity, privacy, and safety.

5. Have students complete a care plan/pathway for an assigned client who is experiencing an alteration in bowel elimination.

Factors influencing bowel elimination
Nursing measures to promote bowel elimination

FACTORS INFLUENCING BOWEL ELIMINATION

Age	
Infection	
Diet	
Fluid Intake	
Physical Activity	
Psychological Factors	
Personal Habits	
Positioning	
Pain	
Pregnancy	
Surgery/Anesthesia	
Medications	
Diagnostic Tests	

Nursing Measure	Specific Details
Regular Bowel Pattern	
Fluid and Food Intake	
Exercise	
Comfort	
Skin Integrity	
Self-Concept	
Positioning	
Ostomies	

CRITICAL THINKING EXERCISES

1. A 17-year-old man with a history of good health and regular exercise is seen by the school nurse. He complains of increasing diarrhea and abdominal cramping. He states that on rare occasions he has noticed blood on the toilet paper he has used. What additional pieces of assessment data do you need?

2. The nursing long-term care center has invited you to come and do a presentation concerning prevention of constipation in their residents. What points of information would you want to include in your presentation?

3. A 22-year-old man is to undergo surgery for Crohn's disease. He will have a new, pouching ileostomy. He and his mother need teaching about what this means for his future elimination needs. What would you tell them?

ANSWERS TO CRITICAL THINKING EXERCISES

1. Additional pieces of data that you should collect include the following: What foods has he eaten recently? Has this ever happened before? Has he been out of the country? What has worked to treat it previously? Is there a history of bowel problems in his family? Is he able to tell whether the blood is in the stool?

2. Information in your presentation should include the need for an adequate fluid intake (intake and output is a must). There are many nonpharmaceutical methods of treating or avoiding constipation, including eating fruits and fiber, and activity; the use of bowel charts is very helpful in identifying problems early. Many clients think that they are drinking enough, when really they are not; be especially attentive to those with dementia or Alzheimer's disease who are unable to recognize the thirst mechanism.

3. Teaching for this family should include the following:
   The anatomical changes associated with this bowel surgery
   The amount of fecal material that the pouch will hold and how often it will need emptying
   The method of evacuating stool from the pouch
   The fact that he will be able to live as he did before; that he can swim, run, participate in any activity that he chooses
   Dietary needs will be important—constipating foods, such as corn, chips, and popcorn, may cause a constipation-like action in the bowel contents

Mobility and Immobility

Chapter 46

CLASSROOM DISCUSSION

1. Review body mechanics and the maintenance of body alignment, balance, coordinated movement, exercise and activity, and friction.

2. Review the body systems involved in the regulation and coordination of body movement.

3. Review how the principles of body mechanics and movement are integrated into nursing care.

4. Review the pathological influences on body alignment and mobility, including postural abnormalities, congenital defects, disorders of the bones, joints, and muscles, CNS damage, and musculoskeletal trauma. Ask students to identify specific pathological problems that may be experienced by clients.

5. Explain the general physiological and psychosocial effects of immobility on the client.

6. Ask students to identify specific growth and development factors that may influence mobility status and place the individual at risk for the hazards of immobility.

7. Guide students in the application of the critical thinking model and the nursing process for clients experiencing alterations in mobility.

8. Review the assessment of client mobility in the following areas:
   a. Joint range of motion
   b. Gait
   c. Exercise and activity tolerance
   d. Body alignment

   Ask students what constitutes expected or abnormal findings in the assessment of mobility.

9. Describe the physical assessment of the immobile client to determine the potential for or the presence of physiological, psychosocial, and developmental hazards.

10. Have students identify which assessment technique or equipment should be used to determine the presence of the following:
    a. Muscle atrophy
    b. Orthostatic hypotension
    c. Thrombosis
    d. Urinary retention
    e. Fecal impaction

11. Ask students what behavioral and psychosocial changes may be experienced by the client, especially the older adult, who is having an adverse response to immobility.

12. Discuss developmentally appropriate nursing measures that may be implemented to reduce or eliminate the negative effects of immobility. Ask students to explain the rationale for these nursing interventions in counteracting the effect of immobility.

13. Have students identify how range-of-motion exercises may be integrated into other nursing care activities.

14. Ask students to identify possible situations in which additional assistance may be needed to position, move, transfer, or ambulate a client.

15. Have students specify the rationale for the use of supports (e.g., trochanter rolls, footboard) for positioning of the client.

16. Invite a physical therapist to speak to the class about measures to prevent the hazards of immobility and appropriate exercises and activities to provide for the immobilized client.

INTERACTIVE EXERCISES

1. Have students identify, verbally or in writing, the influences on mobility for the following client problems:
   a. Post-CVA with resultant right-sided hemiparesis
   b. Scoliosis or kyphosis
   c. Multiple fractures
   d. Osteoarthritis
   e. Paraplegia

2. Have students design teaching plans for the following or similar client situations in which mobility may be compromised:
   a. An 8-year-old child with leukemia who is placed on complete bed rest
   b. An 86 year old who has had a CVA with resultant left-sided hemiplegia
   c. A 32 year old with advanced multiple sclerosis

CLINICAL SKILLS

1. Explain, and demonstrate (using a simulation mannequin/model or volunteer, appropriate equipment, and educational media, as available) specific nursing interventions that may be implemented to promote proper body alignment and mobility and reduce the hazards of immobility, including the following:
   a. Lifting (by the nurse)
   b. Range of motion
   c. Positioning and moving a client in bed
   d. Transfer of a client from bed to chair or stretcher
   e. Applying elastic stockings

2. Have small groups of students practice the skills to promote body alignment and mobility, using the appropriate equipment and supplies and document the procedure and status of the client accordingly. Supervise activities such as client lifting and transfers.

3. Evaluate the students' ability to implement and document selected skills through return demonstration and skill testing before clinical experience.

CLIENT CARE EXPERIENCES

1. Assign students to observe and participate in the nursing care of clients in acute, extended, rehabilitation, or home care settings, with focus placed on the promotion of body alignment and mobility.

2. Discuss expectations of students before the experience, specifically emphasizing client safety and requesting assistance in moving clients.

3. Review the students' assessments, strategies employed, and evaluation of clients' mobility status after the experience.

4. Have students complete a care plan/pathway for an assigned client who is experiencing alterations in physical mobility.

RESOURCE FOR STUDENT ACTIVITIES

Immobility and nursing interventions

Nature of Change	Physiologic Effect of Immobility	Nursing to Minimize Effect
Metabolic		
Respiratory		
Cardiovascular		
Musculoskeletal		
Integumentary		
Elimination		
Psychosocial		

CRITICAL THINKING EXERCISES

1. You are caring for a 57-year-old male client who has just had a bilateral total knee replacement for osteoarthritis. He is 2 days postoperative and beginning to transfer to a chair with help. He is 100 pounds overweight and has a history of deep vein thrombosis. He has compression stockings, continuous passive range of motion, and a heparin lock. Make a list of potential nursing diagnoses.

2. When doing a home visit for a 75-year-old female client, the client's granddaughter runs in and says, "Did you show the nurse the sore on your leg that you got from falling yesterday?" What questions about mobility are important to ask the client? How do you begin your assessment?

3. Your clinical experience is in long-term care. You are working in assisted living. The nurse in charge of the assisted living wing asks you to help her with a program titled, "Lifestyle Choices: Living Life to Its Fullest." She asks you to participate and discuss how regular exercise can be incorporated into activities of daily living. Develop a content outline and a time frame for your presentation.

4. You are caring for a 20-year-old female college student who is immobilized after spinal cord trauma. You note that she is becoming increasingly depressed and withdrawn. What skill is important at this point in the client's care?

ANSWERS TO CRITICAL THINKING EXERCISES

1. Possible nursing diagnoses: Impaired physical mobility related to pain and mobility restrictions secondary to TKR. Risk for trauma (falling) related to impaired mobility. Risk for altered peripheral tissue perfusion–related altered blood flow secondary to obesity, decreased mobility, and platelet agglutination secondary to TKR.

2. Begin your assessment by asking the client about the fall, including why she thinks she fell. How did it happen, where did it happen, and has it happened before? Ask her to show you and to explain her injuries. Has she done anything to correct the cause for the fall? Has she been checked for osteoporosis? Once assessments are made, then begin to work with your client on any corrective actions needed to be taken, including safety assessment for the home (see Chapter 37, p. 193) and a referral for a check for osteoporosis as necessary.

3. Begin your preparation by reviewing Chapters 36 and 46 of *Canadian Fundamentals of Nursing,* Second Edition, paying particular attention to Table 46–3, and Boxes 36–5 and 36–11. Spend 10 minutes discussing the positive effects that exercise can have on the skin and metabolic, respiratory, cardiovascular, musculoskeletal, and urinary systems. Spend 10 minutes with demonstration and return demonstration of how to include exercises into ADLs. You may plan another session on an introduction to Tai Chi Chih or yoga, depending on the receptivity of the group and the availability of someone to teach class.

4. The client who has had an injury of this magnitude must be expected and allowed to grieve. While it is not clear from the description how likely her trauma is to result in permanent damage, it is vital to assess her expected outcomes. Does she have unrealistic expectations of her recovery, of staff, and of family? A clinical nurse specialist may serve as a resource to help further assess the client. A beginning student nurse is in a unique position to use listening skills, which are very important in knowing what is going on. Therapeutic communication techniques (see Chapter 22 of *Canadian Fundamentals of Nursing*, Second Edition) will be vital to this assessment.

Skin Integrity and Wound Care

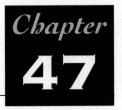

Chapter
47

CLASSROOM DISCUSSION

1. Review the anatomy and physiology of the integumentary system.

2. Review the pathogenesis associated with the development of a pressure ulcer. Show photos, slides, and/or videotapes that depict the stages of pressure ulcers.

3. Discuss the prevalence of pressure ulcers in health care settings and the economic consequences of their development.

4. Identify client risk factors that are associated with the development of pressure ulcers. Have students provide specific client examples of impaired sensation or motor function, altered level of consciousness, and equipment and treatment (e.g., casts, traction) that may increase the risk for pressure ulcer development.

5. Discuss wound classification, using photos/illustrations, models, and other available educational media.

6. Describe wound healing by primary and secondary intention. Identify the phases of primary intention healing. Use photos, illustrations, and/or models to differentiate the two types of wound healing.

7. Describe the following complications of wound healing:
   a. Hemorrhage
   b. Infection
   c. Dehiscence/evisceration
   d. Fistula formation
   e. Delayed wound closure

   Have students specify the etiology and client signs and symptoms for these complications.

8. Explain the assessment tools that may be used to determine a client's risk for pressure ulcer development, including the following:
   a. Norton Scale
   b. Gosnell Scale
   c. Braden Scale

   Ask students to compare the tools and identify similarities and differences in their approaches.

9. Discuss factors that influence the development of pressure ulcers and wound healing, including shearing force/friction, moisture, poor nutrition, anemia, cachexia, obesity, infection, impaired peripheral circulation, and the process of aging. Have students provide the rationale for why each factor contributes to pressure ulcer development.

10. Discuss the potential psychosocial impact that wounds may have on an individual.

11. Describe the staging and identification process for pressure ulcers.

12. Review the physical assessment parameters for determination of possible ulcer development as follows:
    a. Skin
    b. Mobility
    c. Nutritional status
    d. Pain

13. Have students identify how the following clients are at risk for pressure ulcer development:
    a. Unconscious client
    b. Client with restraints in place
    c. Client with a full leg cast
    d. Client with nasal oxygen in place
    e. An incontinent client
    f. A client with hemiplegia or paraplegia

14. Explain the initial and ongoing assessment of wounds in emergency and stable settings.

15. Discuss the possible characteristics of wound drainage and methods to determine the type and amount of drainage.

16. Identify the nursing measures that may be implemented to prevent pressure ulcer development, including the following:
    a. Hygienic care
    b. Positioning
    c. Use of support surfaces
    d. Promotion of nutritional status

17. Discuss the assessment information necessary for the nurse to determine a schedule for positioning and the selection of support surfaces and mattresses.

18. Discuss the newest research and practice of methods to promote pressure ulcer healing, including cleansing, irrigation, and dressings.

19. Invite a nurse who specializes in the treatment of wounds and pressure ulcers to speak to the class about the nurse's role in prevention and promotion of healing. Identify and describe the types of wound drainage systems (e.g., Penrose, Hemovac). Show the students the different types of equipment for evacuation and collection of wound drainage, as available.

20. Discuss the use of sutures and staples for wound closures, using photos, illustrations, and/or models. Identify the nursing care indicated for the different types of closures.

21. Identify and describe nursing interventions for wound care, including first aid, dressings, use of bandages and binders, irrigations, and application of heat and cold therapy.

22. Discuss and demonstrate different types and uses of dressings. Ask students to identify which type of dressing may be indicated for the following wounds:
    a. Infected or necrotic wound
    b. Small, superficial wound
    c. Clean, granulating wound
    d. Moderately deep dermal ulcer
    e. Partial thickness wound
    f. Burn or radiation damage
    g. Clean, surgical wound with small amount of drainage

23. Ask students to identify measures that the nurse may implement to promote client comfort before and during wound care.

24. Have students identify situations in which heat and cold therapy may be used, possible complications of the therapy, and factors that may influence an individual's tolerance to the therapy.

25. Invite an infection control nurse to speak to the class about aseptic technique and wound care.

26. Discuss how wound care may be altered from the acute care to the ambulatory care setting. Ask students to identify creative measures that may be implemented for wound care in the home environment in which some equipment and supplies may not be readily available.

27. Guide students in the application of the critical thinking model and the nursing process for clients who are at risk for or are experiencing impaired skin integrity—pressure ulcers and/or wounds.

INTERACTIVE EXERCISES

1. Provide students with examples of types of wounds, and ask them to identify, verbally and/or in writing, the type of wound and healing process that may be expected.

2. Provide students with photos/illustrations of pressure ulcers, and have them identify and document the stage and/or color, with description of size, drainage, etc. Use sample agency forms for documentation, as available.

3. Provide examples (photos/illustrations) of the following or similar types of ulcers, and have students determine the type of treatment indicated and/or contraindicated:
   a. Heel ulcer with dry eschar
   b. Clean, granulating wound
   c. Infected wound
   d. Deep ulcer with undermining

4. Have students investigate and report on the types of treatment, equipment, supplies, and medication used in an affiliating agency for pressure ulcer prevention and/or healing.

5. Working individually or in small groups, have students design a teaching plan for a family member who will be providing home care for a client who is at risk for developing pressure ulcers. Focus on the areas of skin and hygienic care, nutrition, and/or supportive measures. Have students present the teaching plan to the class.

6. Have students design a teaching plan for a client and/or family member who will be responsible for wound care in the home.

7. Have students complete a care plan/pathway for the following client simulation:

The client is an 82-year-old woman who experienced a CVA and has right-sided hemiparesis. She is frequently incontinent of urine and occasionally incontinent of feces. There are times when she is not fully aware of her surroundings. When she is not in bed, she spends her day in a wheelchair with a soft jacket restraint. The client was admitted to the extended care facility 1 week ago.

CLINICAL SKILLS

1. Using volunteers and/or models, simulate different types of wounds, and have students practice the assessment and treatment of the wound and the documentation of wound care (use a sample form from an affiliating agency, if available).

2. Explain and demonstrate (using a simulation mannequin/model, appropriate equipment and supplies, and available educational media) the following nursing interventions:
   a. Assessment for the risk of pressure ulcer development
   b. Treatment of pressure ulcers
   c. Application of dry and wet-to-dry dressings
   d. Irrigation of wounds
   e. Application of an abdominal or T binder
   f. Application of an elastic bandage
   g. Application of a hot, moist compress to an open wound

3. Have small groups of students, with supervision, practice and document the selected nursing interventions for the assessment, prevention, and treatment of pressure ulcers, and wound care.

4. Evaluate the students' ability, through return demonstration and skill testing to implement and document the risk assessment, prevention, and treatment of pressure ulcers and wound care through return demonstration and skill testing before clinical experience.

CLIENT CARE EXPERIENCES

1. Assign students to observe and participate in the nursing care of clients who are at risk for or are experiencing impaired skin integrity in the acute, restorative, or home care setting.

2. Discuss client assessment and expectations of nursing interventions before the experience. Review orders for specific supportive measures and wound treatment, as indicated. Review and evaluate students' interventions after the experience, focusing on the implementation of strategies to promote skin integrity.

3. Have students complete a care plan/pathway for clients at risk for an impairment in skin integrity.

4. Assign students to observe and participate in the nursing care of clients in acute and home health care settings, with the focus on wound assessment and implementation of wound care techniques.

5. Discuss measures for the prevention and treatment of complications of wounds with the group. Have students identify client educational needs regarding wound care. Assist students in the evaluation of wound healing.

6. Have students complete a care plan/pathway for clients experiencing wounds and/or the complications of wound healing.

RESOURCES FOR STUDENT ACTIVITIES

Assessment tools for risk of pressure ulcer development:
  Norton Scale
  Gosnell Scale: pressure sore risk assessment (parts 1 and 2)
  Braden Scale for predicting pressure sore risk
Wound healing comparison chart
Complications of wound healing

NORTON SCALE

Name	Date	Physical Condition		Mental Condition		Activity		Mobility		Incontinent		
		Good	4	Alert	4	Ambulant	4	Full	4	Not	4	
		Fair	3	Apathetic	3	Walk/help	3	Slightly limited	3	Occasional	3	
		Poor	2	Confused	2	Chair bound	2	Very limited	2	Usually/urine	2	TOTAL
		Very bad	1	Stupor	1	Bed	1	Immobile	1	Doubly	1	SCORE

Modified from Centre for Policy on Ageing: London, England, 1962

GOSNELL SCALE: PRESSURE SORE RISK ASSESSMENT (PART 1)

I.D. _____   Medical Diagnosis: _____

Age _____ Sex _____   Primary _____

Height _____ Weight _____   Secondary _____

Date of Admission _____   Nursing Diagnosis: _____

Date of Discharge _____   _____

Instructions: Complete all categories within 24 hours of admission and every other day thereafter. Refer to the accompanying guidelines for specific rating details.

Date	Mental Status*	Continence*	Mobility*	Activity*	Nutrition*	TOTAL SCORE
	1. Alert 2. Apathetic 3. Confused 4. Stuporous 5. Unconscious	1. Fully controlled 2. Usually controlled 3. Minimally controlled 4. Absence of control	1. Full 2. Slightly limited 3. Very limited 4. Immobile	1. Ambulatory 2. Walks with assistance 3. Chairfast 4. Bedfast	1. Good 2. Fair 3. Poor	

PRESSURE SORE RISK ASSESSMENT MEDICATION PROFILE

Medication	Dosage	Frequency†	Route	Date Begun	Date Discontinued

Courtesy Davina Gosnell, RN, PhD.

*See Part 3, p. 261 for guidelines for rating.

†If prn, record patterns for past 48 hours.

Continued

| | Vital Signs | | | | Diet | 24-Hour Fluid Balance | | Color 1. Pallor 2. Mottled 3. Pink 4. Ashen 5. Ruddy 6. Cyanotic 7. Jaundice 8. Other | General Skin Appearance | | | Interventions | | |
Date	T	P	R	BP		Intake	Output		Moisture 1. Dry 2. Damp 3. Oily 4. Other	Temperature 1. Cold 2. Cool 3. Warm 4. Hot	Texture 1. Smooth 2. Rough 3. Thin/transparent 4. Scaly 5. Crusty 6. Other	No	Yes	Describe

Vital signs: The temperature, pulse, respiration, and blood pressure to be taken and recorded at the time of every assessment rating.

Skin appearance: A description of observed skin characteristics: color, moisture, temperature, and texture.

Diet: Record the specific diet order.

24-hour fluid balance: The amount of fluid intake and output during the previous 24-hour period should be recorded.

Interventions: List all devices, measures, and/or nursing care activity being used for the purpose of pressure sore prevention.

Medications: List name, dosage, frequency, and route for all prescribed medications. If a prn order, list the pattern for the period since last assessment.

Comments: Use this space to add explanation or further detail regarding any of the previously recorded data, patient condition, etc.

or

Describe anything that you believe to be of importance but not accounted for previously.

NOTE: For any item marked "other," please describe.

If any signs of pressure, etc., on bony prominences or other body parts are observed, please describe in detail the location, color, temperature, moisture, texture, and size and any other pertinent items.

Continued

GUIDELINES FOR NUMERICAL RATING OF THE DEFINED CATEGORIES

Rating	1	2	3	4	5
Mental Status An assessment of one's level of response to the environment.	**Alert** Oriented to time, place, and person. Responsive to all stimuli and understands explanations.	**Apathetic** Lethargic, forgetful, drowsy, passive, and dull. Sluggish, depressed. Able to obey simple commands. Possibly disoriented to time.	**Confused** Partial and/or intermittent disorientation to time, place, and person. Purposeless response to stimuli. Restless, aggressive, irritable, anxious, and may require tranquilizers or sedatives.	**Stuporous** Total disorientation. Does not respond to name, simple commands, or verbal stimuli.	**Unconscious** Nonresponsive to painful stimuli.
Continence The amount of bodily control or urination and defecation.	**Fully Controlled** Total control of urine and feces.	**Usually Controlled** Incontinent of urine and/or of feces not more often than once every 48 hours or has Foley catheter and is incontinent of feces.	**Minimally Controlled** Incontinent of urine or feces at least once every 24 hours.	**Absence of Control** Consistently incontinent of both urine and feces.	
Mobility The amount and control of movement of one's body.	**Full** Able to control and move all extremities at will. May require the use of a device but turns, lifts, pulls, balances, and attains sitting position at will.	**Slightly Limited** Able to control and move all extremities but a degree of limitation is present. Requires assistance of another person to turn, pull, balance, and/or attain a sitting position at will but self-initiates movement or requests for help to move.	**Very Limited** Can assist another person, who must initiate movement via turning, lifting, pulling, balancing, and/or attaining a sitting position (contractures, paralysis may be present).	**Immobile** Does not assist self in any way to change position. Is unable to change position without assistance. Is completely dependent on others for movement.	
Activity The ability of an individual to ambulate.	**Ambulatory** Is able to walk unassisted. Rises from bed unassisted. With the use of a device such as cane or walker is able to ambulate without the assistance of another person.	**Walks With Help** Able to ambulate with assistance of another person, braces, or crutches. May have limitation of stairs.	**Chairfast** Ambulates only to a chair, requires assistance to do so or is confined to a wheelchair.	**Bedfast** Is confined to bed during entire 24 hours of the day.	
Nutrition The process of food intake.	Eats some food from each basic food category every day and the majority of each meal served or is on tube feeding.	Occasionally refuses a meal or frequently leaves at least half of a meal.	Seldom eats a complete meal and only a few bites of food at a meal.		

BRADEN SCALE FOR PREDICTING PRESSURE SORE RISK

Patient's Name ——————————— Evaluator's Name ——————————— Date of Assessment ——————————

Sensory Perception Ability to respond meaningfully to pressure-related discomfort	1. Completely limited Unresponsive (does not moan, flinch, or grasp) to painful stimuli due to diminished level of consciousness or sedation. OR Limited ability to feel pain over most of body surface.	2. Very limited Responds only to painful stimuli. Cannot communicate discomfort except by moaning or restlessness. OR Has a sensory impairment which limits the ability to feel pain or discomfort over ½ of body.	3. Slightly limited Responds to verbal commands, but cannot always communicate discomfort or need to be turned. OR Has some sensory impairment that limits ability to feel pain or discomfort in 1 or 2 extremities.	4. No impairment Responds to verbal commands. Has no sensory deficit that would limit ability to feel or voice pain or discomfort.	
Moisture Degree to which skin is exposed to moisture	1. Constantly moist Skin is kept moist almost constantly by perspiration, urine, etc. Dampness is detected every time patient is moved or turned.	2. Very moist Skin is often, but not always, moist. Linen must be changed at least once a shift.	3. Occasionally moist Skin is occasionally moist, requiring an extra linen change approximately once a day.	4. Rarely moist Skin is usually dry, linen only requires changing at routine intervals.	
Activity Degree of physical activity	1. Bedfast Confined to bed.	2. Chairfast Ability to walk severely limited or nonexistent. Cannot bear own weight and/or must be assisted into chair or wheelchair.	3. Walks occasionally Walks occasionally during day, but for very short distances, with or without assistance. Spends majority of each shift in bed or chair.	4. Walks frequently Walks outside the room at least twice a day and inside room at least once every 2 hours during waking hours.	
Mobility Ability to change and control body position	1. Completely immobile Does not make even slight changes in body or extremity position without assistance.	2. Very limited Makes occasional slight changes in body or extremity position but unable to make frequent or significant changes independently.	3. Slightly limited Makes frequent though slight changes in body or extremity position independently.	4. No limitations Makes major and frequent changes in position without assistance.	

Courtesy Barbara Braden and Nancy Bergstrom.

Continued

Nutrition *Usual* food intake pattern	1. Very poor Never eats a complete meal. Rarely eats more than ⅓ of any food offered. Eats 2 servings or less of protein (meat or dairy products) per day. Takes fluids poorly. Does not take a liquid dietary supplement. OR Is NPO and/or maintained on clear liquids or IVs for more than 5 days.	2. Probably inadequate Rarely eats a complete meal and generally eats only about ½ of any food offered. Protein intake includes only 3 servings of meat or dairy products per day. Occasionally will take a dietary supplement. OR Receives less than optimum amount of liquid diet or tube feeding.	3. Adequate Eats over half of most meals. Eats a total of 4 servings of protein (meat, dairy products) each day. Occasionally will refuse a meal, but will usually take a supplement if offered. OR Is on a tube feeding or total parenteral nutrition regimen that probably meets most of nutritional needs.	4. Excellent Eats most of every meal. Never refuses a meal. Usually eats a total of 4 or more servings of meat and dairy products. Occasionally eats between meals. Does not require supplementation.	
Friction and Shear	1. Problem Requires moderate to maximum assistance in moving. Complete lifting without sliding against sheets is impossible. Frequently slides down in bed or chair, requiring frequent repositioning with maximum assistance. Spasticity, contractures, or agitation leads to almost constant friction.	2. Potential problem Moves feebly or requires minimum assistance. During a move skin probably slides to some extent against sheets, chair, restraints, or other devices. Maintains relatively good position in chair or bed most of the time but occasionally slides down.	3. No apparent problem Moves in bed and in chair independently and has sufficient muscle strength to lift up completely during move. Maintains good position in bed or chair at all times.		
				TOTAL SCORE	

Primary Intention	Secondary Intention
Phases:	**Details of Healing:**
Reaction (Inflammatory):	
Regeneration (Proliferative):	
Remodeling (Maturation):	
Types of Wounds:	**Types of Wounds:**

COMPLICATIONS OF WOUND HEALING

Complication	Etiology	Signs/Symptoms	Nursing Assessment and Care
Hemorrhage			
Infection			
Dehiscence			
Evisceration			
Fistula Formation			
Delayed Wound Closure			

CRITICAL THINKING EXERCISES

1. When removing a wet-to-dry dressing, you note that the underlying gauze is wet with saline. The skin surrounding the wound is macerated. What conclusions can you make about the previous dressing? What would you do to avoid recurrence of this type of wet-to-dry application?

2. After changing a client's position, you observe redness over the bony prominences. What type of assessment must you perform to obtain correct information regarding pressure ulcer risk?

3. You have just admitted a client from a nursing home to your division. On initial assessment, you assess a stage III pressure ulcer. How do you determine the type of care and dressing to use with this particular pressure ulcer?

4. You are providing care to an elderly incontinent Hispanic man who is bed-bound. How will you assess for pressure ulcers in this client? What measures will you take to prevent his skin from breaking down?

ANSWERS TO CRITICAL THINKING EXERCISES

1. Increased moisture—the wet-to-dry dressing was applied too wet. Consider re-educating the caregiver on how to correctly apply wet-to-dry dressings. Consider moving to another type of débriding dressing if débridement is still the goal. Use hydrogel or a similar type of dressing.

2. Note length of time of hyperemia. Determine whether it is within normal limits. Palpate skin and underlying tissue for induration. Review the client's turning schedule. Determine the client's ability to change own position.

3. Determine what type of drainage is present. Determine whether the wound is a clean or eschar status. Palpate underlying area to determine other tissue damage. Assess the quality of the non-affected skin surrounding the area. If the wound is clean, the wound will heal through granulation. If the wound is an eschar status, the eschar will lift during the healing process and may need to be cross hatched.

4. The client is at risk because of continency status. You will need to follow AHCPR guidelines for incontinence and use an appropriate product to keep the client's skin dry. Other risks should be determined (e.g., for pressure ulcer development, mental status, ability to independently change positions, and nutritional status).

Sensory Alterations

CLASSROOM DISCUSSION

1. Review the anatomy and physiology of the nervous system, in respect to the major senses: sight, hearing, touch, smell, and taste.

2. Discuss common sensory deficits that the nurse may encounter in client situations.

3. Describe sensory deprivation and overload and its recognition in clients. Ask students to provide examples of possible health care situations that may contribute to sensory deprivation or overload.

4. Discuss factors that influence sensory function.

5. Review the assessment of a client's sensory status, including health promotion behaviors and medical history. Ask students how a client's sensory abilities may be determined through routine observation or communication.

6. Identify clients who are at risk for sensory alterations, including individuals who are older, immobile, engage in particular occupations, have an alteration in mental status, or are isolated.

7. Review the assessment for sensory deficits.

8. Discuss health promotion activities for sensory function:
   a. Screening
   b. Safety and prevention
   c. Assistive devices
   d. Stimulation

9. Discuss methods of communication that may be used by individuals experiencing sensory deficits.

10. Have students specify strategies that may be used to interact and communicate with a client experiencing expressive or receptive aphasia or an inability to speak because of a laryngectomy or placement of an endotracheal tube.

11. Invite a speech and/or occupational therapist to speak to the class about promoting the client's self-care activities and communication.

12. Stimulate a discussion on the importance of promoting sensation and stimulation, especially touch, for the older client in a restorative care setting.

INTERACTIVE EXERCISES

1. Have students complete a sensory assessment on a peer, family member, or friend and report and record the findings.

2. Have students investigate and report on available resources within an affiliating agency to facilitate communication with clients.

3. Organize a role-playing experience for the students based on the following or similar scenarios:
   a. Assisting a visually impaired client to ambulate and independently complete activities of daily living (bathing, dressing, eating)
   b. Communicating with a hearing-impaired or aphasic client
   c. Caring for a client in an intensive care or isolation unit

   Be aware that students simulating sensory deficits may experience an anxiety reaction. Supervision of these exercises is recommended.

CLINICAL SKILL

1. Have students modify a simulated client environment to meet optimum safety and stimulation needs. Students should consider the scheduling of client care activities to avoid overstimulation or understimulation.

CLIENT CARE EXPERIENCES

1. Assign students to observe clients in a health care setting and note the amount and type of stimuli present. If possible, observation in an intensive care, isolation, or burn unit is desirable.

2. Arrange for students to participate in vision and hearing screenings in a community setting, such as a school, clinic, or pediatrician's office.

3. Assign students to observe and participate in the nursing care of clients who may be experiencing sensory or perceptual alterations and/or a risk for injury related to a sensory deficit. Discuss expectations with students before the experience.

4. Focus on the assessment of the client's sensory and perceptual status and the implementation of safety measures, therapeutic communication, and strategies to promote or reduce excessive sensory input.

5. Review and evaluate the students' interactions, noting the degree of sensory stimulation provided and client responses.

6. Have students complete a care plan/pathway for an assigned client with a sensory or perceptual alteration.

Sensory assessment/intervention chart

SENSORY ASSESSMENT/INTERVENTION CHART

Senses	Screening Measures	Prevention and Safety Measures	Enhancement and Assistive Devices	Meaningful Stimuli
Vision				
Hearing				
Touch				
Smell				
Taste				

CRITICAL THINKING EXERCISES

1. Mr. Michaels is 84 years old and is the primary caregiver for his 83-year-old wife. During an initial home visit to the wife, the nurse observed that Mr. Michaels would only respond when he was looking directly at the nurse or standing close. Otherwise, he would not respond to questions or would seem to ignore what was happening or what was being said. What follow-up assessments should be gathered? What interventions would be helpful?

2. The school nurse learns from the fifth-grade teacher that 10-year-old Sue Pieper has been having difficulty with following simple written directions and homework assignments. She seems disinterested when they are assigned to use the computer. The teacher also reports that Sue is showing difficulty with sports such as baseball and soccer—her timing is off—and previously that was not the case. The nurse identifies that Sue has decreased visual acuity. What nursing actions are important to ensure her safety?

3. Mrs. Jones is admitted to the emergency department after being involved in a motor vehicle accident. Assessment reveals severe visual impairment due to bilateral cataracts. Currently she is in stable condition but requires admission. To promote optimal sensory function, what nursing measures should be considered?

ANSWERS TO CRITICAL THINKING EXERCISES

1. Determine whether Mr. Michaels believes that he has a hearing problem, and, if so, assess it thoroughly. If not, spend time talking with him to determine whether there is a loss and what is needed for Mr. Michaels to accept the sensory loss. What has he done to improve his hearing ability? Does he have or use a hearing aid? Has Mrs. Michaels (or others) indicated to Mr. Michaels that he has a hearing problem? The following interventions might be useful: decrease background noise when speaking with Mr. Michaels, and gain his attention by use of a gentle touch to not startle him. Be sure to speak clearly and distinctly. Address Mr. Michaels by name before communicating ideas with him, and, when the client does not respond, attempt to establish eye contact and rephrase information in short, simple terms. Evaluate the appropriateness of the client's responses before continuing further. Encourage the client to have his hearing tested.

2. The nurse should do a vision screening test and contact the parents for a referral to an ophthalmologist. The nurse should request that a report be sent to the school as a follow-up from the physician to assure that the child was seen in a timely manner. The teacher should be encouraged to allow the child to sit closer to the board, and determine if larger print can be available for the student. The nurse should ask that the teacher clearly read materials to assist this student. Safety factors for the play activities should be employed until the vision problem is corrected so that the child does not encounter any injuries. The nurse should follow-up with the referral to the parents since there could be a long lag time.

3. Determine the correct distance for the client to see, then place objects close within her visual field to help her have some independence. Instruct the client on activities that are occurring in the room since she may not be able to distinguish them clearly enough. Instruct the client to shield her eyes from direct front light, and be sure that the nurse uses the overbed light for the client's best vision. Use a broad felt tip marking pen and write largely any information that the client needs to remember. Place dark objects on a light background and vice versa. Instruct the client on the location of equipment and furniture. Organize the environment in a way that is convenient for the client, and have a sign requesting that supplies stay in the same place, if possible, for the convenience of the client.

(Reference: Cleary ME. Helping the person who is visually impaired: concerns, questions, remedies, and resources, *J Ophthalmic Nurs Technol* 14(5):205, 1995.)

Surgical Client

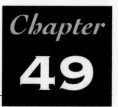

Chapter 49

CLASSROOM DISCUSSION

1. Discuss the highlights of the history of surgical nursing and recent changes in technology (e.g., laser and fiberoptics) and location of surgery (ambulatory centers) that have influenced nursing practice.

2. Discuss the different classifications of surgery and the associated nursing care approaches.

3. Identify client risk factors that, if present, may affect the surgical experience, including the client's age, poor nutritional status, obesity, medical conditions, pregnancy, fluid and electrolyte imbalance, and radiotherapy treatment.

4. Describe the components of a comprehensive preoperative nursing assessment of the client, including the following:
   a. Past medical history
   b. Previous surgeries
   c. Perceptions and understanding of surgery
   d. Medication history
   e. Allergies
   f. Smoking habits
   g. Alcohol/substance abuse
   h. Family support
   i. Occupation
   j. Preoperative pain
   k. Emotional status
   l. Sociocultural background/practices

   Ask students how responses to each area may influence the client's perioperative experience and what the nurse's responsibilities are in relation to follow-up and reporting.

5. Ask students how the nursing assessment and its focus may be altered depending on the location of and circumstances surrounding a client's surgery (e.g., same-day or emergency procedures).

6. Review the physical assessment in relation to preoperative client assessment. Discuss how findings may influence the client's perioperative experience, and determine the nurse's interventions, follow-up, and reporting (e.g., for elevated temperature and decreased respirations).

7. Discuss preoperative laboratory and diagnostic tests that may be used to determine abnormalities before surgery.

8. Describe the general client preparation and education and nursing responsibilities in the preoperative phase. Ask students how these preoperative preparations and nursing interventions may be altered for clients having ambulatory or same-day surgery.

9. Review the legal parameters and nursing accountability associated with informed consent. Ask students what the nurse should do if the client does not demonstrate an understanding of the surgical procedure or if the client is unconscious and requires an emergency procedure.

10. Identify and describe the purposes and advantages of preoperative teaching for the client and family. Discuss the AORN (Association of Operating Room Nurses) criteria for client understanding.

11. Ask students to share personal and/or family perioperative experiences. If the experiences were negative, ask what, if possible, a nurse may have done to improve them.

12. Identify and discuss common expectations of clients in the perioperative phase.

13. Describe common preoperative physical preparation of the client, including promotion of fluid and electrolyte balance, reduction of the risk of surgical wound infection, skin preparation, bowel and bladder preparation, and promotion of rest and comfort. Have students identify any additional specific measures that the nurse may implement to assist the client in the preoperative phase.

14. Review the preparation of the client on the day of surgery, including the following:
    a. Completion of preoperative checklist
    b. Monitoring of vital signs
    c. Provision of hygienic care
    d. Check of hair and cosmetics
    e. Removal/storage of prosthetics and valuables
    f. Preparation of bowel/bladder
    g. Application of antiemboli stockings or compression devices
    h. Implementation of special procedures (e.g., NG tube insertion)
    i. Administration of preoperative medications
    j. Maintenance of client safety and determination of latex allergy

15. Ask students how the preparation for surgery may differ for clients of different ages, who speak other languages, who have no family support, who have specific spiritual or cultural needs, or who have a psychiatric history.

16. Discuss the nurse's responsibility in client transport to the operating room.

17. Discuss the intraoperative phase of the experience, including the immediate preparation of the client, introduction of anesthesia, client positioning, documentation, and roles and responsibilities of the nurse.

18. Identify and describe the different types, uses, risks, and nursing care associated with anesthesia.

19. Discuss the postoperative phase, including transfer to the postanesthesia care unit (PACU), client monitoring, nursing measures to support vital functions, and documentation. Ask students to indicate specific assessments that the nurse in a PACU may conduct to determine overall client status.

20. Have students identify similarities and differences in postoperative/PACU care for clients following inpatient or ambulatory surgery.

21. Discuss discharge criteria for PACU clients returning to an acute care unit or to their home.

22. Discuss postoperative treatment for clients in an acute care setting.

23. Identify nursing interventions for clients in the postoperative phase for the promotion and maintenance of respiratory, circulatory, and neurological function; temperature control; fluid and electrolyte balance; nutrition; elimination; skin integrity; wound healing; rest and comfort; self-concept; and self-care abilities. Have students identify specific examples of nursing measures that assist clients to attain goals in the postoperative phase (see Resources for Student Activities, p. 277).

24. Discuss postoperative complications, their recognition, and subsequent nursing interventions.

25. Invite a nurse who practices in an operating room and/or PACU to speak to the class about client assessment, preparation for surgery or discharge, and nursing responsibilities.

26. Using the following or similar situations, have students identify interventions that the nurse may implement:
    a. A client who has not had blood work or x-ray completed on the day of surgery
    b. A client in the PACU with completely saturated dressings
    c. A client experiencing a rigid, distended abdomen 2 days postoperatively
    d. A client who has an elevated temperature within 2 days after surgery or 5 days after surgery

27. Guide students in the application of the critical thinking model and the nursing process for clients in the preoperative, intraoperative, and postoperative phases.

INTERACTIVE EXERCISE

1. Have students role play the preparation of a client for surgery, including completion of the preoperative checklist.

CLINICAL SKILLS

1. Explain and demonstrate postoperative exercises. Have students practice along with the demonstration in the classroom or skill laboratory. Evaluate the students' ability to perform and teach the postoperative exercises through return demonstration.

2. Have students prepare a simulated client's room for the postoperative phase.

CLIENT CARE EXPERIENCES

1. Assign students to accompany clients (as possible) through the intraoperative phase and to observe surgical asepsis, client preparation, and nursing roles. Have students share their observations after the experience in inpatient and/or ambulatory surgery settings.

2. Assign students to observe and/or participate in the care of clients in a PACU. Have students monitor clients' status and provide and document nursing care, with supervision. Have students collaborate with the nursing staff on client discharge from PACU.

3. Assign students to observe and participate in the nursing care of clients on a postoperative unit in an acute care facility. Work with students to prepare and conduct preoperative client teaching. Discuss the assessment of the client and appropriate nursing interventions for the postoperative period, including reinforcement of postoperative exercises.

4. Have students complete a general care plan/pathway for clients undergoing an operative experience. Have students individualize the care plan/pathway for actual clients with specific preoperative and postoperative needs.

RESOURCES FOR STUDENT ACTIVITIES

Preoperative assessment form
Postoperative nursing interventions
Preoperative/preprocedural checklist

PREOPERATIVE ASSESSMENT FORM

	Assessment Data
Past Medical History	
Previous Surgery	
Medication History	
Allergies	
Smoking Habits	
Alcohol/Substance Abuse	
Family Support	
Occupation	
Preoperative Pain	
Emotional Health	
Sociocultural Factors	

Client Functions	Nursing Interventions
Respiration	
Circulation	
Temperature Control	
Neurological	
Skin Integrity/Wound Healing	
Genitourinary	
Gastrointestinal	
Fluid/Electrolyte Balance	
Pain Management	

A-1c PREOPERATIVE/PREPROCEDURAL CHECKLIST

• File with other A-1c's of same date. •

PROCEDURE: _____

DATE OF PROCEDURE: _____

1. Place initials in appropriate box: YES, NO, N/A (not applicable, or was not ordered). Each item must have an entry.
2. Explain any "No." This can be done in the space after the item or in the "Comments" section. Use back of form, if needed.
3. To give more information on any item, use the space after the item. If more space is needed, use the "Comments" section or back of form.

DATE

HOSP. NO.

NAME

BIRTHDATE

ADDRESS

IF NOT IMPRINTED, PLEASE PRINT DATE, HOSP. NO., NAME AND LOCATION.

YES	NO	N/A	
			Special information (e.g., blind, O$_2$, combative)
			Preoperative orders written.
			(If "NO", Dr. _____ notified at _____ date/time.)
			Consent complete and in medical record.
			Allergies (or NKA) labelled on cover of medical record.
			Specify Allergies:
			Isolation label on cover of medical record. Specify type.
			Ordered lab results in medical record.
			Urinalysis results in medical record.
			Chest x-ray completed. (Report in medical record: Yes____ No____)
			EKG in medical record.
			Type and cross/screen (circle) done. Date drawn:
			History and physical in medical record.
			Forms complete and in medical record:
			1. Nursing documentation with assessment, VS, and wt./ht.
			2. IV Solution Administration Cardex.
			3. Medication Administration Cardex.
			Addressograph plate on cover of medical record. All volumes to procedure, if required.

COMMENTS:

YES	NO	N/A	
			Blood band on patient and legible. Specify location _____ and blood band #_____
			Identification band on patient and legible. Specify location:
			Bathed and in proper attire.
			Nail polish, makeup, and hairpins removed.
			Jewelry removed. Specify item(s) removed and disposition:
			Prosthesis removed: hearing aid, dentures, eye glasses, contact lenses (circle).
			Other: Disposition:
			Anti-embolism stockings on.
			Sequential compression device sleeves on and controller to OR.
			NPO since:
			Teaching completed and documented.
			Preps/tests completed as ordered. Specify:
			Voided/catheterized (circle). Time:
			Medication(s) given.
			Medication(s)/article(s) sent with patient. Specify:

COMMENTS:

Date	Initials	Signature and Title of Individuals Filling Out Form
Date	Initials	Signature of RN Sending Patient to Procedure

41006/4-93/H7528   THE UNIVERSITY OF IOWA HOSPITALS AND CLINICS

Courtesy University of Iowa Hospitals and Clinics.

CRITICAL THINKING EXERCISES

1. Your 82-year-old client is admitted after a fall for repair of a fractured hip. What postoperative complications are seen in the older client undergoing this type of surgery?

2. Mr. B. is a 52-year-old client who will have thoracic surgery. He has a 30-year history of smoking one pack of cigarettes per day. What type of pulmonary preventive measures would you expect Mr. B. to need postoperatively?

3. Your client is of Native American descent. He will be having a cholecystectomy. Describe a potential problem related to pain control and how the problem can be avoided through preoperative teaching.

4. Mrs. C. was admitted for ambulatory surgery for an inguinal hernia repair. What discharge criteria would be used for Mrs. C., and what discharge instructions would she require?

ANSWERS TO CRITICAL THINKING EXERCISES

1. Postoperative complications could include thrombus, embolus, blood loss, atelectasis, dehydration, CHF, pneumonia, activity intolerance, and pressure ulcers.

2. Mr. B. would need to deep breathe, cough, and turn a minimum of every 2 hours. More than likely, either incentive spirometry or PEP therapy would be ordered. Aerosol (nebulizer) treatments with a bronchodilator may be indicated, as well as oxygen therapy.

3. Native Americans are generally stoic when ill. Complaints of pain to the nurse may be in general terms. Preoperative education should emphasize the importance of the need for pain control for both physiological and psychological reasons. Encourage the client to state pain in direct terms to the nurse or family. Encourage the family to communicate when they feel the client is in pain.

4. Discharge criteria would include the following: the ability to void (if applicable); ability to ambulate (if applicable); alert and oriented; no pain medication for 1 hour; minimal nausea and vomiting; no excess bleeding or drainage; received written postoperative instructions and prescriptions; verbalizes understanding of instructions; and is being discharged with a responsible adult. Discharge instructions would include the following: signs and symptoms of infection; medications, including dose, schedule, purpose, and special instructions; activity restrictions (shower, driving, lifting); diet; wound care; and follow-up appointment.

Test Bank

CHAPTER 1

1. All of the following statements accurately reflect the tenets of population health **except:**
   A) Population health is congruent with a socioenvironmental view of health.
   B) "Individual" factors, such as personal health practices, are **foundational** to "collective" factors, such as social and economic environments.
   C) Health is determined by the complex interactions between individual characteristics, social and economic factors, and physical environments.
   D) Important health gains are achieved by focussing interventions on the health of the entire population or significant subgroups, rather than on individuals.

2. The "watershed" document that marked the shift from a lifestyle to a social approach to health was the:
   A) Lalonde Report
   B) Ottawa Charter
   C) Hastings Report
   D) National Forum on Health

3. The **underlying** reason that intersectoral collaboration is a necessary strategy to reach the goal of Health for All is:
   A) The determinants of health are broad
   B) Intersectoral collaboration is cost-effective
   C) Intersectoral collaboration encourages problem solving at a local level
   D) Intersectoral collaboration is less likely to result in conflict

4. The belief that health is primarily an **individual** responsibility is most congruent with the _____ approach to health.
   A) Medical
   B) Behavioural
   C) Socioenvironmental
   D) Public health

5. All of the following statements accurately describe Hamilton and Bhatti's Population Health Promotion Model **except:**
   A) The model suggests that action must be taken on the full range of health determinants
   B) The model incorporates the health promotion strategies of the Ottawa Charter
   C) The model focusses only on interventions at the society level
   D) The model is an attempt to integrate the concepts of population health and health promotion

6. The major determinants of health in a socioenvironmental view of health are:
   A) Psychosocial risk factors and socioenvironmental risk conditions
   B) Physiological risk factors and behavioural risk factors
   C) Behavioural and psychosocial risk factors
   D) Behavioural and socioenvironmental risk factors

7. The most influential determinant of health is now considered to be:
   A) Personal health practices
   B) Income and social status
   C) Health care services
   D) Physical environment

8. Providing immunizations against measles is an example of:
   A) Primary prevention
   B) Secondary prevention
   C) Health promotion
   D) Tertiary prevention

9. Which one of the following statements **does not** characterize health promotion?
   A) Health promotion addresses health issues within the context of the social, economic, and political environment.
   B) Health promotion strategies focus primarily on helping people to develop healthy behaviours.
   C) Health promotion emphasizes empowerment.
   D) Health promotion is political.

10. A community health nurse working with a group of low-income families to effect changes in social assistance policies is an example of:
    A) Advocacy for
    B) Enhancing personal skills
    C) Advocacy with
    D) Personal care empowerment

CHAPTER 2

1. Saskatchewan was the first province to institute:
   A) Medical insurance
   B) Privatization of health care
   C) Health promotion
   D) Routine immunizations

2. Nurses may be most directly influenced by cost control because they:
   A) Constitute a large percentage of the health care budget
   B) Achieve higher salary levels than other health care professionals
   C) Provide direct client care without reimbursement
   D) Deliver the least cost-effective care

3. An example of a health promotion service is a(n):
   A) Immunization clinic
   B) Breast self-examination clinic
   C) Aerobic dance class
   D) Smoking cessation clinic

4. An example of an agency that provides secondary level care is a:
   A) Home health agency
   B) Hospice
   C) Provincially owned psychiatric hospital
   D) Nursing home

5. Which of the following fits within the occupational safety and health categories?
   A) Motorcycle helmets
   B) Firearms safety guidelines
   C) Swimming lessons
   D) Pathogen exposure protocols

6. As an employee of a large corporation, a person's health care not covered by medicare may be paid as an employment benefit by supplementary health insurance. This is an example of a(n):
   A) HMO
   B) PPO
   C) Fee-for-service plan
   D) Third party payment

7. Care management is an innovative approach to delivering health care. The major factor for its success is that it:
   A) Focusses on the process
   B) Allows each discipline to develop a care plan for the client
   C) Is used exclusively in the acute care setting
   D) Allows a high degree of flexibility for the nurse delivering care

8. Case management is one strategy for coordinating health care services. What best describes this caregiving approach?
   A) It is designed for clients requiring minimal to moderate levels of care.
   B) Continuity of care is the primary concern.
   C) The physician is the coordinator of client care.
   D) This focus of care may be more expensive.

9. A client with a sight disability requires support and restorative care in order to return to a prior level of functioning. This client should be referred to a(n):
   A) Community service agency for sight
   B) Ambulatory care centre
   C) Subacute eye care unit
   D) Home health care agency

10. Monitoring of air and water quality is the responsibility of which one of the following?
    A) Volunteer agencies
    B) Federal government
    C) Public health sector
    D) Neighbourhood health centres

11. Restoring a client to normal or near-normal function is the aim of which type of care?
    A) Respite care
    B) Rehabilitative care
    C) Assisted living
    D) Extended care

12. Discharge planning for client begins:
    A) After a diagnosis has been established
    B) Once the long-term needs are identified
    C) When the acute care therapies are completed
    D) Immediately upon admission to a health care facility

CHAPTER 3

1. Community health nursing:
   A) Requires graduate-level educational preparation
   B) Is the same as public health nursing
   C) Focusses on the incidence of disease
   D) Includes direct care and services to subpopulations

2. In working with vulnerable populations, the nurse should:
   A) Be comfortable with diversity
   B) Express his or her own critical beliefs about health care
   C) Focus on only one stressor in the client's environment
   D) Establish goals and priorities for the clients and inform them of how they should be attained

3. Which of the following clients from a vulnerable population is currently at the greatest risk?
   A) A physically abused client in a shelter
   B) An older adult taking medication for hypertension
   C) A schizophrenic client in outpatient therapy
   D) A substance abuser who shares drug paraphernalia

4. A population and a community are each defined as a collection of individuals who share certain characteristics. The key characteristic that distinguishes a population from a community is:
   A) A common identity
   B) A shared interest
   C) A common geographic location
   D) A social or relational connection

5. A client has chronic renal failure and receives peritoneal dialysis in his home. Currently, his family members are disturbed because they do not feel confident about safely managing his therapy. Which of the following statements from his home health nurse reflects a coordinator role?
   A) "This peritoneal dialysis is less disruptive than hemodialysis in the hospital."
   B) "Have you considered a renal transplant?"
   C) "How do you feel about this situation?"
   D) "Let's call the regional dialysis centre and explore options for dealing with your concerns about home dialysis."

6. Community-based primary care is:
   A) A subcategory of home health care
   B) Practised by graduate-prepared nurses
   C) Nurses working with community health care providers
   D) Care for clients who are discharged from an acute care facility

7. The nurse working as an effective facilitator in the community should:
   A) Tell community members how to manage their community health needs
   B) Work with clients and groups to select alternative health care sites and treatments
   C) Make decisions for individual clients regarding their health care options
   D) Provide instruction in the way the community should address health issues

8. A client is being discharged from an acute care facility following a total hip replacement. She will need follow-up regarding her rehabilitation and exercise plan. In addition to a home health care nurse, what referral should be made?
   A) Social worker
   B) Dietician
   C) Physical therapist
   D) Respiratory therapist

9. Which of the following is the largest contributing factor for the increase in the need and use of home care?
   A) Government funding of the home care setting has increased greatly.
   B) The existence of more single-income families has increased the need for their elderly relatives to receive care in the home.
   C) Clients are more acutely ill when discharged from the acute care facility.
   D) There are 7 days/week services for the elderly in home care agencies.

10. The health care climate in Canada and the United States has undergone many changes in recent decades. Conditions that have influenced these changes include all of the following except:
    A) Public control over health care practice
    B) Technological and medical advances in prevention, diagnosis, and treatment
    C) Socioeconomic pressures to reduce government spending
    D) Professional and public support for client participation in health care

CHAPTER 4

1. Changes occur in health care organizations. An example of a transitional change is:
   A) The incorporation of a new computer system for documentation
   B) The move from inpatient to outpatient services
   C) A focus on primary care and improved client outcomes
   D) A reduction in the nursing work force

2. The transformational leader:
   A) Works within the existing culture
   B) Controls and improves current procedures
   C) Provides stability
   D) Uses charisma to motivate others

3. It is necessary for the new nurse manager to delegate tasks to the staff. Which of the following is a requirement for the nurse manager in this delegation process?
   A) Obtaining the employee's voluntary acceptance of the task
   B) Communicating the work assignment in clear terms
   C) Functioning from a laissez-faire style of leadership
   D) Working alongside the staff to evaluate their care

4. As the nurse starts to perform a procedure, a peer says, "I've done that before — would you like me to help?" The peer's leadership style is described as:
   A) Laissez-faire
   B) Coaching
   C) Democratic
   D) Directing

5. A unit manager on a busy multiservice medical nursing unit decides to take responsibility for the direct client care of one of the many new admissions. Later the manager decides she is too busy to give adequate client care. Which of the following situational leadership styles does the nurse manager need to apply?
   A) Coaching
   B) Supporting
   C) Delegating
   D) Directing

6. Which of the following statements best reflects the autocratic style of leadership?
   A) "Everyone knows their work assignment, so let's not meet together unless we have an unexpected crisis."
   B) "Let's discuss this case study thoroughly and decide on a plan of action as a group."
   C) "I'll consider each of your requests, and then give you the guidelines for establishing new acuity ratings for our clients."
   D) "I'll try to pair you in comparable work teams, and we'll evaluate the success of this approach in two weeks."

7. Time management skills for the nurse include:
   A) Meeting all of the client's major needs in the early morning hours
   B) Anticipating possible interruptions by therapists
   C) Doing each of the client's assessments and treatments individually at separate times
   D) Leaving each day unplanned to allow for adaptations in treatments

8. In anticipation of a nursing shortage, the nursing management in a facility investigates a nursing care delivery model that involves the division of tasks, with one nurse assuming the responsibility for particular tasks. This model is called:
   A) Total patient care
   B) Functional nursing
   C) Team nursing
   D) Primary nursing

9. One advantage of a decentralized management structure over a centralized structure is that:
   A) Staff are not responsible for defining their roles
   B) Managers handle the difficult decisions
   C) Each staff member is accountable for evaluating the plan of care
   D) Communication pathways are simplified

10. Indicators in a quality improvement program that evaluate the manner in which care is delivered are:
    A) Structure indicators
    B) Team indicators
    C) Process indicators
    D) Client indicators

CHAPTER 5

1. Which of the following is not a nursing metaparadigm concept?
   A) Environment
   B) Research
   C) Health
   D) Person

2. Which of the following events is not identified as a significant factor influencing the history of theory development in nursing?
   A) A shift from disease care to health care
   B) The rapid influx of scientific and technological development
   C) Changing roles for women in society
   D) Trend toward managed health care

3. Identify the most appropriate reasons for choosing a theory to guide your nursing practice. Check all that apply.
   A) You accept its stated beliefs and values
   B) It avoids technical language
   C) The major components are clearly articulated
   D) It facilitates interpretation of clinical data

4. In needs-based theories, which of the following are true?
   A) There is also a systems approach to make the model operational.
   B) Direction for leadership and administration are made clear.
   C) All needs are hierarchical.
   D) Competing demands of human needs help to explain behavior.

5. Which of the following statements best describes the goal(s) of theoretical knowledge in nursing?
   A) Distinguish nursing from medical practice
   B) Stimulate thinking and create understanding of the discipline
   C) Develop a single model that will represent all facets of practice
   D) Clarify the historical significance of model development in nursing

6. In nursing, the paradigm debates have included:
   A) Defining nursing as an art and not a science.
   B) Developing categories of nursing diagnosis.
   C) The acceptance of a needs-based approach.
   D) Model bashing.

CHAPTER 6

1. A new graduate is able to demonstrate caring behavior toward the client by:
   A) Seeking assistance before attempting a new procedure
   B) Attempting to do new treatments quickly and independently
   C) Being honest and informing clients that the treatments to be done are not familiar
   D) Avoiding situations with clients that may be uncomfortable

2. According to Benner, caring is defined as a:
   A) Central, unifying, and dominant domain necessary for health and survival
   B) New consciousness and moral idea
   C) Nurturing way of relating to a valued other
   D) Person, event, project, or thing that matters to a person

3. Which one of the following activities is an example of Swanson's "enabling" in the caring process?
   A) Staying with the client prior to surgery
   B) Performing a catheterization skillfully
   C) Assessing the client's health history
   D) Teaching the client how to perform self-injection of insulin

4. Riemen's study of nurses' caring behaviors found which one of the following to be a similarity between the perception of male and female clients' behaviors?
   A) Promotion of autonomy
   B) Knowledge of injection technique
   C) Physical presence
   D) Speed of treatment completion

5. The most important aspect for a student nurse to learn in relation to knowing the client is:

A) Establishing a relationship
B) Gathering assessment data
C) Treating discomforts quickly
D) Assuming emotional needs

6. A caring behavior is demonstrated when the nurse does which of the following?
   A) Tells the family about the client's problems
   B) Calls the client by his or her first name
   C) Closes the door and covers the client during a bath
   D) Shares information about the client's responses with other students

7. The nurse manager wants a staff member to enhance the care given to the older clients on the unit. This is best accomplished by the nurse manager:
   A) Telling the staff member how to correctly give baths to the clients
   B) Providing the staff member with good resources to read on bathing older clients
   C) Asking another staff member to provide special skin care
   D) Bringing the staff member into a client's room and demonstrating a gentle bath

CHAPTER 7

1. Cultural behaviour is:
   A) A guide to one's thinking, doing, and being
   B) Biologically defined activities
   C) A unique expression of self-worth
   D) Socially acquired actions in certain situations

2. Ethnicity differs from race in that ethnicity:
   A) Is a unique factor within a cultural group
   B) Includes more than biological identification
   C) Refers to subgroups within a race
   D) Is the set of conflicting values between races

3. Within transcultural nursing, sensitivity to social orientation is the recognition of the client's:
   A) Language usage
   B) Definition of health and health practices
   C) Leisure activities and role in the family
   D) Psychological characteristics and coping mechanisms

4. An example of an efficacious cultural health practice is a client:
   A) Avoiding routine gynecological screenings
   B) Wrapping a newborn tightly to maintain warmth
   C) Using special herbs to reduce headache pain
   D) Positioning a child's crib for maximum positive energy

5. Traditional western medicine, in contrast to alternative therapy, uses:
   A) Medication administration
   B) Guided imagery
   C) Acupuncture
   D) Aromatic touch

6. The nurse is completing an assessment of a Chinese Canadian client. Recognizing that there may be common problems in individuals with this background, the nurse observes for particular signs and symptoms of:
   A) Sickle cell anemia
   B) Stomach cancer
   C) Thalassemia
   D) Diabetes mellitus

7. At a local screening for diabetes mellitus, the nurse is concerned about clients who have been identified in research studies as having the greatest risk for the disease. These individuals are:
   A) Black Canadians
   B) Aboriginal peoples
   C) Chinese Canadians
   D) European Canadians

8. In relating to clients of Chinese Canadian culture, the nurse should be aware that:
   A) The family unit is highly valued
   B) Discrimination practices have been eliminated
   C) Western treatments are initiated at illness onset
   D) Self-concepts are positive and strong

9. Which of the following is an appropriate means of communicating with clients who are not fluent in English?
   A) Interpreting emotional responses as aggressive behaviours
   B) Evaluating intellectual capacity by language used
   C) Responding to the client by his or her first name
   D) Validating nonverbal communication clues

10. The nurse should be aware that Aboriginal people define health as:
    A) Expenditure of much "good" energy
    B) Spiritual peace and tranquility
    C) Living in total harmony with nature
    D) Good luck and a reward from God

11. When planning nursing care for a client with a different cultural background, the nurse should:
    A) Identify how cultural variables affect the health problem
    B) Try to explain how the client can adapt to hospital routines
    C) Speak slowly and clearly to ensure effective communication
    D) Allow the family to provide care during the hospital stay

12. Which of the following is true concerning cultural behaviours?
    A) Environmental control refers to the ability of a group to plan activities that control nature.
    B) Social organization refers to the limitations that exist within a culture.
    C) Nonverbal communication is the same from culture to culture.
    D) Personal space and its meaning are similar from one culture to another.

13. The nurse admits a client she suspects has nontraditional health and illness beliefs. Which of the following is the best approach to determine the use of natural folk medicine by the new client?
    A) "What types of food do you believe are healthy for you?"
    B) "Would you like to continue wearing that gold amulet while in the hospital?"
    C) "Have you been taking any remedies that your family taught you to use?"
    D) "You haven't been eating any of those herbs that people of your culture often eat for this disorder, have you?"

14. Time takes on different meanings from one culture to another. To explore the relationship of time to nursing interventions, the nurse should:
    A) Avoid using set times to do procedures, if possible
    B) Maintain a flexible attitude and not become upset when the client desires that procedures be performed at "awkward times"
    C) Encourage clients to set their own times when they would like the nurse to perform nursing care activities, regardless of the nurse's schedule
    D) Disregard the usual adherence to time schedules for medications

CHAPTER 8

1. Which of the following is a current trend in families or family living?
    A) People marrying earlier
    B) A reduction in the divorce rate
    C) People having more children
    D) More people living alone

2. Which one of the following trends or concerns represents the greatest current health care challenge to nurses?
    A) "New homelessness"
    B) Single-parent families
    C) "Sandwiched generation"
    D) Alternate relationship patterns

3. For the following examples, which assessment views the "family as context"?
    A) The family's ability to support the client's dietary and recreational needs
    B) The client's ability to understand and manage his own dietary needs
    C) The family's demands on the client based on his role performance
    D) The adjustment of the client and family to changes in diet and exercise

4. Assessment of the healthy family should find that:
    A) Change is viewed as detrimental to family processes
    B) There is a passive response to stressors
    C) The structure is flexible enough to adapt to crises
    D) Minimum influence is exerted on the environment

5. In completing a client's family assessment, the nurse should begin by:
    A) Gathering the health data from all family members
    B) Testing the family's ability to cope
    C) Evaluating communication patterns
    D) Determining the family's form and attitudes

6. In implementing family-centered care, the nurse:
   A) Provides his or her own beliefs on how to solve problems
   B) Assists family members to assume dependent roles
   C) Works with clients to help them accept blame for their interactions
   D) Offers information about necessary self-care abilities

7. A client with severe arthritis is returning home after having had a colostomy. The client is unable to perform the colostomy care. The nurse should first:
   A) Inform the client that an alternate way of managing the colostomy must be learned
   B) Arrange for a private duty nurse to take care of the client
   C) Investigate whether or not someone else in the family or neighborhood will be able to do the colostomy care
   D) Refer the client to a colostomy self-help support group

8. Effective communication within the family promotes:
   A) Problem solving and psychological support
   B) Role development of individual members
   C) Socialization among individual members
   D) Better financial conditions for the family

9. Family-centered nursing is concerned with:
   A) Strengthening the family unit
   B) Promoting the health of the family as a unit and the health of the individual member
   C) Caring for the expectant family
   D) Providing care outside the hospital for family members

10. The nurse has recently been employed in a long-term care facility and must learn gerontological principles related to families. Which of the following is one of those principles?
    A) Members of later-life families do not have to work on developmental tasks.
    B) The caregivers are often not members of the family.
    C) Role reversal is usually expected and well-accepted by the elderly client.
    D) Social support systems are likely to differ from those for clients in younger age groups.

CHAPTER 9

1. A genetic theory of aging focuses on:
   A) Cellular changes and loss of effectiveness
   B) Programmed cell death
   C) Organ impairment
   D) Stress and the immune system

2. A nurse who wants to apply a theory that relates to moral development should read more about:
   A) Kohlberg
   B) Piaget
   C) Freud
   D) Erikson

3. The nurse using Erikson's theory to assess a 20-year-old client's developmental status expects to find which of the following behaviors?
   A) Coping with physical and social losses
   B) Enjoyment of a sense of freedom and participation in the community
   C) Development of a sense of industry
   D) Overcoming a sense of guilt or frustration

4. Freud's theory approaches development by looking at:
   A) Cognitive development
   B) Moral reasoning
   C) Logical maturity
   D) Psychosexual aspects

5. According to Piaget, a preschool child (3 to 5 years old) is expected to exhibit which of the following behaviors?
   A) Exploration of the environment
   B) Thinking with the use of symbols and images
   C) Cooperation and sharing
   D) Organization of thoughts and far-reaching problem-solving

6. In applying Havighurst's theory, the nurse expects the client to begin to achieve social and civic responsibility in:
   A) Adolescence
   B) Early adulthood
   C) Middle adulthood
   D) Older adulthood

7. A common behavioral task or critical event for the older adult client is:
   A) Selecting a mate
   B) Rearing children
   C) Finding a congenial social group
   D) Adjusting to decreasing physical strength

8. The nurse who wishes to learn more about a developmental theory that focuses on the adult years should select a theory proposed by:
   A) Gould
   B) Chess and Thomas
   C) Freud
   D) Piaget

9. Which of the following statements about growth and development is correct?
   A) Development ends with adolescence.
   B) Growth refers to qualitative events.

C) Developmental tasks are age-related achievements.
D) Cognitive theories focus on emotional development.

10. In Kohlberg's moral development theory, an individual who reaches Level II (Conventional Thought) is expected to exhibit:
    A) Absolute obedience to authority
    B) Reasoning based on personal gain
    C) Personal internalization of other's expectations
    D) Self-chosen ethical principles, universality, and impartiality

11. According to Piaget, the infant is in the first period of development, which is characterized by:
    A) Sensorimotor intelligence
    B) Concrete operations
    C) Identity versus role confusion
    D) Preoperational thought

CHAPTER 10

1. Which of the following items is the most important for the nurse to assess in caring for a woman in her second trimester of pregnancy?
   A) The amount of weight gained in the last 2 weeks
   B) The use of alcohol, tobacco, or medications
   C) How many times the baby has moved during the last 24 hours
   D) Confirmation of the mother's desire to breast feed

2. A 6-month-old child is brought to the clinic for a well-baby examination. Which one of the following newborn reflexes should the nurse be able to elicit at this visit?
   A) Babinski
   B) Extrusion
   C) Startle
   D) Moro

3. Which of the following findings is appropriate for growth and development during infancy?
   A) Birth height increases 1 inch each month for the first 6 months
   B) The anterior fontanel closes 4 to 8 weeks after birth
   C) Birth weight triples by 6 months
   D) The chest circumference is larger than the head circumference at 12 months

4. A 6-month-old child is seen for a well-baby examination. Which of the following gross motor behaviors would the nurse expect the child to perform?
   A) Assuming a sitting position independently
   B) Pulling self to a standing position
   C) Rolling completely over
   D) Creeping on all four extremities

5. Which of the following characterizes the cognitive development of a 2-year-old child?
   A) Using short sentences to express independence
   B) Initiating play with other children
   C) Recognizing right and wrong
   D) Having a vocabulary of at least 1000 words

6. An 18-month-old child is admitted for a hernia procedure. In planning nursing care for this child, the nurse should know what predominant developmental characteristic of children this age?
   A) Imaginary playmates
   B) Parallel play
   C) Peer pressure
   D) Mutilation anxiety

7. A 5-year-old child is about to have his tonsils removed. Which of the following should his nurse remember?
   A) Explaining which behaviors are "right" in the hospital
   B) Responding to overwhelming separation anxiety

C) Allowing him to handle and look at the movements when using B/P equipment
D) Recognizing complaints of vague negative feelings

8. A parent of a 3-year-old states that she is concerned because the child was potty trained before hospitalization but now refuses to use the toilet. What is the best response by the nurse?
   A) "You may need to include the staff in using discipline because children easily lose the ability to be toilet trained during hospitalization."
   B) "This is a common behavior that is expressed when the child is stressed or anxious."
   C) "Your son was probably not ready to be potty trained, and you may want to continue the training for the next 6 months."
   D) "Your son is probably feeling neglected, and you should make an effort to spend more time with him."

9. A 4½-year-old child is crying from pain related to her fractured leg. Which of the following is the most appropriate nursing statement for her alteration in comfort?
   A) "Please try to not move your leg, and that will make it feel better."
   B) "I'll give you a shot that will help take the pain away."
   C) "It's OK to cry—would you like to hold your favorite doll?"
   D) "Would you like to hold this needle and tell me where you want me to give you your shot?"

10. The nurse is going to teach the parents of a 3-month-old child about basic infant safety. The nurse should emphasize:
    A) Placing gates or fences at stairways
    B) Keeping bathroom doors closed
    C) Giving large teething biscuits
    D) Removing bibs at bedtime

11. The parents of a 3-month-old child ask the nurse what behavior they should expect. The nurse informs the parents that the child will be able to:
    A) Smile responsively
    B) Differentiate a stranger
    C) Say "Da-da"
    D) Play peekaboo games

12. A client in her first trimester of pregnancy asks the nurse about how the baby is growing. The nurse responds by telling the client which of the following?
    A) "The organ systems are beginning to develop."
    B) "Fingers and toes are differentiated clearly."
    C) "The sex of the baby can be determined."
    D) "There is a fine hair that covers the body."

13. The nurse assists the family of a 9-year-old with nutritional information. A recommended snack for a child of this age is:
    A) Bite-sized candy
    B) Thick milkshake
    C) Potato chips
    D) Plain popcorn

14. Which of the following statements accurately describes physical development during the school-aged years?
    A) The child grows an average of 1 to 2 inches per year.
    B) The child's weight almost triples.
    C) Few physical differences are apparent among children at the end of middle childhood.
    D) Fat gradually increases, contributing to the child's heavier appearance.

15. An 8-year-old child is hospitalized for treatment for asthma. Which of the following toys would be appropriate to help this child resolve the crisis of hospitalization?
    A) Crayons and a book to color in
    B) A 500-piece puzzle to complete
    C) Cassette player with soothing tapes to listen to
    D) Velcro darts to throw at a soft board

16. A 7-year-old child is attending the second grade. Which of the following is an expected statement for a child from this age group?
    A) "I wonder what the poem that my teacher read means."
    B) "I like to play with Craig—can I meet him at the park?"
    C) "I would never talk to someone that I don't know because they might try to hurt me."
    D) "I know that I should always practice safe sex when I grow up."

17. Which of the following statements is correct regarding the developmental stage of preadolescence?
    A) It signals the development of secondary sex characteristics.
    B) It appears 2 years earlier in boys than in girls.
    C) Intimate feelings about school and friends are confided in the parents.
    D) Interest in the opposite sex is still greatly decreased.

18. A possible warning sign that a teenager is considering suicide is:
    A) A sudden interest in school activities
    B) Increase in appetite
    C) Increased sleepiness
    D) Verbalization of suicidal thoughts

19. Which of the following statements most accurately describes the stage of development for a 15-year-old?
   A) He is likely to not become any taller, but his voice may continue to deepen in tone.
   B) Communication of in-depth feelings with his peers should be encouraged.
   C) He will probably continue to adhere to his parents' and teachers' wishes without outwardly questioning their advice.
   D) He will probably make decisions about his own health care practices.

20. A 14-year-old female is visiting the county health center for "birth control help." Which of the following is the most appropriate question that the nurse could ask her?
   A) "Have you told your parents that you are sexually active?"
   B) "Are any of your friends participating in sexual behaviors?"
   C) "What can you tell me about your past sexual activities?"
   D) "Have you been protecting yourself with safe sex measures?"

21. Which of the following behaviors is expected for a 13-year-old individual?
   A) Confidence with peer group acceptance
   B) Concern about the approval from teachers
   C) Enjoyment in assisting younger siblings with homework
   D) Seeking advice from parents before trying new experiences

CHAPTER 11

1. A client thinks that she might be pregnant. Which first trimester physiological changes would most likely indicate this?
   A) Amenorrhea and nausea
   B) Braxton Hicks contractions
   C) Breast tenderness
   D) Edematous ankles and dyspnea

2. A 29-year-old single parent of three children comes into the well-child clinic for a prenatal visit. Which of the following is the best question by the nurse performing her assessment?
   A) "Have you ever been married?"
   B) "Has anyone ever taught you the principles of contraception?"
   C) "Who is your greatest support during this pregnancy time?"
   D) "Where do you work, and how does this pregnancy affect your employment?"

3. A 45-year-old adult most likely experiences which of the following physiological changes related to normal aging?
   A) Decreased hearing acuity
   B) Decreased strength of abdominal muscles
   C) Decreased function of the cranial nerves
   D) Decreased sense of smell

4. A 49-year-old client is experiencing problems with depression. She has come to the clinic showing signs of malnutrition and fatigue. Which of the following is the best approach for the nurse to take in the assessment phase?
   A) "Your depression is somewhat uncommon—can you tell me what has happened recently to cause it?"
   B) "Have you recently been experiencing menopausal symptoms?"
   C) "Depression is something to expect at your age, and with assistance you will get better."
   D) "How much weight have you lost over the past month?"

5. Which of the following is the best strategy in client teaching for positive health habits?
   A) Teaching the client to abstain from alcohol consumption
   B) Demonstrating how to take an accurate blood pressure measurement
   C) Determining an effective daily exercise schedule
   D) Describing the types of medications commonly used in the treatment of depression

6. Young adult clients are generally expected to:
   A) Continue their physical growth
   B) Experience severe illnesses
   C) Ignore physical symptoms
   D) Seek frequent medical care

7. A young adult client is at the greatest ongoing risk from which one of the following?
   A) Smoking
   B) Poor hygiene
   C) Lack of exercise
   D) Stress

8. A nurse is preparing an education program on safety for a young adult group. Based on the major cause of mortality and morbidity for this age group, the nurse should focus on:
   A) Birth control
   B) Automobile safety
   C) Avoidance of substance abuse
   D) Prevention of heart disease

9. The primary concern for a nurse assessing a young adult is the individual's:
   A) Lifestyle and leisure activities
   B) Experience with chronic disease
   C) Marital status
   D) History of childhood immunizations

10. The middle adult years may be influenced by chronic illness resulting in:
    A) Decreased health care tasks
    B) Reinforcement of previous family roles
    C) Changed sexual behavior
    D) Improved family relationships

11. Which of the following is an anticipated finding during a physical assessment of a middle adult client?
    A) Reduced pupillary reaction to light
    B) Palpable thyroid lobes
    C) Decreased skin turgor
    D) Increased range of joint motion

CHAPTER 12

1. A 77-year-old male client is currently in a long-term care facility. According to Lueckenotte, which of the following data for assessing the elderly is most important in assessing the client's health?
   A) Focus on the physiological status of the client's well-being
   B) Identify the deficits in his ability to adapt to stressors
   C) Recognize the fact that he is probably not independent in most of his activities
   D) Attempt to assess those areas in which he does not appear normal for his age group

2. An 82-year-old woman lives at home with her husband. A home health nurse visits her weekly. Which of the following statements by the nurse is appropriate for this client?
   A) "I need to obtain permission from your children to see you next week."
   B) "I will review the side effects of this medication next week."
   C) "Does your husband think that you should continue to take the medication?"
   D) "You probably can't see this size print, so I'll have the prescription enlarged for you by next week."

3. A 76-year-old client has been widowed for the past 11 years. His children are saying, "He looks much older since the loss of his wife, and he won't do things with us like he used to." Which aging theory best explains his behavior?
   A) Continuity theory
   B) Nonstochastic theory
   C) Stochastic theory
   D) Activity theory

4. A 70-year-old client is to have her blood pressure checked each shift. She asks the nurse to explain her hypertension. An appropriate response would be that older clients often experience hypertension because of:
   A) Vascular changes and the accumulation of plaque on arterial walls, both of which reduce contractility
   B) A reduction in physical activity
   C) Ingestion of processed foods that are high in sodium
   D) Arterial walls becoming thin and fragile

5. Which of the following statements related to cognitive functioning in the older client is true?
   A) Reversible systemic disorders are often implicated as a cause of delirium.
   B) Cognitive deterioration is an inevitable outcome of aging.
   C) Delirium is easily distinguished from irreversible dementia.
   D) Therapeutic drug intoxication is a common cause of senile dementia.

6. A client has been diagnosed recently with Alzheimer's disease. When teaching the family about the prognosis, the nurse must explain that:
   A) It progresses gradually with deterioration of function
   B) Many individuals can be cured if the diagnosis is made early

C) Diet and exercise can slow the process considerably
D) Few clients live more than 3 years after the diagnosis

7. Which of the following statements describes the health concerns of older adults?
   A) Approximately 50% of adults over the age of 65 have two chronic health problems.
   B) Cancer is the most common cause of death among older adults.
   C) Minimum nutritional needs for older adults are essentially the same as for younger adults.
   D) Adults over the age of 65 make up the highest percentage of prescription medication consumers.

8. Which of the following statements related to the use of therapeutic modalities with the older client is true?
   A) The major purpose of reality orientation is to prevent confusion.
   B) Resocialization is primarily intended to promote independence.
   C) Reminiscence therapy uses the past to assign new meanings to present experiences.
   D) The goal of validation therapy is to alleviate disorientation and inappropriate behaviors.

9. The nurse works with elderly clients in a wellness screening clinic on a weekly basis. Which of the following is the best statement made to clients in the older adult age group?
   A) "Your shoulder pain is normal for your age."
   B) "Continue to exercise any arthritic joints."
   C) "Don't worry about taking that combination of medications because your doctor has prescribed them."
   D) "Why don't you begin walking 2 to 3 miles a day, and we'll evaluate how you feel next week."

10. A long-term care facility sponsors a discussion group on the administration of medications. Which of the following is the best statement by a nurse at this meeting?
   A) "Don't worry about the medication's name, if you can identify it by its color and the way it looks."
   B) "Please feel free to ask your physician why you are receiving the medications that are ordered for you."
   C) "Remember that the hepatic system is primarily responsible for the pharmacotherapeutics of your medications."
   D) "Unless you have severe side affects from taking your medications, don't worry about the minor changes in the way you feel."

11. Older adults may deny the effects of aging by:
   A) Reducing cosmetic use
   B) Spending more time with other older adults
   C) Refusing assistance with certain activities
   D) Overstating their actual ages

12. In a physical assessment of an older adult, the nurse anticipates finding which of the following normal physiological changes of aging?
   A) Increased perspiration
   B) Increased audio pitch discrimination
   C) Increased salivary secretions
   D) Increased respiratory rate

13. The nurse recognizes which of the following as a musculoskeletal change in the older adult?
   A) Older men have a greater problem with osteoporosis.
   B) Muscle fibers increase in size and become tight.
   C) Exercise reduces the loss of bone mass.
   D) Muscle strength does not diminish as much as muscle mass.

14. The nurse, preparing to discharge an 81-year-old client, recognizes that the majority of older adults:
   A) Require institutional care
   B) Are unable to afford any medical treatment
   C) Have no social or family support
   D) Are capable of taking charge of their own lives

15. In order to assist older adults to meet their needs for sexuality, the nurse should recognize that:
   A) Therapeutic medications may alter sexual function
   B) Physiological changes do not adversely influence sexual activity
   C) Sexual interest declines and fades with age
   D) Prevention of sexually transmitted diseases is no longer an issue with this age group

16. The nurse is providing recommendations regarding nutritional intake for a group of older adults. The nurse should recommend:
   A) Reduced fiber
   B) Reduced protein
   C) Reduced vitamin A
   D) Reduced refined sugars

17. Which of the following foods meets the recommended nutritional guidelines for older adults?
   A) Grilled chicken
   B) Baked potato with cheese and bacon bits
   C) Hamburger and french fries
   D) Hot dog with pickle relish

CHAPTER 13

1. Which of the following statements best reflects the philosophy of critical thinking as taught by a nurse educator to a nursing student?
   A) "Don't draw subjective inferences about your client—be more objective."
   B) "Please think harder—there is a single solution for which I am looking."
   C) "Trust your feelings—don't be concerned about trying to find a theory to support your decision."
   D) "What are several interventions that you could use with this client?"

2. The second component of critical thinking in the "critical thinking model" is:
   A) Competencies
   B) Experience
   C) Specific knowledge
   D) Diagnostic reasoning

3. The nurse is using critical thinking skills in approaching newly diagnosed oncological pediatric clients. To decrease the parents' anxiety, she decides to first ask open-ended questions when talking to them about the new diagnosis. Which type of critical thinking competency is she using?
   A) Decision making
   B) Problem solving
   C) General critical thinking
   D) Diagnostic reasoning

4. The nurse manager has developed a staff protocol for peer evaluation. The nurses on her surgical unit are nervous about using her instrument. If the nurse manager continues to implement the new strategy, which of the following critical thinking attitudes is she portraying?
   A) Accountability
   B) Thinking independently
   C) Risk taking
   D) Humility

5. The client is experiencing syncope when first ambulating. The nurse decides to assess the client using Gordon's functional health patterns. The nurse accurately labels the subjective and objective data from their conversation. Which component of critical thinking best describes the nurse's approach?
   A) Experience in nursing
   B) Critical thinking competencies
   C) Critical thinking attitudes
   D) Standards for critical thinking

6. Which of the following examples reflects use of the scientific method in the nursing process?
   A) "My instincts tell me that the client is getting depressed."
   B) "The client seems to be having more pain today than yesterday."
   C) "The client's blood pressure is elevated, which makes me suspect that his pain level is increasing."
   D) "The client's husband told me that she is feeling uncomfortable."

7. The nurse decides to administer tablets of Tylenol instead of the intramuscular Demerol she has been giving one of her orthopedic clients. Which step of the nursing process does this address?
   A) Assessment
   B) Planning
   C) Implementation
   D) Nursing diagnosis

8. Reflection is one way in which critical thinking skills may be reviewed. Which one of the following is a specific example of reflection?
   A) Using particular nursing terminology
   B) Going with a feeling without the use of conscious reasoning
   C) Framing one's thoughts
   D) Writing a journal

9. An example of critical thinking at the complex level is:
   A) Following a procedure for catheterization step-by-step
   B) Giving a medication only at the time ordered
   C) Discussing alternative pain management techniques
   D) Supporting the client's decision to refuse chemotherapy

10. The nurse is deciding on the type of dressing to use for a client. Which step of the decision-making process is being used when the nurse observes the absorbency of different dressing brands?
    A) Defining the problem
    B) Considering consequences
    C) Testing possible options
    D) Making final decisions

11. Which of the following examples demonstrates the critical thinking attitude of responsibility and accountability?
    A) Offering an alternative approach
    B) Looking for a different treatment option
    C) Sharing ideas about nursing interventions
    D) Reporting client difficulties

12. Use of the intellectual standard of critical thinking implies that the nurse:
    A) Questions the physician's order
    B) Recognizes conflicts of interest
    C) Approaches assessment logically and consistently
    D) Listens to both sides of the story

CHAPTER 14

1. The three phases of an interview are:
   A) Introduction, assessment, conclusion
   B) Orientation, documentation, data base
   C) Introduction, controlling, selection
   D) Orientation, working, termination

2. The client states that he has trouble breathing at night. In obtaining the review-of-systems data the nurse should question the client about:
   A) The onset and duration of his present breathing problem
   B) His smoking and exercise practices
   C) Any family members who have heart disease
   D) Changes in other body systems

3. When validating data, which of the following questions does the nurse seek to answer?
   A) Did the client have an allergic reaction to a penicillin injection?
   B) Do I have all of the equipment for the catheterization?
   C) Is the medication record completed?
   D) What is needed to complete the QI project?

4. When looking for relationships between factors and symptoms in the database the nurse:
   A) Clusters data
   B) Validates data
   C) Formulates a problem statement
   D) Performs a peer review

5. The client recently became febrile and stated that he "felt hot." You take the client's temperature and find it to be 38.2° C. In addition, his pulse is 88/min and his blood pressure is 168/80. Which of these data are subjective data?
   A) Pulse of 88/min
   B) The client's statement about feeling hot
   C) Blood pressure of 168/80
   D) The fact that the client became febrile

6. The nurse decides to interview the client using the open-ended question technique. Which of the following statements reflects this type of questioning?
   A) "Is your pain worse or better than it was an hour ago?"
   B) "Do you believe that your nausea is from the new antibiotic?"
   C) "What do you think has been causing your depression?"
   D) "What symptoms have you had from the chemotherapy, and what have you done to alleviate them?"

7. The nurse is gathering a nursing health history on the client. The client tells the nurse that he just lost his job and that his son has newly diagnosed juvenile-onset diabetes. Which of the following categories best fits the loss of the job?
   A) Psychosocial history
   B) Family history
   C) Environmental history
   D) Biographical history

8. The client has a loud abdominal aortic bruit. This abnormality can be heard with a stethoscope, visually seen with the client lying flat, and felt with the hand. Which physical examination technique of the abdominal bruit is the least invasive?
   A) Inspection
   B) Palpation
   C) Percussion
   D) Auscultation

9. The client is found to have an activity and exercise abnormality. Which of the following organizing formats has probably been used?
   A) Review of systems
   B) Nursing health history
   C) Gordon's functional health patterns
   D) Biographical information

10. Which of the following is classified as objective data?
    A) Pain in the left leg
    B) Elevated blood pressure
    C) Fear of surgery
    D) Discomfort on breathing

11. The primary source of information when completing an assessment is:
    A) A family member
    B) An experienced nurse on the unit
    C) The client
    D) The physician

12. The first step that the nurse takes in data collection is the:
    A) Interview
    B) Physical exam
    C) Review of medical records
    D) Discussion with other health team members

13. During an interview, the nurse requires specific information about the signs and symptoms of a health problem. The nurse should use:
    A) Open-ended questions
    B) Closed-ended questions
    C) Back channeling
    D) Problem-seeking responses

14. Which response by the nurse is an example of the clarifying technique of communication?
    A) "I understand how you must feel."
    B) "This medication is used to lower your blood pressure."
    C) "You appear anxious. You're wringing your hands constantly."
    D) "I'm not sure that I understand. Could you give me an example of how the pain feels?"

CHAPTER 15

1. Nursing diagnoses are used because:
   A) They assist the nurse to distinguish medical from nursing problems
   B) Nursing education is required for accreditation purposes
   C) Client problems all become more easily and quickly resolved with their use
   D) They identify the domain of nursing

2. A 53-year-old client is seen at the clinic for a yearly physical examination. In evaluating the client's weight, the nurse also considers his age and height. This is an example of:
   A) Defining the client characteristics
   B) Recognizing gaps in data assessment
   C) Comparing data with normal health patterns
   D) Drawing conclusions about the client's response

3. The client, a coal miner, had a cholecystectomy yesterday. Potential health care risks are related primarily to what information in the database?
   A) Complaints of pain
   B) Complaints of hunger
   C) Level of anxiety
   D) Breathing coal dust

4. Which of the following nursing diagnosis statements is formulated correctly?
   A) Cardiac output decreased related to motor vehicle accident
   B) Potential for injury related to improper teaching in the use of crutches
   C) Ineffective airway clearance related to increased secretions
   D) Risk for change in body image related to cancer

5. The nurse has diagnosed the client's problem as altered elimination. From the database the nurse identifies which one of the following as appropriate etiology for this diagnosis?
   A) Increased fiber intake
   B) Limited fluid intake
   C) Total hip replacement (surgery)
   D) Intestinal polyps

6. The nurse is concerned that atelectasis may develop as a postoperative complication. Which of the following is an appropriate label for this problem should it occur?
   A) Airway clearance, ineffective
   B) Gas exchange, impaired
   C) Cardiac output, decreased
   D) Ventilation, inability to sustain spontaneous

7. Which of the following is true with regard to the formulation of nursing diagnoses?
   A) The etiology of the diagnosis must be within the scope of the health care team's practice.
   B) The diagnosis must remain constant during the client's hospitalization.
   C) The diagnosis should include the problem and the related contributing conditions.
   D) The diagnosis should identify a "cause-and-effect" relationship.

8. A likely source for a nursing diagnosis error is that the nurse:
   A) Validates the assessment information in the database
   B) Uses the NANDA list of diagnoses as a source
   C) Formulates a diagnosis too closely resembling a medical diagnosis
   D) Distinguishes the nursing focus instead of other health care disciplines

9. Identify the defining characteristics in the following nursing diagnosis: altered speech related to recent neurological disturbance, as evidenced by inability to speak in complete sentences.
   A) "Altered speech"
   B) "Inability to speak in complete sentences"
   C) "Recent neurological disturbances"
   D) "As evidenced by"

10. The primary purpose of a nursing diagnosis is to:
    A) Support the medical plan of care
    B) Provide a standardized approach for all clients
    C) Recognize the client's response to an illness or situation
    D) Offer the nurse's subjective view of the client's behaviors

11. Which one of the following is an appropriate etiology for a nursing diagnosis?
    A) Abnormal blood gas levels
    B) Myocardial infarction
    C) Increased airway secretions
    D) Cardiac catheterization

12. Which of the following is an appropriate etiology for a nursing diagnosis?
    A) Need to offer bedpan frequently
    B) Incisional pain
    C) Inadequate prescription of medication by the physician
    D) Poor hygienic practices

13. One advantage of using a nursing diagnosis is the:
    A) Communication with other nurses
    B) Use of familiar nursing jargon
    C) Ability to label the client
    D) Application in a malpractice lawsuit

14. Which one of the following is a NANDA nursing diagnosis label?
    A) Parental role conflict
    B) Abnormal hygienic care practices
    C) Coughing and dyspnea
    D) Frequent urination

15. Which of the following is an example of a diagnostic error in interpreting?
    A) Using inaccurate data
    B) Clustering data incorrectly
    C) Failing to consider cultural influences
    D) Using the client's condition as a collaborative problem

CHAPTER 16

1. The client wants to have her hair shampooed. Which of the following is the correct label with regard to prioritizing her request?
   A) Intermediate priority
   B) An unmet need
   C) Low priority
   D) A safety and security need

2. The client is a tailor who was admitted for eye surgery. A long-term goal for this client should include:
   A) Preventing ocular infection
   B) Returning to sewing
   C) Performing daily activities this week
   D) Administering eyedrops on time in the hospital

3. The nurse writes the following goal for a client who is hypertensive: "Client will maintain a blood pressure within acceptable limits." Which of the following would be an acceptable outcome criterion?
   A) Client will request pain medication as needed.
   B) Client will identify at least two things that cause stress.
   C) Client will have a 7 AM blood pressure reading of less than 140/90.
   D) Client will experience no headache or dizziness.

4. Which of the following nursing interventions is considered physician- or prescriber-initiated?
   A) Teaching a client to administer his or her insulin injection
   B) Assisting a new mother with breast-feeding
   C) Notifying the nutritionist of a client's dietary preferences
   D) Giving an enema in preparation for radiological testing

5. The intervention statement "Nurse will apply warm, wet soaks to the patient's leg each shift while awake" lacks which of the following components?
   A) Method
   B) Quantity
   C) Frequency
   D) Person who will perform action

6. Which of the following is a purpose of nursing care plans?
   A) Organizing information for legal actions
   B) Ordering nursing supplies
   C) Identifying nursing actions to be delivered
   D) Documenting the activities of other health care team members

7. The client is receiving postural drainage from physical therapy and intermittent breathing treatments from respiratory therapy. Which type of care plan would be the ideal method to document interventions for this client?
   A) Nursing Kardex
   B) Computerized care plan
   C) Critical pathway
   D) Standardized care plan

8. The nurse is involved in requesting a management consultation for personnel-related issues. Which of the following is true regarding the consultation process in which the nurse is involved?

A) The problem area is usually identified by another member of the health care team.
B) Consultation is often used when the exact problem remains unclear.
C) Detailed feelings about the problem should be described to the consultant by the nurse.
D) The problem area should be totally delegated to the consultant.

9. Which of the following client needs should take priority in planning care?
   A) An impending divorce
   B) A nutritional deficit
   C) Difficulty breathing
   D) Financial problems

10. Which is the best example of a goal or outcome statement?
    A) Nursing assistant will ambulate the client in the hallway three times each day
    B) Lungs will be clear to auscultation and respiratory rate will be 20/minute
    C) Vital signs will return to normal
    D) Urinary output will be at least 100 cc/hour within 24 hours

11. In goal setting, which of the following factors is associated with available client resources and motivation? This factor is:
    A) Client-centered
    B) Observable
    C) Measurable
    D) Realistic

12. An example of a nurse-initiated intervention is:
    A) Providing client teaching
    B) Administering medication
    C) Ordering a CAT scan
    D) Referring a client to physical therapy

13. Which one of the following is an example of a physician-initiated intervention?
    A) Taking vital signs
    B) Providing support to a family
    C) Changing a dressing two times each day
    D) Measuring intake and output

14. Which one of the following interventions selected by the nurse is classified as Level 2, Domain 2 (Physiological: complex)?
    A) Maintaining regular bowel elimination
    B) Promoting the health of the family
    C) Managing restricted body movement
    D) Restoring tissue integrity

15. Critical pathways differ from nursing care plans in their:
    A) Multidisciplinary approach
    B) Nursing interventions
    C) Client outcomes
    D) Client assessment

16. Which of the following is the best example of a nursing intervention? The nurse will:
    A) Offer fluids to the client q2h
    B) Irrigate the nasogastric tube q2h with 30 ml of normal saline
    C) Observe the client's respirations
    D) Change the client's dressing daily

17. Which of the following is the best example of a nursing intervention? The nurse will:
    A) Turn the client as needed
    B) Apply dry abdominal dressing with two 4" × 4" gauze pads t.i.d.
    C) Take vital signs
    D) Refer the client to a therapist

CHAPTER 17

1. The client comes to the family planning clinic for birth control. The nurse obtains a health history and performs a pelvic examination and Pap smear. The nurse is functioning according to:
   A) Protocol
   B) Quality improvement guidelines
   C) Nursing care plan
   D) Intervention strategy

2. The client is given an injection of an antibiotic. Shortly afterward she says that she has hives and is "itchy." The nurse administers an antihistamine to counteract the effect of the antibiotic. The nurse is using which of the following intervention methods?
   A) Compensation for adverse reactions
   B) Preventive measures
   C) Assisting with ADLs
   D) Preparing for special procedures

3. The client is scheduled to receive Coumadin (an anticoagulant) at 9:00 AM. His morning laboratory results show him to have a high partial thromboplastin time (PTT). His nurse decides to withhold the Coumadin. Which step of the implementation process is she using?
   A) Modifying the nursing care plan
   B) Reassessing the client
   C) Revising the nursing diagnosis
   D) Stating an expected outcome

4. The nurse notes that a narcotic is to be administered "per epidural cath." The nurse, however, does not know how to perform this procedure. Which aspect of the implementation process should be followed?
   A) Reassess the client
   B) Seek assistance
   C) Use interpersonal skills
   D) Critical decision making

5. The nurse recognizes the discharge needs of a client following a hip replacement. This is an example of which type of nursing skill?
   A) Cognitive
   B) Interactive
   C) Psychomotor
   D) Communication

6. A client in the adolescent clinic is having difficulty accepting the diagnosis of cancer. The nurse talks with the client about la summer camp especially for teenage cancer patients. This activity by the nurse is:
   A) Managing
   B) Teaching
   C) Communicating
   D) Counseling

7. An enterostomal nurse shows a client's significant other how to assist with the supplies for and manipulation of the ostomy equipment. In which implementation method is the nurse participating?
   A) Managing
   B) Teaching
   C) Communicating
   D) Counseling

8. The client normally ambulates with assistance. Today, while walking with the nurse, the client becomes lightheaded from an antihypertensive medication and must be safely assisted to a chair. This was considered a(n):
   A) Activity of daily living
   B) Intervention to achieve predetermined client goals
   C) Adverse reaction
   D) Psychomotor skill

9. While performing range-of-motion exercises with a client following knee surgery, the nurse tells the client that the exercises need to be done four times a day after discharge. Which of the following is the nurse trying to achieve?
   A) Achievement of realistic goals
   B) Preventive measures
   C) Client adherence
   D) Assistance with activities of daily living

10. For a client with a nursing diagnosis of impaired physical mobility related to bilateral arm casts, the nurse should select which of the following methods of nursing intervention?
    A) Counseling
    B) Teaching
    C) Compensating for adverse reactions
    D) Assisting with activities of daily living (ADLs)

11. An example of a lifesaving measure that the nurse may implement is:
    A) Restraining a violent client
    B) Administering daily insulin
    C) Initiating stress-reduction therapy
    D) Teaching the client how to take his/her pulse

CHAPTER 18

1. The client smokes two packs of cigarettes per day. The nurse works with the client, and they agree that he will smoke one cigarette less each week until he is down to one pack per day. In 3 weeks, the client is smoking two and a half packs of cigarettes per day. This is an example of:
   A) An unrealistic goal
   B) A noncompliant client
   C) A negative evaluation
   D) A nonmeasurable goal

2. The nurse formulates a diagnosis of knowledge deficit related to complications of pregnancy. One outcome criterion is that the client can state five symptoms that indicate a possible problem that should be reported. The client is able to tell the nurse three symptoms. The evaluation statement would be:
   A) Goal met; client able to state three symptoms
   B) Goal partially met; client able to state three symptoms
   C) Goal not met; client unable to list five symptoms
   D) Goal not met; client able to list three symptoms

3. A standard gives the following information:
   A) Goals to be reached
   B) Competencies of clients
   C) A basis for judging
   D) Needs to be modified

4. The nurse manager asked each nurse on the cardiac care unit to provide evidence that they had updated their skills through an advanced life support course. This is an example of:
   A) Agency structure
   B) Evaluation of care
   C) Agency liability
   D) Threshold for evaluation

5. The client has an abdominal surgical incision and is currently febrile and tachycardic. In addition, her back "is sore from lying in bed." Which nursing intervention is the best quality indicator?
   A) Back massage
   B) Careful monitoring of the vital signs
   C) Sterile technique in dressing the wound and observing for specific signs and symptoms of infection
   D) Therapeutic communication regarding her statements of being uncomfortable in bed

6. The nurse writes the following in the nursing care plan: "Goal not met; client unable to perform activities of daily living (ADLs) because of pain." Which area of quality improvement does this address?
   A) Establishing standards for evaluation
   B) Developing quality indicators
   C) Analyzing data
   D) Resolving problems

7. The nurse begins to auscultate the client's lungs. While listening, the nurse notices fresh bloody drainage oozing from the abdominal dressing. The nurse stops auscultating and applies direct pressure to the wound site. This is an example of:
   A) Performing the appropriate nursing action
   B) Critically analyzing the data and effectively implementing the safest nursing action
   C) Analyzing the data
   D) Setting realistic goals and implementing nursing interventions

8. The client is able to ambulate without signs or symptoms of shortness of breath. Which statement by the nurse is an objective evaluation of the client's goal attainment?
   A) "Client has no pain after ambulating."
   B) "Client has no manifestations of nausea while up in hall."
   C) "Client has no evidence of respiratory distress when ambulating."
   D) "Client walked well and did not have any problem when up."

9. When modifying a care plan to meet a client's changing needs, the nurse should:
   A) Re-do the entire care plan
   B) Focus only on the nursing diagnoses and the goals that have changed
   C) Perform a complete reassessment of all client factors
   D) Add more nursing interventions from a standardized plan of care

10. Which of the following is an appropriate evaluative measure for a client outcome of "erythema will be reduced in 2 days"?
    A) Assess respiratory rate during exercise
    B) Palpate radial pulse
    C) Review client's dietary habits
    D) Inspect color of pressure ulcer

CHAPTER 19

1. Contemporary nursing practice is based on knowledge generated through nursing theories. Nightingale's theory introduced the concept that nursing care focusses on:
    A) Manipulating the client's environment
    B) Promoting the client's psychological needs
    C) Maintaining a maximum level of wellness
    D) Developing interpersonal interactions with the client

2. Florence Nightingale has been described as the first nurse:
    A) Epidemiologist
    B) Researcher
    C) Theorist
    D) All of the above

3. The history of organized nursing has been the history of a profession seeking to:
    A) Define and control its own body of knowledge and practice
    B) Win recognition, respect, and just reward for its contribution
    C) Assert itself
    D) All of the above

4. Nursing education programs may seek voluntary accreditation through:
    A) International Council of Nurses
    B) Canadian Association of University Schools of Nursing
    C) Canadian Nurses Association
    D) Provincial associations

5. The educational preparation for a nurse practitioner is:
    A) Diploma
    B) Baccalaureate degree
    C) Master's degree
    D) Certificate

6. A group that lobbies at the national level for advancement of the nurse's role and economic interest, and health care is:
    A) Canadian Nurses Association
    B) HEAL
    C) National Federation of Nurses' Unions
    D) Canadian Hospital Association

7. A nurse moves from Ontario to Alberta to seek employment at the University of Alberta Hospital. The most important factor for the nurse is:
    A) Standards of Practice for nurses in Alberta
    B) Registration by the Alberta Association of Registered Nurses
    C) Review of policies and procedures of the hospital
    D) Continuing education at the hospital

8. A nurse is caring for a client who has congestive heart failure. The client is experiencing intense fatigue and has knowledge deficit related to the therapy he will be receiving at home. The nurse states, "We will do everything to return you to the optimal level of self-care." This is an example of a nurse fulfilling which role?
    A) Caregiver
    B) Teacher
    C) Rehabilitator
    D) Communicator

9. Isabel Hampton and Adelaide Nutting, two Canadian nurses working in the United States were instrumental in the development of:
   A) American Society of Superintendents of Training Schools
   B) St. Catharine's General and Marine Hospital
   C) Nurses Associated Alumnae of the United States and Canada
   D) International Council of Nurses

10. A registered nurse is seeking certification in Cardiovascular Nursing. He or she will have to complete:
    A) An examination and minimum practice requirements
    B) An examination given to all nurses seeking certification
    C) A graduate degree in nursing
    D) A request for CNA approval

11. In the Standards of Professional Practice, the "nurse provides, facilitates, and promotes the best possible professional service. The nurse responds to the needs of consumers in a way that fosters trust, respect, collaboration, and innovation." The major indicator is:
    A) "Collaborates with the consumer and health team members to provide professional service"
    B) "Creates environments that are conducive to meeting professional practice standards"
    C) "Supports the evaluation and use of research relevant to the profession"
    D) "Ensures that resources are used efficiently and effectively to protect consumer interest"

12. The majority of nurses in Canada practise in:
    A) Tertiary settings
    B) Long-term care
    C) Ambulatory care
    D) Home care

13. A 35-year-old male patient who is employed as a mechanic in a nuclear plant has recently been diagnosed with multiple sclerosis. He seeks assistance in the type of training he will need to change jobs whereby safety is not an issue. To which allied health care professional will you refer this patient?
    A) Respiratory therapist
    B) Physiotherapist
    C) Occupational therapist
    D) Social worker

14. According to the data presented in the 1998 *RN Data Statistics*, the majority of nurses in Canada have attended which of the following educational programs?
    A) Diploma programs
    B) Baccalaureate degree programs
    C) Certification programs
    D) Continuing education

CHAPTER 20

1. The client states that she needs to exercise regularly, watch her weight, and reduce her fat intake. This demonstrates that the client:
   A) Believes she will have a heart attack
   B) Values health promotion activities
   C) Believes she will not become sick
   D) Has unrealistic expectations for herself

2. A client has actively picketed for gun control. During a robbery of his business, he was shot in the leg. As the nurse assists him with morning care, which statement would the nurse expect him to make?
   A) "Individuals should arm themselves for protection."
   B) "Firearms may have a place in our society."
   C) "Prosecution should be the maximum for that felon."
   D) "Protection is a necessary evil for the good guy."

3. A secondary-school teacher with advanced multiple sclerosis insists on teaching from a wheelchair and being treated the same as other colleagues. The teacher is demonstrating which of the following?
   A) Choosing from alternatives
   B) Considering all consequences
   C) Prizing her choice
   D) Acting with a pattern of consistency

4. Values clarification interventions are beneficial for the client when:
   A) The client and nurse have different beliefs
   B) The client is experiencing a values conflict
   C) The nurse is unsure of a client's values
   D) The client has rejected normal values

5. Values clarification is a three-step process that allows an individual to identify personal values. These steps are:
   A) Choosing, prizing, evaluation
   B) Choosing, prizing, acting
   C) Reflecting, choosing, acting
   D) Reflecting, prizing, acting

6. A nurse might examine her values because:
   A) She wants to align her values closer with those of others
   B) Examining values provides answers to ethical dilemmas
   C) Examining values helps a nurse to reach a higher level of moral reasoning
   D) Examining values reveals a clearer picture of one's value system that never changes

7. Which of the following statements best reflects the moralizing mode of values transmission?
   A) "I learned to dislike smoking from my grandmother."
   B) "I finally decided to abstain from alcohol when I learned how many traffic deaths drinking caused."
   C) "I want my child to be taught about safe sex."
   D) "I want my son to learn from his mistakes and then make the right decision on his own."

8. A 68-year-old Oriental client recently admitted for esophageal reflux wants the nurses to assist her in using a religious undergarment. Which essential value is the professional nurse recognizing?
   A) Human dignity
   B) Esthetics
   C) Altruism
   D) Freedom

9. *The Code of Ethics for Registered Nurses:*
   A) Defines the entitlements of employers and employees
   B) Is the sole guide for ethical and legal nursing practice
   C) Outlines which values take priority over others
   D) Provides advisory guidance in ethical dilemmas

10. A student nurse realizes that she has administered the wrong dose of medication to a patient. She immediately informs her clinical instructor. This student nurse is described as:
    A) Honest
    B) Trustworthy
    C) Compliant
    D) Accountable

11. Which of the following is the best sequence for resolving ethical problems?
    A) Examine one's own values, evaluate, identify the problem
    B) Evaluate the outcomes, gather data, consider actions
    C) Gather facts, verbalize the problem, consider actions
    D) Recognize the dilemma, evaluate, gather information

12. A nurse is ambivalent as to the need to vigorously suction a terminal client in a comatose state. Which of the following is an appropriate statement by the nurse in regard to processing an ethical dilemma?
   A) "I need to know the legalities of the living will of this client."
   B) "My spiritual beliefs mandate that I continue to provide all the interventions in my scope of practice."
   C) "I cannot derive a right solution to this dilemma and therefore need to collect more data."
   D) "I just feel like I should not suction this client."

13. Which of the following statements best illustrates the deontological ethical theory?
   A) "I believe this disease was allowed by a supreme being."
   B) "He has become a stronger individual through experiencing the loss of his father."
   C) "It would never be right for a person to stop CPR efforts."
   D) "The chemotherapy did not cure this person, but it provided a better life for him."

14. On admission to a hospital, a terminal cancer patient says he has a living will. This document functions to state the client's desire to:
   A) Receive all means of technical assistance and equipment used to prolong his life
   B) Have his wife make decisions regarding his care
   C) Be allowed to die without life-prolonging techniques
   D) Have a lethal injection administered to relieve his suffering

15. A nurse has stopped at an accident scene and begun to provide emergency care for the victims. Her actions are best labelled as:
   A) Respect for persons
   B) Beneficence
   C) Nonmaleficence
   D) Triage

16. A primary role of a hospital ethics committee is to:
   A) Serve as a resource for specific situations that may occur
   B) Interview all persons involved in a case
   C) Illustrate circumstances that demonstrate malpractice
   D) Examine similar previous instances for comparison of outcome decisions

17. You are assigned to care for two patients that have many complex problems. Which ethical principle are you applying in determining how you will divide your time and resources?
   A) Autonomy
   B) Beneficence
   C) Fidelity
   D) Justice

18. An example of the ethical principle of autonomy is:
   A) Learning how to do a procedure safely and effectively
   B) Returning to speak to a client at an agreed upon time
   C) Preparing the client's room for comfort and privacy
   D) Supporting a client's right to refuse therapy

19. Which of the following statements is an example of the essential nursing value of human dignity?
    A) "I'm concerned that decreased funding may affect the outpatient program."
    B) "I'm going to put some flowers in the client's room."
    C) "I cannot share that information with you about the client."
    D) "I need to get more information about the client's health history."

CHAPTER 21

1. A nurse accidentally administers an incorrect dosage of morphine sulfate to a client. Which source of law best addresses this situation?
    A) Civil law
    B) Criminal law
    C) Common law
    D) Administrative law

2. A junior nursing student prepares to give her client an injection. What standard of care applies to the student nurse's conduct when providing care normally performed by a registered nurse (RN)? The student is held to:
    A) A standard of care of an unlicensed person
    B) The same standard of care as an RN
    C) A standard similar to but not the same as the staff nurse with whom the student is assigned to work
    D) No special standard of care because the faculty member is responsible for the student's conduct

3. Treating a patient without his or her consent is considered:
    A) Battery
    B) Negligence
    C) Implied consent
    D) Presumed consent

4. An unconscious client with a head injury needs surgery to live. His wife speaks only French, and the health care providers are having a difficult time explaining his condition. Which of the following is the most correct answer regarding this situation?
    A) Two licensed health care personnel should witness and sign the preoperative consent indicating their hearing an explanation of the procedure given in English.
    B) An institutional review board needs to be contacted to give their emergency advice on the situation.
    C) A friend of the family could act as an interpreter, but the explanation could not provide details of the client's accident, due to confidentiality laws.
    D) The health care team should continue with the surgery after providing information in the best manner possible.

5. A physician asks a family nurse practitioner to prescribe a medication that the nurse practitioner knows is incompatible with the current medication regimen. If the nurse practitioner follows the physician's desire, which of the following is the most likely result?
    A) The nurse practitioner will be liable for malpractice.
    B) Good Samaritan laws will protect the nurse.
    C) If the nurse practitioner has developed a good relationship with the client, there probably will not be a problem.
    D) The nurse practitioner should get malpractice insurance.

6. A registered nurse interprets a medication order scribbled by the attending physician as 25 mg. The nurse administers 25 mg of the medication to a client, then discovers that the dose was incorrectly interpreted and should have been 2.5 mg. Who would ultimately be responsible for the error?
   A) Attending physician
   B) Assisting resident
   C) Pharmacist
   D) Nurse

7. Because of an influenza epidemic among nursing staff, a nurse has been moved from the eye unit to a general surgical floor. The nurse recognizes that he is inexperienced in this specialty. The nurse's initial recourse is to:
   A) Politely refuse to move, take a leave-of-absence day, and go home
   B) Ask to work with another general surgery nurse
   C) Fill out a report noting his dissatisfaction
   D) Notify the provincial/territorial board of nursing of the problem

8. Which of the following is true concerning the legalities of death and dying issues?
   A) Withholding life-prolonging treatment is illegal in all provinces.
   B) Organ donation must be attempted if it will save the recipient's life.
   C) Assisted suicide is a constitutional right.
   D) Artificial feedings may be refused by individuals who are unable to feed themselves.

9. The nurse has a responsibility to file an incident report when a client:
   A) Leaves the floor to eat in the cafeteria with his family
   B) Complains of feeling dizzy and starts itching after an injection of penicillin

C) Reports soreness after a treatment of warm soaks to her leg
D) Climbs over the side rail and falls

10. Which of the following statements is correct concerning revocation of a nursing license?
    A) The hearings are usually held in court.
    B) Due process rights are waived by the nurse.
    C) There must be an opportunity to defend against any charges.
    D) The federal government becomes involved in the procedures.

11. Which one of the following is an example of an unintentional tort?
    A) Leaving the side rails down and the client falls out of bed
    B) Restraining a client who refuses care
    C) Taking photos of a client's surgical wounds
    D) Talking about a client's history of sexually transmitted diseases

12. Which one of these individuals may legally give informed consent?
    A) A 16-year-old mother for her newborn child
    B) A sedated 42-year-old client
    C) The friend of an 84-year-old married client
    D) A 56-year-old client who does not understand the proposed treatment plan

13. The nurse's signature as a witness on an informed consent indicates that the client:
    A) Fully understands the procedure
    B) Agrees with the procedure to be done
    C) Has authorized the physician to continue with the treatment
    D) Has voluntarily signed the form

CHAPTER 22

1. A nurse is working with an alcohol-dependent client and is discussing support groups and Alcoholics Anonymous. The information that the nurse gives to this client would correspond to which of the following terms?
   A) Channel
   B) Symbolism
   C) Feedback
   D) Referent

2. When using nonverbal communication in a nurse-client relationship, the nurse must be most aware of:
   A) Ethnic background
   B) Nervous hand movements
   C) Contradictions to the client
   D) The client's developmental level

3. The nurse formulates a diagnosis of impaired verbal communication for a client in the hospital. Related factors for this diagnosis apparent to the nurse during assessment include:
   A) Inadequate situational support
   B) Changes in life setting
   C) Cultural differences
   D) Maturational crisis

4. The client draws back when the nurse reaches over the side rails to take his blood pressure. To promote effective communication, the nurse should:
   A) Sit at the bedside and explain the reason for taking a blood pressure reading every hour
   B) Rotate the nurses who are assigned to take the client's blood pressure
   C) Convey confidence and gentleness when performing the procedure
   D) Apologize for startling the client and explain the need for close contact

5. A staff nurse in the intensive care unit, explains to the client's wife the types of monitoring devices they will be using for her husband, and then there is silence. The nurse uses silence as a communication technique to:
   A) Give both communicators time to relax
   B) Allow time for reorganization of thoughts
   C) Allow the client's wife to have time for herself
   D) Build up emotional tension

6. During the assessment phase of the nursing process, the nurse may uncover data that help to identify communication problems. An example of these data might be:
   A) Extreme dyspnea or shortness of breath
   B) Urinary frequency and pain
   C) Chronic stomach pain
   D) Lack of appetite

7. A nurse tells an advanced nurse practitioner that the client is "slipping a little" in reference to hemodynamic pressures. The nurse is using:
   A) Brevity
   B) Pacing and control
   C) Connotative meaning
   D) Relevance

8. A client is admitted for a CAT scan (diagnostic test) of the cranium. As the nurse explains this diagnostic test, the client moves away from the nurse. This is an example of what influencing factor in communication?
   A) Gender
   B) Space and territoriality
   C) Sociocultural background
   D) Environment

9. Which of the following statements by a nurse best conveys empathy?
A) "I can appreciate your desire to not use any form of blood products."
B) "Do you mean you would like to talk to the new family nurse practitioner?"
C) "Good morning. How did you sleep last night?"
D) "Can you describe what the pain in your abdomen feels like?"

10. Which of the following is the greatest barrier to effective communication?
A) Giving an opinion when asked
B) Being defensive
C) Using assertiveness techniques
D) Using too much nonverbal language

11. A parent tells the pediatric nurse practitioner, "I've never told anyone this information about my son." This is an example of:
A) Identifying problems and goals
B) Building trust
C) Clarifying roles
D) Revealing

12. Discussing the client's follow-up dietary needs immediately prior to the client's surgery is an error in:
A) Denotative meaning
B) Pacing
C) Intonation
D) Timing and relevance

13. The zone of personal space and touch that extends the farthest from an individual is the:
A) Personal zone
B) Social zone
C) Consent zone
D) Vulnerable zone

14. Communication is used throughout the nursing process. In the evaluation phase, the nurse:

A) Delegates activities to other staff members
B) Validates the client's health needs
C) Documents expected outcomes and planned interventions
D) Acquires verbal and nonverbal feedback

15. Which of the following is an example of an interpersonal variable that may influence the client's communication?
A) Postoperative discomfort
B) An extremely warm room
C) A talkative roommate
D) A loud television

16. Which of the following statements regarding nonverbal communication is correct?
A) Gestures alone are meaningless.
B) The nurse's appearance can influence interactions.
C) Personal space needs are predictable for adult clients.
D) Eye contact should be maintained with all clients.

17. The nurse is establishing a helping relationship with the client. In addressing the client, the nurse should:
A) Use the client's first name
B) Touch the client right away to establish contact
C) Sit far enough away from the client
D) Knock before entering the client's room

18. In using communication skills with clients, the nurse evaluates which response as being therapeutic?
A) "Why don't you stick to the special diet?"
B) "We can't continue talking about your financial problems right now. It's time for your bath."
C) "I noticed that you didn't eat lunch. Is something wrong?"
D) "I think you need to find another physician that you'll like more than this one."

19. What communication technique may be used most effectively with toddlers or preschoolers?
    A) Using analogies to explain health-related ideas
    B) Allowing manipulation of equipment to be used
    C) Moving quickly and minimizing contact to avoid distress
    D) Focusing on what other children have done

20. For a client with aphasia, the nurse may enhance communication by:
    A) Speaking loudly
    B) Using open-ended questions
    C) Using a speech therapist to communicate with the client
    D) Using visual cues

CHAPTER 23

1. The client has been informed that he can be discharged once he can irrigate his colostomy independently. The client requests that the nurse observe his irrigation technique. Which of the following learning motives is the client displaying?
   A) Physical need
   B) Social activity
   C) Task mastery
   D) Evaluation stance

2. Which of the following age-groups is correctly matched with the developmental characteristic?
   A) A toddler expresses feelings more through words.
   B) To a preschooler, play is more formal and imaginative.
   C) A school-age child is easily intimidated by adults outside of the family.
   D) An adolescent fears loss of self-concept and body image.

3. An industrial nurse is planning to give an informative talk on hypertension to employees in honor of Heart Month. He plans to teach individuals how to take their blood pressure. Which information is essential for him to ask the planning committee before this presentation?
   A) Specific ages of the people involved
   B) Number of individuals with high blood pressure in this group
   C) Type of room available for the meeting
   D) The names of employees who are married

4. The nurse established the following objective for the client who was unable to void. "The client's intake will be at least 1000 ml between 7 AM and 3:30 PM." Feedback indicating success would be the client doing which of the following?
   A) Voiding at least 1000 ml
   B) Verbalizing abdominal comfort without pressure
   C) Having adequate intake and output
   D) Drinking 240 ml of fluid, five or six times

5. The nurse has important information to share with a parent who has brought his child to the emergency room. The nurse discovers that the parent has just learned that his son will require surgery. The most effective teaching approach is:
   A) Participating
   B) Entrusting
   C) Telling
   D) Group teaching

6. A client is taught the clinical manifestations of inflammation so that she can detect a complication of her surgical wound. The client states, "I will look at the wound four times a day and tell my surgeon if it looks red or swollen." Her statement is an example of:
   A) Attitudes
   B) Effective communication
   C) Analysis
   D) Application

7. The client continues to ask questions about her surgical wound. The client states, "I think I would like help the first time I look at my wound." This is an example of:
   A) Guided response
   B) Adaptation
   C) Perception
   D) Organizing

8. The nurse assesses the client's readiness to learn insulin injection sites. The most important factor for the nurse to assess is the:
   A) Previous knowledge level of the client
   B) Willingness of the client to want to learn the injection sites
   C) Adaptation of the client to the new need for injections
   D) Intelligence and developmental level of the client

9. The nurse is demonstrating to the client how to put on antiembolytic stockings. In the middle of the lesson, the client asks, "Why have my feet been swelling?" The nurse should adhere to which one of the following teaching principles?
   A) Timing
   B) Setting priorities
   C) Building on existing knowledge
   D) Organizing teaching materials

10. Which of the following is an example of an evaluation of a psychomotor skill?
    A) The client is able to state the side effects of medication.
    B) The client responds appropriately to eye contact.
    C) The client planned an exercise program.
    D) The client uses the cane correctly.

11. Which of the following is a topic that would be covered under health maintenance/illness prevention?

A) Limitations on function
B) Self-help devices
C) Stress management
D) Environmental alterations

12. An example of an evaluation of a client's attainment of a cognitive skill is:
    A) The client takes the medication with meals to avoid gastric upset
    B) The client looks at the surgical incision without prompting
    C) The client uses crutches appropriately to go up and down stairs
    D) The client dresses him/herself after breakfast

13. The nurse evaluates which of the following statements as an indication that the client is not ready to learn at this time?
    A) "I need to understand more about the reason for the colostomy."
    B) "I will find out when the support group meets."
    C) "There's no sense in showing me. I'm too sick right now."
    D) "Tell me if I am doing this correctly."

14. In planning to teach an older adult client, the nurse should incorporate which teaching method or principle into the plan?
    A) Teach in the early morning or late evening.
    B) Keep teaching sessions short.
    C) Put as much as possible into each teaching session.
    D) Focus on teaching a family member.

15. Which of the following nursing diagnoses indicates a need to postpone teaching?
    A) Knowledge deficit regarding impending surgery
    B) Activity intolerance related to pain
    C) Ineffective management of treatment regimen
    D) Noncompliance with prescribed exercise plan

16. Which teaching method is best applied to a cognitive learning need?
    A) Computer-assisted instruction
    B) Demonstration of a procedure
    C) Modeling of behavior
    D) Discussion of feelings

17. For a functionally illiterate client, the nurse particularly focuses on:
    A) Using intricate analogies and example
    B) Avoiding return demonstrations
    C) Incorporating familiar terminology
    D) Spending longer sessions with the client

CHAPTER 24

1. Which of the following should the nurse include in an intershift report to nursing colleagues?
    A) The client's family history
    B) All routine care procedures required by the client
    C) Audit of client care procedures
    D) Instructions given to the client in a teaching plan

2. The correct reporting of an incident involves which of the following?
    A) The completion of a report by the nurse who witnessed the client injury
    B) A subjective description of the details of the incident
    C) An explanation of the possible cause for the incident
    D) A notation in the medical record that an incident report was prepared

3. Which of the following chart entries is written correctly?
    A) "09:00 Demerol given for lower abdominal pain"
    B) "12:30 Client's vital signs taken"
    C) "07:00 Client drank adequate amount of fluids"
    D) "08:30 Increased IV fluid rate to 100 mL/h according to protocol"

4. The nurse makes an entry in a client's record. Which of the following is the best example of how to document this type of situation?
    A) "08:30 Client received Percodan (1 tablet) PO an hour before going to radiology"
    B) "13:15 I gave the client morphine 10 mg IM at 11:10, but did not document it then"
    C) "14:45 ASA 500 mg given for temperature of 38.1°C"
    D) "20:30 Abdominal dressing change at 19:30. No s/s of infection, and wound edges approximating well"

5. "Client is wheezing and experiencing some dyspnea upon exertion" is an example of:
    A) The "S" in SOAP documentation
    B) Focus charting
    C) The "E" of PIE
    D) Charting by exception

6. Recording a nurse's description of how a client is to perform a procedure involving self-care is likely to be found in a(n):
    A) Kardex
    B) Nursing history form
    C) Discharge summary form
    D) Incident report

7. When the nurse discovers that an error has been made in the chart, which is the best approach?
    A) Draw a straight line through the error and initial it.
    B) Erase the error and write over the material in the same spot.
    C) Use a dark color marker to cover the error and continue immediately after that point.
    D) Footnote the error at the bottom of the page.

8. A client receives daily tracheostomy care and suctioning by a home health nurse. The nurse's documentation should:
   A) Clearly identify the criteria necessary for the client needing readmission to acute care
   B) Include the percentage of the daily care covered by family
   C) Specify teaching concepts communicated to the client's family concerning the performed skills
   D) Not identify any other health care team member currently assisting with client care

9. The nurse uses computerized documentation in a community health nurse role. An advantage is:
   A) Improved auscultation skills
   B) A laptop computer may be used in the home
   C) Increased confidentiality
   D) Documentation tasks are less repetitive

10. A physician phones the nurse to obtain electrolyte levels of a client. The physician is using a:
    A) Transfer report
    B) Telephone order
    C) Telephone report
    D) Distance communication order

11. A characteristic of a problem-oriented record that distinguishes it from a source-oriented record is that the problem-oriented record:
    A) Includes progress notes
    B) Includes initial information obtained from a patient
    C) Is organized around a patient's health problem
    D) Is considered to be an acceptable legal document

12. The client developed a slight hematoma on his left forearm. The nurse labels the problem as an infiltrated intravenous (IV) line. The nurse places hot packs around the forearm. The client states, "My arm feels better." What is documented as the "R" in focus charting?
    A) "My arm feels better"
    B) "Slight hematoma on left forearm"
    C) "Infiltrated IV line"
    D) "Placement of hot packs"

13. Which of the following is evaluated as a legally appropriate notation?
    A) "Dr. Green made an error in the amount of medication to administer."
    B) "Client verbalized sharp, stabbing pain along the left side of chest."
    C) "Nurse Williams spoke with the client about the surgery."
    D) "Client upset about the physical therapy."

14. In order to avoid legal risks associated with computerized documentation, many programs currently have:
    A) All nursing staff use the same access code
    B) Use of data only by centralized medical records
    C) Thumbprint identification restrictions
    D) Periodic changes in staff passwords

CHAPTER 25

1. Knowledge that is organized into general laws and theories in order to describe, explain and predict phenomena is known as:
   A) Esthetics
   B) Ethics
   C) Empirics
   D) Personal

2. Which of the following is an expected research role for the baccalaureate-prepared nurse?
   A) Assumes the role of a clinical expert
   B) Identifies clinical nursing problems in nursing practice
   C) Develops methods of inquiry relevant to nursing
   D) Acquires funding for research projects

3. A nurse researcher distributes an explanatory information sheet about the purpose of the study to subjects solicited for participation in her study. Which of the following ethical principles that guide research is this researcher using?
   A) Protection of subjects
   B) Freedom from harm
   C) Confidentiality of subjects
   D) Informed consent

4. Which of the following violates an ethical responsibility associated with informed consent? The researcher must:
   A) Provide alternatives, including the right of refusal and standard practices
   B) Give information about the study, withholding knowledge of treatment to avoid study bias
   C) Explain the possibility of risks when appropriate
   D) Adhere to verbal and written agreements

5. Which of the following does not apply to planning a nursing research investigation for a Level III question?
   A) Hypothesis
   B) Correlational tests
   C) Differences between means
   D) Test of theory

6. A sample of orthopedic clients varies greatly in their requests for post-surgical analgesics. Which type of research design would best determine which factors affect comfort in a group of clients?
   A) Quasi-experimental design
   B) Phenomenological design
   C) Grounded theory design
   D) Descriptive survey design

7. Which of the following has the least priority in nursing research?
   A) Developing instruments to measure nursing outcomes
   B) Classifying nursing practice phenomena
   C) Promoting health practices in self-care across social groups
   D) Describing methods of curing chronic diseases

8 A nurse researcher has completed a study involving the use of intravenous analgesics for post-surgical discomfort. The description of the 16 clients used in the study would best be placed in which of the following areas of the research report?
   A) Analysis
   B) Purpose
   C) Design
   D) Sample

9. A nurse works on a neurological nursing unit. She has read a study report on the effects of early stimulation with clients who have had head injuries. In which of the following designs are statistical techniques used to test for significant relationships among the variables?
   A) Descriptive survey design
   B) Experimental designs
   C) Exploratory descriptive designs
   D) Phenomenological designs

10. Which one of the following is an example of qualitative research?
    A) Determination of how well a new hospital policy works
    B) Study of the relationship between pre-operative teaching and postoperative anxiety
    C) Determination of the effectiveness of pain-management techniques
    D) Interview of clients about the experience of mechanical ventilation

11. Identify which of the following is a Level III question.
    A) Why is guided imagery effective in reducing stress levels?
    B) How often do stress reactions occur?
    C) What does guided imagery mean to clients?
    D) What creates increases in stress levels?

CHAPTER 26

1. The client has just learned that his motorcycle accident has resulted in his left leg being amputated. When helping this client form goals and strategies for achieving goals, the nurse needs to assess the client's:
   A) Interests and past accomplishments
   B) Intellectual and spiritual strengths
   C) Involvement with significant others
   D) Ideal and perceived self-concept

2. A client experiencing depersonalization might manifest:
   A) Distorted thinking
   B) Escape behavior
   C) Withdrawal from activities
   D) Self-destruction

3. A 76-year-old client who recently lost his wife is admitted for surgery. Which of the following behaviors would alert the nurse that the client has an alteration in the integrity stage of his psychosocial development?
   A) Accepting his own limitations
   B) Verbalizing fear about the surgery
   C) Demanding unnecessary assistance from his daughter
   D) Expressing his opinions about his care

4. A client has been hospitalized for months while receiving therapies for lung cancer. The client has become very depressed, refuses to participate in personal grooming, and does not want visitors. To assist in achieving resolution of the client's problem, the nurse should have the client:
   A) Think positively instead of negatively
   B) Contact a support group and explore a psychological consultation
   C) Get washed and dressed
   D) Become more independent and return to prior activities

5. The client is on the orthopedic unit following back surgery. He states, "I feel like I can't do anything anymore—and I won't be able to continue my landscaping business." This is predominantly an example of a problem in which of the following components of self-concept?
   A) Body image
   B) Self-esteem
   C) Identity
   D) Roles *performance*

6. A recently divorced client comes to the clinic. She has custody of her two teenagers and is an established lawyer. She states, "I can't keep working so hard and raise my children the way I would like." This is an example of:
   A) Role ambiguity
   B) Role strain
   C) Role conflict
   D) Gender role stereotype

7. A prostitute, with HIV and severe complications, is being cared for on a medical unit. The nurse is seeking to develop a therapeutic relationship with the client. Which of the following statements best reflects the nurse's attempt to support the client's self-exploration?
   A) "Don't be embarrassed by your former occupation."
   B) "Who do you go to for support?"
   C) "On what type of schedule do you think you could realistically eat your meals without being nauseated?"
   D) "The people who work here are professionals, and we don't judge your past actions."

8. A school-aged client has just been diagnosed with juvenile diabetes. The client is very angry about her new disease. Which of the following statements is most appropriate for the nurse counselor working with this client?
   A) "Try not to be angry because you are receiving the best care possible."
   B) "It is all right to be angry with your friends, but try not be angry with your parents."
   C) "Tell me what you do when you get angry."
   D) "You learn quickly and will probably handle the treatment very well."

9. A client is most concerned about the interactions that she has with her family, and she is in the process of establishing a positive view of herself. This client is meeting the developmental needs of the:
   A) 12- to 20-year-old age-group
   B) Early 20s to mid-40s age-group
   C) Mid-40s to mid-60s age-group
   D) Late 60s and older age-group

10. In developing role behavior, the child learns which of the following through substitution?
    A) Avoiding unacceptable behavior because it is punished
    B) Engaging in an acceptable behavior instead of another unacceptable one
    C) Internalizing beliefs and values of role models
    D) Refraining from behavior even though tempted

11. Which developmental task associated with self-concept is expected in an assessment of an individual from the 12- to 20-year-old age-group?
    A) Distinguishing oneself from the environment
    B) Identifying with a gender
    C) Exploring goals for the future
    D) Feeling positive about one's life achievements

12. Which of the following questions should the nurse use to assess a client's perception of identity?
    A) "How would you describe yourself?"
    B) "What changes would you make in your appearance?"
    C) "What activities do you enjoy doing?"
    D) "What is your usual day like?"

CHAPTER 27

1. The preschooler's interest in gender sexuality is characterized by an interest in:
   A) His or her genitalia
   B) Learning how and why his or her anatomy differs from that of other children
   C) Playing and developing friendships with children of the opposite sex
   D) Spending most of his or her time with the parent of the opposite sex

2. When a male client acts out sexually to a female nurse caring for him, the nurse should:
   A) Immediately report the incident to the client's physician
   B) Tell the client that his behavior is offensive and leave the room
   C) Have a male nurse assume care for this client
   D) Review and define the nurse-client relationship

3. A client states that she is afraid that she and her husband will not be able to maintain a healthy sexual relationship now that they have a baby in the house. To assist these clients, it would be helpful to know:
   A) If they have similar parenting beliefs
   B) How comfortable they are in communicating their feelings to each other
   C) How well they have approached other role changes
   D) The level of knowledge they have regarding healthy sexual relationships

4. A married client has a fulfilling intimate relationship with his wife. In addition, he enjoys male friendships and practices warm, affectionate embraces with members of both sexes. This is an example of:
   A) Gender dysphoria
   B) Homosexuality
   C) Heterosexuality
   D) Transsexuality

5. An adolescent female student, who is sexually active, visits the office of the school nurse. Which of the following statements best reflects her understanding of the effective use of contraception devices?
   A) "My boyfriend is able to withdraw prior to ejaculation, and that prevents me from getting pregnant."
   B) "I take my temperature every morning, and when it goes down for at least two days, we have unprotected sex."
   C) "We use 'foam' before each time that we have sex and I haven't gotten pregnant yet."
   D) "I use a diaphragm and contraceptive cream."

6. A school nurse is responsible for teaching adolescents about sexually transmitted diseases (STDs). Which of the following is the best statement the nurse could make regarding prevention of STDs?
   A) HIV is best prevented with the use of condoms and foam.
   B) Herpes simplex is detected easily and therefore symptom education is very necessary.
   C) Communicate with your sexual partners and assess their sexual behaviors before having intimate relationships.
   D) Many STDs are transmitted to the fetus through the bloodstream from the placenta.

7. The nurse is conducting a sexual history with a client who is scheduled for cardiac surgery. The client tells the nurse that he is nervous about resuming sexual activities. Which of the following statements by the nurse best reflects an understanding of obtaining this type of data?
   A) "You can have sexual intercourse after your surgery, but there are predictable risks."
   B) "Your partner will be nervous about resuming sexual activities, but that is normal."
   C) "In about 2 months you will be able to return to your normal sexual patterns."
   D) "You are expressing a very normal concern—perhaps we could discuss your feelings further."

8. The nurse is teaching sexuality to a group of senior adults. Which of the following comments by a participant reflects an understanding of the topic?
   A) "So, sexual intercourse will be more painful for my wife and we should have sex less frequently?"
   B) "We have recently seen the need to begin using a lubricant — is that because we make love less often?"
   C) "My orgasms seem to not last as long, but John and I are probably more satisfied now than when we were younger."
   D) "I don't understand why our children think we shouldn't talk about sexual feelings at our age."

9. The parents of a 10 year old are interested in knowing if his use of inappropriate language is "normal." The nurse explains that children of this age group:
   A) Imitate their parents' actions
   B) Explore romantic relationships
   C) Engage in aggressive gender activity
   D) Engage in limit testing

10. A 58-year-old woman asks the nurse what she can do to promote healthy sexual relations. Considering the client's age, what would be an appropriate response?
    A) "Continue what you've been doing. Nothing should have changed."
    B) "I will refer you to a sexual therapist to better assist you."
    C) "Using a water-based lubricant may be helpful."
    D) "Reducing the frequency of intercourse may help you."

11. In preparing a presentation on the prevention of sexual abuse, the nurse incorporates which of the following statements?

A) Approximately 25 to 50% of females experience some type of sexual abuse.
B) Sexual abuse is found primarily in lower socioeconomic groups.
C) Abusers fit into easily identified, classic profiles.
D) Most of the incidents occur with strangers or unknown assailants.

12. To increase the tone and sensation of the pelvic floor for a female client, the nurse teaches:
    A) Sensate focus exercises
    B) Kegel exercises
    C) Vaginal dilation
    D) Stop-start techniques

CHAPTER 28

1. A client is scheduled for abdominal surgery tomorrow. During his preparation for surgery, the client reminds the nurse that he is a Jehovah's Witness. There is a need to consider that a person of this religion:
   A) Receives Holy Communion before surgery
   B) Has a religious leader present during surgery
   C) Is opposed to blood transfusions
   D) Must have any removed body parts buried

2. An aspect of caring that plays a tremendous role in the promotion of a client's spiritual well-being is:
   A) Using intuition to select nursing interventions
   B) Establishing a nursing presence
   C) Identifying spiritual cues
   D) Making decisions for the client

3. Which of the following statements best exemplifies what the nurse should say after her client has a near-death experience (NDE)?
   A) "This is a common experience that is easily explained."
   B) "Did you experience anything frightening from your NDE?"
   C) "Have you ever heard of other persons having NDEs?"
   D) "What was your NDE like, and how did it make you feel?"

4. A 76-year-old client has just been admitted to the nursing unit with "terminal cancer of the liver." Which of the following is the best nursing statement in assessing the client's spirituality?
   A) "I notice you have a Bible—is that a source of spiritual strength to you?"
   B) "What do you believe happens to your spirit when you die?"
   C) "We will allow members of your church to visit you whenever you desire."
   D) "Does your terminal condition make you not have the same spiritual beliefs?"

5. A client with diabetes is being cared for in her home by a home health nurse and a family member. The client asks you if eating a vegetarian diet will conflict with the disease. The client is most likely a member of which one of the following religions?
   A) Hinduism
   B) Buddhism
   C) Islam
   D) Sikhism

6. Hope may be used effectively with clients who have terminal diseases. Hope provides a:
   A) Relationship with a divinity
   B) System of organized beliefs
   C) Cultural connectedness
   D) Meaning and purpose

7. While working with a client to assess and support spirituality, the nurse should first:
   A) Refer the client to the agency chaplain
   B) Determine the client's perceptions and belief system
   C) Assist the client to use faith to get well
   D) Provide a variety of religious literature

8. If a client is following the traditional health care beliefs of Judaism, the nurse should prepare to incorporate the following into care:
   A) Observance of the Sabbath
   B) Faith healing
   C) Ongoing group prayer
   D) A fatalistic view of health

9. The nurse is conferring with the nutritionist about the needs of a Native American. The nurse anticipates that the client will:
   A) Follow a strict vegetarian diet
   B) Avoid the use of alcohol and tobacco
   C) Avoid pork products
   D) Follow a diet according to individual beliefs

10. Which of the following nursing diagnoses most indicates a need to plan for a client's spiritual needs?
    A) Health maintenance, altered
    B) Coping, ineffective individual
    C) Memory, impaired
    D) Adaptive capacity, decreased: intracranial

11. The nurse is working in the labor and delivery area with parents who are members of the Shinto and Buddhist religions. The nurse expects that after the birth of the child:
    A) Baptism will be performed immediately
    B) Special prayers will be said over the child
    C) Special preparations will be made for the umbilical cord and placenta
    D) No particular rituals will be performed in the immediate postpartum period

320   Test Bank

CHAPTER 29

1. According to Engel, three phases are involved in the grieving process. By experiencing these steps, a person is believed to:
   A) Die with dignity
   B) Develop self-awareness
   C) Accept the inevitable
   D) Help family members

2. Anticipatory grieving can be beneficial to a client or family because it can:
   A) Be done in private
   B) Draw a family closer to help care for each other more
   C) Be discussed with others
   D) Help a person progress to a healthier emotional state

3. A newly graduated nurse is assigned to his first dying patient. The nurse is best prepared to care for this client if he:
   A) Has completed a course dealing with death and dying
   B) Is able to control his own emotions about death
   C) Has developed a personal understanding of his own feelings about death
   D) Has experienced the death of a loved one

4. When caring for a dying client who is in pain, the nurse should provide:
   A) Pain medication on a regular schedule
   B) Frequent bathing and skin care
   C) An environment that is quiet and limits visitors
   D) Backrubs and positioning every 2 hours

5. The nurse is assigned to a client who was recently diagnosed with a terminal illness. During morning care, the client asks about organ donation. The nurse should:
   A) Have the client first discuss the subject with his family
   B) Suggest that the client delay making a decision at this time
   C) Assist the client to obtain the information necessary to make this decision
   D) Contact the client's physician in order to obtain consent from the family

6. A client has been diagnosed with terminal cancer of the liver and is receiving chemotherapy on a medical unit. In an in-depth conversation with the nurse, the client states, "I wonder why this happened to me?" Which stage is this associated with?
   A) Anxiety
   B) Denial
   C) Confrontation
   D) Depression

7. A client is dying from an unexplained condition of the bone marrow. Which of the following is true for the client's family in this situation?
   A) Family members should be told to be emotionally controlled and to be a source of support for the client.
   B) Children should not be told how serious the client's condition is until the client has stabilized his/her own emotions.
   C) The client's spouse should be given information that explains how he/she may go through stages of grief in a different manner from the client.
   D) The spouse should be expected to react in the same manner as in other crises that have occurred in the past.

8. Which of the following is the primary concern of the nurse for providing care to a dying client? The nurse should:
   A) Attempt to assess hope in the client and to be a source of encouragement to the client
   B) Intervene in the client's activities of daily living and promote as near normal functions as possible
   C) Allow the client to be alone and expect isolation on the part of the dying person
   D) Promote dignity and self-esteem in as many interventions as possible

9. Which of the following is true concerning hospice nursing care?
   A) It is designed to meet the client's individual wishes, as much as possible.
   B) It usually aims at offering curative treatment for the dying client.
   C) It involves learning how to provide postmortem care.
   D) It offers quality care to clients with good third party payment plans.

10. An 11 year old is seeing a counselor to help her deal with the death of a maternal grandmother. The counselor should expect this child to make which of the following statements?
    A) "I wonder if Grandma will ever come back."
    B) "I think I'll start going to church with Mom now."
    C) "I'm not ever going to die—it makes everyone too sad."
    D) "I wonder if I'll die of a heart attack, too."

11. To maintain the client's sense of self-worth during the end of life, the nurse should:
    A) Leave the client alone to deal with final affairs
    B) Call upon the client's spiritual advisor to take over care
    C) Plan regular visits throughout the day
    D) Have a grief counselor visit

12. A nursing intervention to assist the client with a nursing diagnosis of *Sleep pattern disturbance related to the loss of spouse and fear of nightmares* should be:
    A) Administer sleeping medication per order
    B) Refer the client to a psychologist or psychotherapist
    C) Complete a sleep pattern assessment
    D) Sit with the client and encourage verbalization of feelings

13. To promote comfort specific to nausea and vomiting for the terminally ill client, the nurse:
    A) Provides prompt mouth care
    B) Offers high protein foods
    C) Increases the fluid intake
    D) Administers analgesics

14. A nurse-initiated activity for promotion of respiratory function in a terminally ill client is:
    A) Positioning the client upright
    B) Reducing narcotic analgesic use
    C) Limiting fluids
    D) Administering bronchodilators

15. The client yells at the nurse, "Do things look that bad?" The nurse should respond by saying which of the following?
    A) "I'll be back when you are able to talk reasonably."
    B) "Do you think that you are dying?"
    C) "I'll tell the doctor how you feel."
    D) "Tell me how you feel right now."

CHAPTER 30

1. A recommended intervention for a lifestyle stress indicator is:
   A) Regular physical exercise
   B) Attendance at a support group
   C) Self-awareness skill development
   D) Time management

2. A nonspecific response of the body to a demand is:
   A) Stress
   B) Distress
   C) Adaptation
   D) Homeostasis

3. A child and his mother have gone to the playroom on the pediatric unit. His mother tells him he cannot have a toy another child is playing with. The child cries, throws a block, and runs over to kick the door. This child is using a mechanism known as:
A) Displacement
B) Compensation
C) Denial
D) Conversion

4. The nurse goes in to check on a client before scheduled surgery. The client states that she is nervous, and her respiratory and pulse rates are elevated. The client is experiencing which type of anxiety?
A) Mild anxiety
B) Moderate anxiety
C) Severe anxiety
D) Panic

5. During the intershift report the nurse notes that a client had been very nervous and preoccupied during the evening and that no family visited. To determine the amount of anxiety that the client is experiencing, the nurse should ask which of the following questions?
A) "Would you like for me to call a family member to come support you?"
B) "Would you like to go down the hall and talk with another client who had the same surgery?"
C) "How serious do you think your illness is?"
D) "You seem worried about something. Would it help to talk about it?"

6. A 23-year-old client who recently had a head injury from a motor vehicle accident is in a state of unconsciousness. Which of the following physiological adaptations is primarily responsible for his level of consciousness?
A) Medulla oblongata
B) Reticular formation
C) Pituitary gland
D) External stress response

7. A client is having psychological counseling for problems in communicating with his mother. Which of the models of stress would her nurse benefit the most from in reference to this stressor?
A) Adaptation model
B) Stimulus-based model
C) Transaction-based model
D) Selye's model of stress

8. The nurse is working with a client who recently developed a staphylococcal infection in a postoperative abdominal wound. The client's abdominal muscles are weakened from the surgery and for the past 8 hours the client has been febrile. Which of the following responses is probably responsible for this febrile condition?
A) Delayed reponse
B) Reflex pain response
C) Generalized response to stress
D) Inflammatory response

9. A 72-year-old client is in a long-term care facility after having had a cerebrovascular accident. The client is non-communicative, enteral feedings are not being absorbed, and respirations are becoming labored. Which of the stages of the GAS is the client experiencing?
A) Resistance stage
B) Exhaustion stage
C) Reflex pain response
D) Alarm reaction

10. A client recently lost a child in a severe case of poisoning. The client tells the nurse, "I don't want to make any new friends right now." This is an example of which of the following indicators of stress?
A) Emotional behavioral indicator
B) Spiritual indicator
C) Sociocultural indicator
D) Intellectual indicator

11. A corporate executive works 60 to 80 hours/week. The client is experiencing some physical signs of stress. The practitioner teaches the client to "include 15 minutes of biofeedback." This is an example of which of the following health promotion interventions?
   A) Structure
   B) Relaxation technique
   C) Time management
   D) Regular exercise

12. The client is assessed by the nurse as experiencing a crisis. The nurse plans to:
   A) Allow the client to work through independent problem-solving
   B) Complete an in-depth evaluation of stressors and responses to the situation
   C) Focus on immediate stress reduction
   D) Recommend ongoing therapy

CHAPTER 31

1. A client has developed pneumonia, and his temperature has increased to 37.7° C. The client is shivering and "feels uncomfortable." Which of the following is true concerning the physiology of heat production in this client?
   A) The increased BMR is probably causing the febrile condition.
   B) Encouraging the client to ambulate would help decrease heat production.
   C) The shivering is likely the cause of the increased temperature.
   D) The client may need to consume more nutrients during the febrile condition.

2. A 74-year-old client currently has a temperature reading of 36° C. The client walks 1 mile every day and takes naps during the day. Which of the following is most likely the reason for the lowered body temperature?

   A) The lowered temperature is a natural result of the aging processes.
   B) Increased stress from exercise has probably reduced the temperature.
   C) The individual circadian rhythm requiring daytime naps lowers the temperature.
   D) Hormone levels are the most probable cause of the hypothermic condition.

3. A construction worker comes to the emergency room with low blood pressure, normal pulse, cool skin temperature, diaphoresis, and weakness. These are clinical signs of:
   A) Heat exhaustion
   B) Heat stroke
   C) Heat cramp
   D) Hypothermia

4. The nurse is ready to take vital signs on a 6-year-old child. The child has just enjoyed a grape popsicle. An appropriate action would be to:
   A) Take the rectal temperature
   B) Take the oral temperature as planned
   C) Have the child rinse out the mouth with warm water
   D) Wait 30 minutes and take the oral temperature

5. The client's pulse is 72/minute, easily palpated. In addition, the pedal pulses are equal in strength in both feet. To best assess for an irregularity in the pulses, the nurse should:
   A) Determine the rate of the pedal pulses
   B) Auscultate for the strength of the apical pulse
   C) Examine the electrocardiogram's reading
   D) Ask the client if there is a pulsation that is abnormal

6. Which of the following is an appropriate site for taking the pulse of a 2-year-old?
   A) Radial
   B) Apical
   C) Femoral
   D) Pedal

7. The client begins to breathe rapidly. The nurse should:
   A) Ask the client if there have been any stressful visitors
   B) Measure the oxygen saturation level
   C) Count the rate of respirations
   D) Take the radial pulse

8. A client complains of pain and asks the nurse for pain medication. The nurse first assesses vital signs: blood pressure, 134/92; pulse, 100; and respiration 32. The nurse's most appropriate action is to:
   A) Ask if the client is anxious
   B) Check the client's dressing for bleeding
   C) Give the medication
   D) Recheck the client's vital signs in 30 minutes

9. If measuring blood pressure is necessary in the leg, the nurse expects the diastolic pressure to be:
   A) 10 to 40 mm Hg higher than in the brachial artery
   B) 20 to 30 mm Hg lower than in the brachial artery
   C) 50 mm Hg higher than in the brachial artery
   D) Essentially the same as that in the brachial artery

10. An 84-year-old diabetic client is admitted for insulin regulation. Which of the following blood pressure, pulse, and respiration measurements, respectively, is considered within the expected limits for this client?
    A) 148/90, 68, 16
    B) 94/52, 68, 30
    C) 108/80, 112, 15
    D) 132/74, 90, 24

11. The student nurse is assessing the vital signs of a 10-year-old client. The expected values for this client are:
    A) P, 140; R, 50; BP, 80/50
    B) P, 100; R, 40; BP, 90/60
    C) P, 80; R, 22; BP, 110/70
    D) P, 60; R,12; BP, 160/90

12. Which of the following vital sign readings is outside of the expected range for a 30-year-old client?
    A) T , 37.4° C
    B) P, 110
    C) R, 20
    D) BP, 120/76

13. In teaching a client at home to accurately assess the axillary temperature of a 1½ -year-old child with a glass thermometer, the nurse should tell the parent to:
    A) Hold the thermometer at the bulb end
    B) Clean the thermometer in hot water
    C) Leave the thermometer in place for 3 to 5 minutes
    D) Let the child hold the thermometer

14. The postoperative vital signs of an average size adult client are: BP, 110/68; P, 54; R, 8. The client appears pale, disoriented, and has minimal urinary output. The nurse should:
    A) Take the vital signs again in 30 minutes
    B) Administer oxygen
    C) Continue with care as planned
    D) Notify the physician

15. A client has just gotten out of bed to go to the bathroom. As the nurse enters the room, the client says, "I feel dizzy." The nurse should:
    A) Take the client's blood pressure
    B) Go for help
    C) Assist the client to sit
    D) Tell the client to take deep breaths

16. A false high blood pressure reading may be assessed if the nurse:
    A) Wraps the cuff too loosely around the arm
    B) Deflates the cuff too quickly
    C) Presses the stethoscope too firmly in the antecubital fossa
    D) Repeats the blood pressure assessment too soon

17. The client's temperature needs to be reduced. The nurse anticipates that which of the following therapies will be initiated?
    A) Alcohol and water bath
    B) Ice packs to the axillae and groin
    C) Cool, plain water sponges
    D) Cooling blanket

18. The nurse is alert to which of the following factors that lowers the blood pressure?
    A) Anxiety
    B) Heavy alcohol consumption
    C) Cigarette smoking
    D) Diuretic administration

CHAPTER 32

1. The position that maximizes the nurse's ability to assess the client's body for symmetry is:
    A) Sitting
    B) Supine
    C) Prone
    D) Dorsal recumbent

2. When examining a dark-skinned client, what part of the body would the nurse assess for pallor?
    A) Buccal mucosa of the mouth
    B) Dorsal surface of the hands
    C) Ear lobe
    D) Sclera

3. A 48-year-old client has cancer of the liver. The skin is jaundiced, and the turgor is poor. Which of the following is true concerning an integumentary assessment for this client?
    A) The skin turgor is probably poor because of the client's age.
    B) Petechiae could be seen in this condition.
    C) Erythema probably exists due to the moist condition of the skin.
    D) The jaundice discoloration would best be assessed on the extremities.

4. A client in the clinic has been having severe headaches and some visual disturbances. The nurse performs an eye examination. Which of the following is true concerning this assessment?
    A) To evaluate the lower eyelids, the nurse uses a syringe with sterile water.
    B) The client's lacrimal apparatus is best assessed by using a dull object to stimulate her normal reflex conditions.
    C) Accommodation is tested by asking the client to comply with the nurse's requests.
    D) The red reflex should be assessed with the ophthalmoscope.

5. A 66-year-old client is having an annual physical examination. The nurse is currently assessing the ears. Which of the following is accurate regarding this assessment?
    A) The auricle should be pulled down and back when using the otoscope.
    B) The cochlea could be responsible for a gradual loss of hearing.
    C) The nurse should palpate the outer ear for any unusual pulsations.
    D) If an internal examination reveals excessive cerumen, it is best removed with a small syringe.

6. The client has an enlarged thyroid gland and is currently admitted to a medical nursing unit. Which of the following is accurate regarding a neck assessment for this client?
    A) Swallowing should cause the lateral aspect of the thyroid gland to rise.
    B) The postauricular nodes should be examined visually.
    C) The sternocleidomastoid muscle is best assessed when hyperextending the neck.
    D) A soft bruit over the thyroid area indicates infected and potentially enlarged lymph nodes.

7. A normal vesicular sound is a:
   A) Medium-pitched blowing sound with inspiration equaling expiration
   B) Loud, high-pitched hollow sound with expiration longer than inspiration
   C) Soft, breezy, low-pitched sound with longer inspiration
   D) Sound created by air moving through small airways

8. The nurse could best auscultate the point of maximum impulse (PMI) in an 8-year-old child at the:
   A) Fourth intercostal space, left of the midclavicular line
   B) Fifth intercostal space, left of the midclavicular line
   C) Second intercostal space, right of the midclavicular line
   D) Third intercostal space, left of the midclavicular line

9. Which of the following signs and symptoms indicate vascular disease?
   A) Headache, dizziness, tingling of a body part
   B) Diplopia, floaters, headache
   C) Leg cramps, numbness of extremities, edema
   D) Pain and cramping in lower extremities relieved by walking

10. A 21-year-old woman asks when she should perform a breast self-examination during the month. The nurse should state which of the following?
    A) "Any time you think of it."
    B) "At the same time each month."
    C) "On the first day of your menstrual period."
    D) "On the last day of your menstrual period."

11. The client has abdominal pain of unknown origin. During the abdominal examination, which of the following is most accurate?

A) The palpation should be performed first.
B) Auscultation is best done with the client in the sitting position.
C) Bowel sounds should be heard by examining each quadrant for 5 minutes.
D) A paralytic ileus would result in low, growling sounds.

12. Asking a client to explain the meaning of the phrase, "Every cloud has a silver lining," measures:
    A) Knowledge
    B) Judgment
    C) Association
    D) Abstract thinking

13. Measurement of the client's ability to differentiate between sharp and dull sensations over the forehead tests which cranial nerve?
    A) Optic
    B) Trigeminal
    C) Facial
    D) Oculomotor

14. Assessment of the skin reveals a fluid-filled circumscribed elevation of 0.4 cm. The nurse identifies this as a:
    A) Nodule
    B) Macule
    C) Vesicle
    D) Wheal

15. The expected appearance of the oral mucosa in a light-skinned adult is:
    A) Pinkish-red, smooth, and moist
    B) Light pink, rough, and dry
    C) Cyanotic with rough nodules
    D) Deep red with rough edges

16. In the assessment of a 90-year-old client, the nurse documents an exaggeration of the posterior curvature of the thoracic spine as:
    A) Lordosis
    B) Osteoporosis
    C) Scoliosis
    D) Kyphosis

17. If a mitral valve problem is suspected, the best position for the nurse to place the client in to auscultate the apical site is:
    A) Sitting up
    B) Standing
    C) Lying on the left side
    D) In the dorsal recumbent position

18. The nurse wants to assess the client's balance. The test that should be administered is the:
    A) Weber test
    B) Allen test
    C) Romberg test
    D) Rinne test

19. Part of the neurological exam is evaluating the response of the cranial nerves. To test cranial nerve VIII, the nurse should:
    A) Ask the client to read printed material
    B) Assess the directions of the gaze
    C) Assess the client's ability to hear the spoken word
    D) Ask the client to say "ah"

20. A student nurse is working with a client who has asthma. The primary nurse tells the student that wheezes can be heard on auscultation. The student expects to hear:
    A) Coarse crackles and bubbling
    B) High-pitched musical sounds
    C) Dry, grating noises
    D) Loud, low pitched rumbling

21. The protocol for testicular self-examination is for men to:
    A) Perform the exam annually after age 35
    B) Perform the exam prior to bathing or showering
    C) Contact the physician if a cordlike structure is felt on the top and back of the testicle
    D) Use both hands to roll the testicles and feel the consistency

22. A recommended annual screening for female adults aged 40 years and up is:
    A) A complete eye examination
    B) Total skin examination
    C) A complete hearing check
    D) A mammogram

23. The nurse uses olfaction in the client's assessment. If a sweet, fruity smell is noticed in the oral cavity, the nurse suspects:
    A) Diabetic acidosis
    B) Gum disease
    C) Malabsorption syndrome
    D) Stomatitis

CHAPTER 33

1. The client has a 6-inch laceration on his right forearm that develops an infection. Which of the following is a sign of an acute inflammatory process?
    A) A decrease in the number of white blood cells
    B) A release of histamine that adds to the pain response
    C) A blanching of the skin
    D) A decrease in temperature at the site

2. A child receives a vaccine for measles, mumps, and rubella. The client has experienced which type of immunity?
    A) Natural immunity
    B) Artificial immunity
    C) Passive immunity
    D) Complete immunity

3. Which of the following could contribute to causing a nosocomial infection?
    A) Washing hands before applying a dressing
    B) Taping a plastic bag to the bed rail for tissue disposal
    C) Placing a Foley catheter bag on the bed when transferring a client
    D) Using Betadine to cleanse the skin before starting an intravenous line

4. Which of the following clients is most susceptible to infection?
   A) A 29-year-old postpartum client
   B) A 42-year-old client with a recent uncomplicated appendectomy
   C) A 76-year-old client with a hip fracture
   D) An 18-year-old athlete with repair of torn knee ligaments

5. A 78-year-old client admitted to the medical unit is at risk for infection because of the following physiological changes:
   A) Increased cough reflex
   B) Thicker, more elastic skin
   C) Increase in stomach acid
   D) Reduced salivary production

6. The nurse shows that he understands the psychological implications of isolation when he plans care to control the client's risk of:
   A) Denial
   B) Depression
   C) Regression
   D) Aggression

7. The nurse employs surgical aseptic technique when:
   A) Placing soiled linen in moisture-resistant bags
   B) Inserting an intravenous catheter
   C) Disposing of syringes in puncture-proof containers
   D) Washing his or her hands before changing a dressing

8. The client has a large abdominal incision that requires a dressing. The incision is packed with half-inch iodoform packing (soaked in Betadine) and covered with a dry sterile 4 × 4 inch gauze. When changing the dressing, the nurse accidentally drops the packing onto the client's abdomen. The nurse should:

A) Add more Betadine to the packing and insert it into the incision
B) Throw the packing away, and prepare a new one
C) Pick up the packing with sterile forceps, and gently place it into the incision
D) Rinse the packing with sterile water, and put the packing into the incision with sterile gloves

9. A client has a viral infection. Which of the following is typical of the illness stage of the course of the infection?
   A) There are no longer any acute symptoms.
   B) The client was first exposed to the infection 2 days ago but has no symptoms.
   C) An oral temperature reveals a very febrile condition.
   D) The client "feels sick" but is able to continue her normal activities.

10. Medical asepsis is applied when the nurse:
    A) Completes handwashing before care
    B) Prepares an intramuscular injection
    C) Changes a postoperative dressing
    D) Suctions a tracheostomy

11. The nurse recognizes that special care must be taken in the handling of which of the following in order to prevent the transmission of hepatitis A?
    A) Blood
    B) Feces
    C) Vaginal secretions
    D) Saliva

12. The use of acid-reducing medications may lead to an overgrowth of gastrointestinal organisms. The nursing staff should be alert to the possibility that this could contribute to:
    A) Urinary tract infection
    B) Hepatitis
    C) Nosocomial pneumonia
    D) Cellulitis

13. The parent of a preschool child asks the nurse how chickenpox (varicella zoster) is transmitted. The nurse explains that the virus is:
    A) Carried through the air in droplets after sneezing or coughing
    B) Transmitted through person to person contact
    C) Carried by a vector organism
    D) Acquired through contact with contaminated objects

14. Vulnerable clients with which of the following have the greatest risk for infection?
    A) Second-degree burns
    B) Diabetes mellitus
    C) Multiple sclerosis
    D) Emphysema

15. While working with clients in the postoperative period, the nurse is very alert to the results of laboratory tests. Which one of the following results is indicative of an infectious process?
    A) Iron 80 g/100 ml
    B) White blood cells (WBC) 18,000/mm³
    C) Erythrocyte sedimentation rate (ESR) — 15 mm/hr
    D) Neutrophils — 65%

16. A nursing intervention that reduces a reservoir of infection for a client is:
    A) Covering the mouth and nose when sneezing or coughing
    B) Wearing disposable gloves
    C) Isolating the client's articles
    D) Changing soiled dressings

17. The single most important technique to prevent and control the transmission of infections is:
    A) The use of disposable gloves
    B) Handwashing
    C) The use of isolation precautions
    D) Sterilization of equipment

18. A client with active tuberculosis requires implementation of which of the following guidelines?
    A) Airborne precautions
    B) Droplet precautions
    C) Contact precautions
    D) Basic precautions

19. Which of the following is an appropriate technique for sterile asepsis?
    A) Clean forceps may be used to move items on the sterile field.
    B) Sterile fields may be prepared well in advance of the procedures.
    C) The first small amount of sterile solution should be poured and discarded.
    D) Wrapped sterile packages should be opened starting with the flap closest to the nurse.

CHAPTER 34

1. A client is nauseated, has been vomiting for several hours, and needs to receive an antiemetic (antinausea) medication. Which of the following is accurate?
   A) An enteric-coated medication should be given.
   B) No medication will be absorbed easily because of the nausea
   C) A parenteral route is the route of choice.
   D) A rectal suppository must be administered.

2. The client receiving an intravenous infusion of morphine sulfate begins to experience respiratory depression and decreased urine output. This effect is described as:
   A) Therapeutic
   B) Toxic
   C) Idiosyncratic
   D) Allergic

3. The client is to receive a sedative via the buccal route. Which of the following is true?
   A) The medication is placed under the tongue.
   B) This route is probably more expensive than the intramuscular route.
   C) The nurse should offer the client a glass of orange juice after taking the sedative.
   D) This method of administration would be avoided in the event of facial injuries.

4. The physician orders a grain and a half of secobarbital to help a client sleep. The label on the medication bottle reads secobarbital 100 mg. How many capsules should the nurse give the client?
   A) ½
   B) 1
   C) 1½
   D) 2

5. The physician has ordered 6 mg morphine sulfate every 3 to 4 hours prn for a client's postoperative pain. The unit dose in the medication dispenser has 15 mg in 1 mL. How much solution should the nurse give?
   A) 0.2 ml
   B) 0.3 ml
   C) 0.4 ml
   D) 0.25 ml

6. To determine the proper drug dosages for children, the most precise calculations are made on the basis of the child's:
   A) Weight
   B) Height
   C) Age
   D) Body surface area

7. The nurse uses a mortar and pestle to crush a medication before giving it to one of her clients. Which of the five rights is the nurse ensuring?

A) The right route
B) The right client
C) The right time
D) The right drug

8. A 76-year-old client lives alone and takes medications without supervision. Which of the following is the most appropriate question for his home health nurse to ask in regard to his medication regimen?
   A) "How much do you weigh?"
   B) "What medications are you currently taking?"
   C) "We'll have to take away your sedatives if you keep taking them during the day."
   D) "Have you been taking substances other than those ordered by the physician?"

9. In preparing two different medications from two vials, the nurse must:
   A) Inject fluid from one vial into the other
   B) Uncap the syringe and wipe the needle with an alcohol preparation before inserting it into either vial
   C) Discard the medication from vial number two if medication from vial number one is pushed into it
   D) Insert air into the first vial, but not the second vial

10. The nurse is preparing 10 U of regular insulin and 5 U of NPH insulin. Which of the following statements is the most accurate?
    A) The NPH insulin is the shortest-acting form of insulin.
    B) Air is injected first into the regular insulin, then into the NPH.
    C) The insulin vial should be discarded if there are any bubbles in it.
    D) This medication order is given via the subcutaneous route.

11. A 73-year-old client who is very obese requires an intramuscular injection of Demerol 100 mg. Which of the following is least appropriate for the administration of this medication?
    A) A $5/8$-inch needle used at a 45-degree angle to the skin
    B) Pinching the skin before administration
    C) Aspirating the syringe before injecting the medication
    D) Using a 25-gauge needle

12. The student nurse reads the order to give a 1-year-old client an intramuscular injection. The appropriate and preferred muscle to select for a child would be the:
    A) Deltoid
    B) Dorsogluteal
    C) Ventrogluteal
    D) Vastus lateralis

13. The nurse administers the intramuscular medication of iron by the **Z**-track method. The medication was administered by this method to:
    A) Provide faster absorption of the medication
    B) Reduce discomfort from the needle
    C) Provide more even absorption of the drug
    D) Prevent the drug from irritating sensitive tissue

14. The client is ordered to have eyedrops administered daily to both eyes. Eyedrops should be instilled on the:
    A) Outer canthus
    B) Cornea
    C) Lower conjunctival sac
    D) Opening of the lacrimal duct

15. Following the administration of ear drops to the left ear, the client should be placed in which of the following positions?
    A) Sitting up
    B) Prone
    C) Right lateral
    D) Dorsal recumbent with hyperextension of the neck

16. The order is for eye medication, ii gtts OD. The nurse administers:
    A) 2 cc to the right eye
    B) 2 drops to the left eye
    C) 2 drops to the right eye
    D) 2 drops to both eyes

17. In the acute care environment, the most effective way to determine the client's identity prior to administering medications is to:
    A) Ask the client's name
    B) Check the name on the chart
    C) Ask the other caregivers
    D) Check the client's name band

18. An order is written for Demerol 500 mg IM q3-4h prn for pain. The nurse recognizes that this is significantly more than the usual therapeutic dose. The nurse should:
    A) Give 50 mg IM as was probably intended to be written
    B) Refuse to give the medication and notify the nurse manager
    C) Administer the medication and watch the client carefully
    D) Call the prescriber to clarify the order

19. An order is written for 80 mg of a medication in elixir form. The medication is available in 80 mg/5 mL strength. The nurse prepares to administer:
    A) 2 mL
    B) 5 mL
    C) 10 mL
    D) 15 mL

20. Which of the following angles of injection is appropriate for an intradermal injection?
    A) 15 degrees
    B) 30 degrees
    C) 45 degrees
    D) 90 degrees

21. The nurse prepares an intradermal injection for the administration of medication for:
    A) Pain
    B) Allergy sensitivity
    C) Anticoagulant therapy
    D) Low-dose insulin requirements

22. The nurse is evaluating the integrity of the ventrogluteal injection site. The nurse finds the site by locating the:
    A) Middle third of the lateral thigh
    B) Head of the femur, anterior iliac spine, and iliac crest
    C) Greater trochanter of the femur, posterior iliac spine, and iliac crest
    D) Acromion process and axilla

23. Heparin is usually administered to the client in the:
    A) Scapular region
    B) Vastus lateralis
    C) Posterior gluteal region
    D) Abdomen

CHAPTER 35

1. Therapeutic touch may be most effective for which of the following clients?
   A) Unstable premature infant
   B) Headache sufferer
   C) Pregnant woman
   D) Psychiatric client

2. A nurse giving a presentation about herbal therapies to a community group should inform them that herbal medicines:
   A) Have fewer side effects than allopathic medicines
   B) Are natural plants and are therefore safe to ingest

C) Are of a consistent quality due to adherence to standards of quality control
D) Should be used with caution by pregnant and nursing mothers

3. The client asks the nurse about a herbal remedy that may relieve her insomnia. Information may appropriately be provided on:
   A) Ginkgo biloba
   B) Ginger
   C) Echinacea
   D) St. John's wort

4. When assessing a client's history of use of CAM therapies, the nurse should ask:
   A) "What herbal supplements have you taken?"
   B) "What remedies, diet, or other habits do you employ in your daily life to ensure a sense of well-being?"
   C) "Have you ever used relaxation or other biobehavioural therapy?"
   D) "Do you use holistic treatments?"

5. Which of the following statements is correct regarding CAM in Canada?
   A) Fifty percent of Canadians reported using alternative therapies in 1996.
   B) Physicians frequently suggest patients with chronic conditions explore complementary therapies.
   C) In a 1997 telephone survey, 44 percent of those using CAM therapies found them effective.
   D) CAM and its therapies are fully covered by publicly funded provincial health insurance.

6. A benefit that the client can gain from relaxation therapy is a decrease in:
   A) Receptivity
   B) Peripheral skin temperature
   C) Oxygen consumption
   D) Alpha brain activity

7. A client who may benefit the most from the passive type of relaxation is one who is experiencing:
   A) Hypertension
   B) Dysfunctional grieving
   C) Terminal cancer
   D) Work-related stress

8. A client who has Raynaud's disease with intermittent peripheral ischemia may benefit the most from:
   A) Relaxation therapy
   B) Imagery
   C) Biofeedback
   D) Acupuncture

9. A nurse needs to be alert to possible negative effects of meditation for some clients. Clients may experience:
   A) Aggressive feelings
   B) Delusions
   C) Insomnia
   D) Loss of control

10. Practitioners of traditional Chinese medicine base their understanding of the human body on the primary concept of:
   A) Yin and yang
   B) Twelve meridians
   C) Six evil senses
   D) Acupressure points

CHAPTER 36

1. The nurse assists a very tall, obese male client to a standing position each morning. The nurse should:
   A) Keep her feet close together
   B) Move slightly away from the client as he begins to stand
   C) Stand on her tiptoes when the client is in a standing position to keep their center of gravity closer together
   D) Assess the client's weight and consider asking another nurse to assist her

2. What is the first step in assessing the body alignment of an alert and mobile client?
   A) Determine activity tolerance.
   B) Determine range of joint motion.
   C) Observe gait.
   D) Put the client at ease.

3. A male client of average size has right-sided hemiparesis. The nurse helps this client to walk by:
   A) Standing at his left side and holding his arm
   B) Standing at his left side and holding one arm around his waist
   C) Standing at his right side and holding his arm
   D) Standing at his right side and holding one arm around his waist

4. The nurse is working with a client who has left-sided weakness. After instructing the client in proper use of a cane the nurse watches the client ambulate in order to evaluate his use of the cane. Which action indicates that the client knows how to use the cane properly?
   A) After advancing the cane, the client moves the right leg forward.
   B) The client keeps the cane on the left side.
   C) Two points of support are kept on the floor at all times.
   D) There is a slight lean to the right when the client is walking.

5. A client with a fractured left femur has been using crutches for the past 4 weeks. The physician tells the client to begin putting a little weight on the left foot when walking. Which of the following gaits should the client use?
   A) Two-point
   B) Three-point
   C) Four-point
   D) Swing-through

6. The client needs to use crutches at home and will have to manage going up and down a short flight of stairs. The nurse evaluates the use of an appropriate technique if the client:
   A) Uses a banister or wall for support when descending
   B) Advances the affected leg after moving the crutches to descend the stairs
   C) Uses one crutch for support while going up and down
   D) Advances the crutches first to ascend the stairs

7. While ambulating in the hallway of a hospital, the client complains of extreme dizziness. The nurse, alert to a syncopal episode, should first:
   A) Support the client and walk quickly back to the room
   B) Lean the client against the wall until the episode passes
   C) Lower the client gently to the floor
   D) Call for help

8. The nurse correctly teaches the client which one of the following principles of range-of-motion exercises?
   A) Flex the joint to the point of discomfort
   B) Work from proximal to distal joints
   C) Move the joints quickly
   D) Provide support for distal joints

9. Which principle of body mechanics should the nurse incorporate into client care?
   A) Flex the knees and keep the feet wide apart
   B) Assume a position far enough away from the client
   C) Twist the body in the direction of movement
   D) Use the strong back muscles for lifting or moving

10. The nurse is presenting a teaching session on exercise for a group of corporate executives. An appropriate recommendation is that:
    A) Continuous activity is required in order for the exercise to be worthwhile
    B) 3000 to 4000 calories may be easily expended each week
    C) Lower-intensity activities need to be done more often for value
    D) Only formal exercise activities are counted in a regular plan

CHAPTER 37

1. In regard to safety, which of the following statements is most accurate?
   A) Bacterial contamination of foods is uncontrollable.
   B) Fire is the greatest cause of unintentional death.
   C) Temperature extremes seldom affect the safety of clients in acute care facilities.
   D) Carbon monoxide levels should be monitored in home settings.

2. A 76-year-old client lives alone at home. Which of the following is the highest priority question for his home health nurse to ask regarding his safety?
   A) "Do you use softglow light bulbs in your front room lamps?"
   B) "At what temperature is your thermostat set?"
   C) "Why don't you consider selling your two-story home and buying a house without stairs?"
   D) "Do any of your medications cause you to be physically unsteady?"

3. Which of the following questions has the highest priority for the nurse when talking with parents about the safety of a 4 year old?
A) "Can you talk to the parents of your child's friend to find out why they are getting in fights?"
B) "Would the families in your neighborhood share your concern about reporting strangers when they see them?"
C) "Do you have the kitchen cleaning supplies locked in the cupboard?"
D) "Does your child have the appropriate protective equipment for the games he plays?"

4. The best overall rule for avoiding accidents with equipment in the hospital is for the nurse to:
A) Always lock wheels on movable equipment
B) Never operate equipment without prior instruction
C) Always unplug equipment when moving the client
D) Never use equipment without a person to assist you

5. A 4-year-old child is scheduled to receive an IV line. The most appropriate type of restraint to use for this client to prevent removal of the IV line would be a(n):
A) Wrist restraint
B) Jacket restraint
C) Elbow restraint
D) Mummy restraint

6. A 79-year-old resident in a long-term care facility is known to "wander at night" and has fallen in the past. Which of the following is the most appropriate nursing intervention?
A) A loose abdominal restraint should be placed on the client during sleeping hours.
B) The caregivers should check the client frequently during the night.

C) A radio should be left playing at the bedside to assist in reality orientation.
D) Reassign the client to a room that is close to the nursing station.

7. The workmen cause an electrical fire when installing a new piece of equipment in the intensive care unit. A client is on a ventilator in the next room. The first action the nurse should take is to:
A) Attempt to extinguish the fire
B) Pull the fire alarm
C) Call the physician to obtain orders to take the client off the ventilator
D) Use an Ambu bag and remove the client from the area

8. In a nursing home an elderly client drops his burning cigarette in a trash can and starts a fire. The most appropriate type of fire extinguisher for the nurse to use is the:
A) Type A
B) Type B
C) Type C
D) Type D

9. A frantic grandmother calls the emergency room to report that her grandson took some of her medicine and that she is unable to arouse him. The nurse should instruct her to:
A) Induce vomiting with syrup of ipecac
B) Provide fluids to dilute the toxin
C) Hyperextend his head
D) Bring the medicine bottle to the hospital

10. In teaching parents how to promote infant safety, the nurse tells them to:
A) Place the infant on its abdomen for sleeping
B) Use small toys sized for the infant
C) Place the infant in a highchair or swing when the child must be unattended
D) Ensure crib sheets fit very snugly

11. Which of the following statements by the parent of a child indicates that further teaching by the nurse is required?
    A) "Now that my child is 2 years old I can let her sit in the front seat of the car with me."
    B) "I make sure that my child wears a helmet when he rides his bicycle."
    C) "I have spoken to my child about safe sex practices."
    D) "My child is taking swimming classes at the community center."

12. The nurse assesses that the client may need a restraint and recognizes that:
    A) An order for a restraint may be implemented indefinitely until it is no longer required by the client
    B) Restraints may be ordered on a prn basis
    C) No order or consent is necessary for restraints in long-term care facilities
    D) Restraints are to be removed periodically to have the client re-evaluated

CHAPTER 38

1. The client has a red, raised skin rash. Which of the following is most important when cleansing the skin?
   A) Assess for further inflammatory reactions
   B) Discuss the body image problems created by the presence of the rash
   C) Wash the skin thoroughly each day with hot water and soap
   D) Moisturize the skin to prevent drying

2. The nurse is caring for a client who is paralyzed on the right side. Which of the following factors is most likely to result in decubitus ulcer formation?
   A) Poor nutrition
   B) Immobility
   C) Reduced hydration
   D) Skin secretions

3. When giving a bath to a newborn, the nurse should:
   A) Use mild soap such as Ivory
   B) Use powder after the bath
   C) Put baby oil in the water
   D) Wash with water only

4. The nurse delegates morning care to a new certified nursing assistant. Which of the following actions by the assistant would appropriate?
   A) Placing the client's dentures in a tissue while the are not being worn
   B) Cutting the client's nails with scissors
   C) Washing the client's legs with long strokes from the ankle to the knee
   D) Using soap to cleanse the client's eye orbits

5. A 61-year-old client with diabetes mellitus has physician's orders for meticulous foot care. Which of the following is the best rationale for this order?
   A) The aging process causes increased skin breakdown.
   B) There is increased neuropathy with diabetes mellitus that places the client at risk.
   C) The client probably has a history of poor hygienic care.
   D) The lower extremities are difficult to see and are therefore hard to maintain with good hygiene.

6. The client is unable to rest even after medication. The nurse decides to give the client a backrub. Which of the following strokes should the nurse use when finishing the backrub?
   A) Long firm strokes down the back
   B) Light strokes while moving up the back in a circular motion
   C) Kneading movements toward the sacrum
   D) Circular motion upward from buttocks to shoulders

7. The nurse should avoid using lemon-glycerin swabs on a client's tongue and mucous membranes because regular use of this product:
   A) Erodes tooth enamel
   B) Reduces adhesion to the mucous membrane
   C) Swells gums and mucous membranes
   D) Destroys normal mouth bacteria

8. To administer oral care to a semi-comatose client, the nurse should place the client in which of the following positions?
   A) Reverse Trendelenberg
   B) High Fowler's with the head to the side
   C) Side-lying with the head turned toward the nurse
   D) Supine with the neck slightly forward

9. The client is unable to perform self-care for the hair. Which of the following is accurate when performing hair care?
   A) Brushing the hair distributes the natural oils evenly.
   B) Using a hot comb may be very helpful for straight and oily hair.
   C) Very tight braids keep the hair in good condition.
   D) Shampooing should be done daily.

10. A client has recently experienced difficulty hearing out of both ears. Which of the following is the best nursing response to the client?
    A) "Can you turn your head toward me when I am talking to you?"
    B) "Your hearing aid should not need a new battery for at least 3 months."
    C) "Let's irrigate your ears with cool water."
    D) "Try to avoid putting a Q-Tip (cotton-tipped applicator) into your ears."

11. An adolescent client with acne should be taught by the nurse to:

A) Apply antiseptic sprays or creams
B) Wash the face and hair daily with hot water and soap
C) Use a depilatory to remove excess hair
D) Add moisture with the use of a humidifier

12. A client who is unable to complete a bath because of right-sided weakness has a nursing diagnosis of:
    A) Knowledge deficit of hygiene practices
    B) Powerlessness
    C) Self-care deficit
    D) Tissue integrity impairment

13. A different approach to traditional hygienic care is the "bag bath." The best rationale for using this approach is that it:
    A) Is less expensive than the traditional method
    B) Takes less time to complete
    C) Leaves the skin softer
    D) Reduces the risk of infection

14. The position of choice for female perineal care is:
    A) Dorsal recumbent
    B) Side-lying
    C) Supine
    D) Prone

15. A client suspected of having vascular insufficiency to the lower extremities is assessed by the nurse to have a(n):
    A) Increased hair growth on the legs and feet
    B) Dull appearance of the skin
    C) Erythema on elevation of the feet
    D) Diminished pedal pulses

16. In teaching a client about proper foot care, the nurse should emphasize:
    A) Using scissors to cut the nails straight
    B) Soaking the feet daily in warm water
    C) Changing socks regularly
    D) Applying heating pads to promote circulation

17. If a male client has an erection during perineal care, the nurse should:
    A) Continue with the procedure
    B) Tell the client it's okay and just to relax
    C) Ask the client to try and do the care as well as he can
    D) Defer the care until a little later in the procedure

18. For a client with stomatitis, the nurse advises the use of:
    A) A commercial mouthwash
    B) An alcohol and water mixture
    C) Normal saline rinses
    D) A firm toothbrush

CHAPTER 39

1. Which of the following is true concerning the physiology of the cardiovascular system?
    A) Stimulating the parasympathetic system would cause the heart rate to go up.
    B) When a person has heart muscle disease, the heart muscles stretch as far as is necessary to maintain function.
    C) The QRS interval on the electrocardiogram represents the electrical impulses passing through the ventricles.
    D) When stroke volume decreases, there is a resultant decrease in heart rate.

2. The client has emphysema from smoking. During a respiratory system assessment the nurse anticipates finding:
    A) Abnormal palpation signs in the upper thorax
    B) Dull sounds on percussion
    C) A depressed sternum on inspection
    D) Moist breath sounds on auscultation

3. A 64-year-old client is seen in the emergency room for palpitations and mild shortness of breath. The ECG reveals a normal P wave, P-R interval, and QRS complex with a regular rhythm and rate of 108. The nurse should recognize this cardiac dysrhythmia as:
    A) Sinus dysrhythmia
    B) Sinus tachycardia
    C) Supraventricular tachycardia
    D) Ventricular tachycardia

4. A client recently fractured his spinal cord at the C-3 level and is at great risk for developing pneumonia primarily because:
    A) The resulting paralysis immobilizes him, and secretions will increase in his lungs
    B) Innervation to the phrenic nerve is absent, preventing chest expansion
    C) The resulting abnormal chest shape disallows efficient ventilatory movement
    D) Trauma decreases the ability of his red blood cells to carry oxygen

5. The client has experienced a myocardial infarction damaging the right ventricle. Which of the following is a likely complication he would experience?
    A) Jugular neck vein distention
    B) Pulmonary congestion
    C) Peripheral edema
    D) Liver enlargement

6. On admitting a client, the nurse finds that there is a history of myocardial ischemia. The most disconcerting dysrhythmia for electrocardiography to reveal is:
    A) Sinus bradycardia
    B) Paroxysmal supraventricular tachycardia
    C) Ventricular tachycardia
    D) Premature ventricular contractions

7. A client develops acute renal failure and a resulting metabolic acidosis. The respiratory system compensates by:
   A) Hypoventilating and increasing the bicarbonate in the bloodstream
   B) Alternating periods of deep versus shallow breaths to maintain homeostasis of the serum pH
   C) Hyperventilating to decrease the serum CO_2 and thereby raise the pH
   D) Expanding the lung tissues to their fullest, which increases the inspiratory reserve volumes to provide more oxygen to the tissues

8. For a client who is having respiratory symptoms of unknown etiology, the diagnostic test that is most invasive is:
   A) Pulse oximetry to determine oxygen saturation levels
   B) Throat cultures with sterile swabs
   C) Bronchoscopy of the bronchial trees
   D) Computed tomography of the lung fields

9. The nurse identifies that the client is unable to cough to produce a sputum specimen and must be suctioned. Which suctioning route is preferred?
   A) Nasopharyngeal
   B) Nasotracheal
   C) Oropharyngeal
   D) Orotracheal

10. To help the client prevent postoperative pulmonary complications, preoperatively the nurse should:
    A) Ask the physician to order nebulizer treatments
    B) Teach the client to do leg exercises
    C) Teach the client to use a flow-oriented incentive spirometer
    D) Tell the client that if he does not cough, he may need to be suctioned

11. A client has recently had a mitral valve replacement. To prevent excess serosanguinous fluid buildup, the best form of management is:
    A) Frequent chest physiotherapy
    B) Incentive spirometry on a regularly scheduled basis
    C) Chest tube placement in the thoracic cavity
    D) Increased oxygen therapy

12. A common symptom of a pneumothorax is:
    A) Dyspnea
    B) Eupnea
    C) Fremitus
    D) Orthopnea

13. Which of the following nursing interventions is indicated for the client with a nasal cannula in place?
    A) Assess nares for skin breakdown every 6 hours
    B) Check patency of the cannula every 2 hours
    C) Inspect the mouth every 6 hours
    D) Check oxygen flow and orders every 24 hours

14. A 15-year-old client requires cardiopulmonary resuscitation. The nurse who is delivering the cardiac compressions should compress the sternum 1½ to 2 inches (4 to 5 cm) with one hand at the rate of:
    A) 40 to 60 times/min
    B) 60 to 80 times/min
    C) 80 to 100 times/min
    D) 100 to 120 times/min

15. One of the early signs of hypoxia that the nurse can assess in a client is:
    A) Cyanosis
    B) A decreased respiratory rate
    C) A decreased blood pressure
    D) Restlessness

16. Which of the following abnormal assessment findings represents the most serious indication of decreased oxygenation?
    A) Decreased skin turgor
    B) Clubbing of the nails
    C) Central cyanosis
    D) Pursed-lip breathing pattern

17. In teaching a client about an upcoming diagnostic test, the nurse identifies that which of the following uses an injection of contrast material?
   A) Electrophysiological study (EPS)
   B) Echocardiography
   C) Cardiac catheterization
   D) Exercise stress test

18. The nurse should implement which of the following techniques for pulse oximetry?
   A) Use the nasal site for clients with low perfusion status.
   B) Move the sensors every 8 to 12 hours to an alternate site.
   C) Set the alarm for low oxygen levels only.
   D) Avoid aligning the photoelectron and light-emitting diode.

19. At a community health fair, the nurse informs the residents that the influenza vaccine is recommended for clients:
   A) In any age group who are currently experiencing flu-like symptoms
   B) Aged 40 to 60 years of age
   C) In any age group who have a chronic disease
   D) Above the age of 65

20. The unit manager is orienting a new staff nurse and evaluates which of the following as an appropriate technique for nasotracheal suctioning?
   A) Placing the client in a supine position
   B) Preparing for a clean or nonsterile technique
   C) Suctioning the oropharyngeal area first, then the nasotracheal area
   D) Applying intermittent suction for 10 seconds during catheter removal

21. In working with a client who has chest tubes in place, the nurse should:
   A) Clamp off the tubes except during client assessments
   B) Remove the tubing from the connection to check for adequate suction power
   C) Milk or strip the tubes every 15 to 30 minutes to maintain drainage
   D) Coil and secure excess tubing next to the client

22. Which of the following is a priority for the nurse teaching a family about home oxygen therapy?
   A) Pathophysiology of the client
   B) Use of the equipment
   C) PaO_2 levels of the client
   D) Length of time the oxygen is to be used

CHAPTER 40

1. When a deficit of body fluid exists in the intravascular compartment, which one of the following signs can be expected?
   A) Rales
   B) A bounding pulse
   C) Engorged peripheral veins
   D) An elevated hematocrit level

2. A client was recently jogging in 90° F temperatures, suffered dehydration fatigue, and was hospitalized. Which of the following fluid losses is most difficult to measure?
   A) Urinary output
   B) Sodium and potassium levels
   C) Insensible water loss
   D) Major cation and anion losses

3. When a client's serum sodium level is 120 mEq/L, the priority nursing assessment is to monitor the status of which body system?
   A) Neurological
   B) Pulmonary
   C) Hepatic
   D) Gastrointestinal

4. An 8-year-old is admitted to the pediatric unit with pneumonia. On assessment the nurse notes that the child is warm and flushed, is lethargic, has difficulty breathing, and has moist rales. The nurse determines that the child is suffering from:
A) Metabolic acidosis
B) Respiratory acidosis
C) Respiratory alkalosis
D) Metabolic alkalosis

5. A client with a serum pH, 7.48; CO_2, 42; and HCO_3, 32 is evidencing which one of the following acid-base imbalances?
A) Metabolic acidosis
B) Respiratory acidosis
C) Respiratory alkalosis
D) Metabolic alkalosis

6. Which of the following compensating mechanisms is most likely to occur in the presence of respiratory acidosis?
A) Hyperventilation to decrease the CO_2 levels
B) Hypoventilation to increase the CO_2 levels
C) Retention of HCO_3 by the kidneys to increase the pH level
D) Excretion of HCO_3 by the kidneys to decrease the pH level

7. Which of the following clients is most at risk for fluid volume deficit?
A) A 6-month-old learning to drink from a cup
B) A 12-year-old who is moderately active in 80° F weather
C) A 42-year-old with severe diarrhea
D) A 90-year-old with frequent headaches

8. A client experiences a loss of intracellular fluid. Which of the following IV concentrations should be used to replace this loss?
A) Hypotonic solution
B) Hypertonic solution
C) Isotonic solution
D) An electrolyte composition

9. The client has been experiencing right flank and lower back pain. Which of the following laboratory values would be the most desirable to know?
A) Serum potassium
B) Serum sodium
C) Serum magnesium
D) Serum calcium

10. The physician orders 1000 ml of D_5RL with 20 mEq KCl to run for 8 hours. Using an infusion set with a drop factor of 15 gtt/ml, the nurse calculates the flow rate to be:
A) 12 drops/minute
B) 22 drops/minute
C) 32 drops/minute
D) 42 drops/minute

11. Which of the following is important in the site selection for a new intravenous line?
A) Starting with the most proximal site
B) Looking for hard, cordlike veins
C) Using sites away from a dialysis graft
D) Selecting the dominant arm

12. A client has intravenous therapy for the administration of antibiotics and is stating that the "IV site hurts and is swollen." Which of the following data should confirm phlebitis, as opposed to infiltration?
A) Intensity of the pain
B) Warmth of integument surrounding IV site
C) Amount of subcutaneous edema
D) Skin discoloration of a bruised nature

13. A client complains of a headache and nausea and vomiting during a blood transfusion. Which one of the following actions should the nurse take immediately?
A) Check the vital signs.
B) Stop the blood transfusion.
C) Slow down the rate of blood flow.
D) Notify the physician and blood bank personnel.

14. For a nursing diagnosis of "fluid volume excess," the nurse is alert to which one of the following signs and symptoms?
   A) Weak, thready pulse
   B) Hypertension
   C) Dry mucous membranes
   D) Flushed, dry skin

15. A client is currently taking Lasix and digoxin. As a result of the medication regimen, the nurse is alert to the presence of:
   A) Cardiac dysrhythmia
   B) Diarrhea
   C) Hyperactive reflexes
   D) Peripheral cyanosis

16. A rapid infusion of citrated blood has been given to the client. The nurse observes for:
   A) Diaphoresis
   B) Anxiety
   C) Chvostek's sign
   D) Nausea and vomiting

17. For a child who has ingested the remaining contents of an aspirin bottle, the nurse suspects:
   A) Metabolic acidosis
   B) Metabolic alkalosis
   C) Respiratory acidosis
   D) Respiratory alkalosis

18. The single best indicator of fluid status is the nurse's assessment of the client's:
   A) Intake and output
   B) Serum electrolyte levels
   C) Skin turgor
   D) Daily body weight

19. The nurse evaluates that the client has an understanding of the fluid restriction when the client states which of the following?
   A) "Three-quarters of my total fluid should be taken between 8 AM and 12 noon."
   B) "Frequent mouth care is necessary."

C) "Only actual liquids should count in my restriction."
   D) "At least 4 ounces should be held aside for each time medications are taken."

20. An IV of 125 ml is to be infused over a 1-hour period. A microdrip infusion set will be used. The nurse calculates the infusion rate as:
   A) 32 gtt/min
   B) 60 gtt/min
   C) 125 gtt/min
   D) 250 gtt/min

CHAPTER 41

1. The physiology of sleep is complex. Which of the following is the most appropriate statement in regard to this process?
   A) Ultradian rhythms occur in a cycle longer than 24 hours.
   B) Nonrapid eye movement (NREM) refers to the cycle that most clients experience when in a high stimulus environment.
   C) The reticular activating system is partly responsible for the level of consciousness of a person.
   D) The bulbar synchronizing region causes the rapid eye movement (REM) sleep in most normal adults.

2. The client's wife is staying in the intensive care waiting room so she can visit her husband for a few minutes every 3 hours. What effect will this have on her sleep cycle?
   A) Increase REM sleep
   B) Increase stage 2 NREM sleep
   C) Increase stage 3 NREM sleep
   D) Increase stage 4 NREM sleep

3. When a client is deprived of sleep, the nurse might assess such symptoms as:
   A) Elevated blood pressure and confusion
   B) Confusion and mistrust
   C) Inappropriateness and rapid respirations
   D) Decreased temperature and talkativeness

4. The parents of a newborn wonder when she should start to sleep through the night. The nurse's response should be that infants usually develop a nighttime pattern of sleep by:
   A) 6 weeks
   B) 2 months
   C) 3 months
   D) 6 months

5. The mother of a 2 year old tells the nurse that the child has started crying and resisting going to sleep at the scheduled bedtime. The nurse should advise the parent to:
   A) Offer the child a bedtime snack
   B) Maintain the same bedtime ritual
   C) Eliminate one of the naps during the day
   D) Allow the child to sleep longer in the mornings

6. A child in middle school is currently experiencing sleep-related fatigue during classes. Which of the following is most appropriate for the school nurse counseling the child's parents?
   A) "What are the child's usual sleep patterns?"
   B) "Establish bedtimes for the child and withhold his allowance whenever those times are not adhered to."
   C) "We need to explore other health-related problems, because sleep problems are not likely the cause of his fatigue."
   D) "The bulbar synchronizing region of the child's central nervous system is causing these insomniac problems."

7. In describing the sleep patterns of older adults, the nurse recognizes that they:
   A) Are more difficult to arouse
   B) Require more sleep than middle-aged adults
   C) Take less time to fall asleep
   D) Have a decline in stage 4 sleep

8. The nurse should inform the client who is currently taking a diuretic that he/she may experience:
   A) Reduced REM sleep
   B) Nocturia
   C) Nightmares
   D) Increased daytime sleepiness

9. Which of the following is the most significant difference between narcolepsy and insomnia?
   A) Narcolepsy occurs as an obstructive disorder of the muscles of the oral cavity.
   B) Insomnia is a dyssomnia.
   C) Narcolepsy causes vivid dreaming states.
   D) Insomnia may be voluntarily managed.

10. A 74-year-old client has been having sleeping difficulties. Which of the following reflects the most appropriate nursing response?
    A) "What do you do just prior to going to bed?"
    B) "Let's make sure that your bedroom is completely darkened at night."
    C) "Why don't you try napping more during the daytime?"
    D) "You should always eat something just before bedtime."

11. Which of the following information provided by the client's bed partner is most often associated with sleep apnea?
    A) Restlessness
    B) Talking during sleep
    C) Somnambulism
    D) Excessive snoring

12. In teaching methods to promote positive sleep habits at home, the nurse instructs the client to:
    A) Use the bedroom for sleep or sexual activity only
    B) Eat a large meal 1 to 2 hours before bedtime
    C) Exercise vigorously before bedtime
    D) Stay in bed if sleep does not come after ½ hour

CHAPTER 42

1. Which of the following nursing interventions for a client in pain is based on the gate-control theory?
    A) Giving the client a back massage
    B) Changing the client's position in bed
    C) Giving the client a pain medication
    D) Limiting the number of visitors

2. The client has chronic back pain, and the nurse is assessing the subjective symptoms of his discomfort. Which of the following represents the most important data in the assessment?
    A) Incongruence between the objective signs and the subjective symptoms
    B) Presence or absence of a sympathetic response of hypertension
    C) The quality of facial grimacing that the client is making
    D) The cultural and family background as they relate to his outward manifestations of the pain

3. The client tells the nurse about a burning sensation in the epigastric area. The nurse should describe this type of pain as:
    A) Referred
    B) Radiating
    C) Deep visceral
    D) Superficial or cutaneous

4. The nurse must frequently assess a client who is experiencing pain. When assessing the intensity of the pain, the nurse should:
    A) Ask about what precipitates the pain
    B) Question the client about the location of the pain
    C) Offer the client a pain scale to objectify the information
    D) Use open-ended questions to find out about the sensation

5. A 75-year-old client is experiencing bladder spasms on a frequent basis. Which of the following is the most likely reason for the client to withhold information regarding this pain? The client:
    A) Knows that no one in the family will listen to verbal complaints of pain
    B) Is fearful that the pain could indicate a more severe problem
    C) Has grown up in a culture that prohibits the elderly from showing emotions of pain and discomfort
    D) Does not want to draw attention to this problem

6. The client will be going home on medication administered through a PCA (patient-controlled analgesia) system. To assist the family members with an understanding of how this therapy works, the nurse explains that the client:
    A) Has control over the frequency of the IV analgesia
    B) Can choose the dosage of the drug received
    C) May request the type of medication received
    D) Controls the route for administering the medication

7. A client requests holistic approaches in the management of chronic pancreatic pain. Which of the following is the best statement for the nurse to make to the client?
   A) "Therapeutic touch is a better form of treatment than acupressure in your condition, because it is less invasive."
   B) "Guided imagery focuses on your ability to use your imagination."
   C) "We will want to make sure and evaluate the effects of the therapy you choose by monitoring your blood pressure and pulse."
   D) "Some of these pain relief measures may sound strange, but we want to encourage whatever works."

8. The nurse tells the client to "be prepared for the Foley catheter insertion to feel uncomfortable." This is most accurately an example of:
   A) Distraction
   B) Reducing pain perception
   C) Anticipatory response
   D) Self-care maintenance

9. Which of the following clients is best suited for PCA management? A client who:
   A) Has psychogenic discomfort
   B) Is recovering after a total hip replacement
   C) Experiences renal dysfunction
   D) Recently experienced a cerebrovascular accident (stroke)

10. A client with chronic back pain has an order for a TENS unit for pain control. The nurse should instruct the client to:
    A) Keep the unit on high
    B) Use the unit when pain is perceived
    C) Remove the electrodes at bedtime
    D) Use the therapy without medications

11. A terminally ill client with liver cancer is experiencing great discomfort. A realistic goal in caring for the client is to:
    A) Increasingly administer narcotics to oversedate the client and thereby decrease the pain
    B) Continue to change the analgesics until the right narcotic is found that completely alleviates the pain
    C) Adapt the analgesics as the nursing assessment reveals the need for specific medications
    D) Use hospice personnel who have been trained to relieve painful conditions

12. A client is having severe, continuous discomfort from kidney stones. The nurse anticipates which of the following findings in the client's assessment?
    A) Tachycardia
    B) Diaphoresis
    C) Pupil dilation
    D) Nausea and vomiting

13. Nurses working with clients in pain need to recognize and avoid common misconceptions and myths about pain. In regard to the pain experience, which of the following is correct?
    A) The client is the best authority on the pain experience.
    B) Chronic pain is mostly psychological in nature.
    C) Regular use of analgesics leads to drug addition.
    D) The amount of tissue damage is accurately reflected in the degree of pain perceived.

14. A nonpharmacological approach that focuses on promoting pleasurable and meaningful stimuli is:
    A) Acupressure
    B) Distraction
    C) Biofeedback
    D) Hypnosis

15. In caring for the client who is receiving epidural analgesia, the nurse:
    A) Changes the tubing every 48 to 72 hours
    B) Changes the dressing every shift
    C) Secures the catheter to the outside skin
    D) Uses a bulky occlusive dressing over the site

CHAPTER 43

1. While performing a nutritional assessment of a low-income family, the community health nurse determines that the family's diet is inadequate in protein content. The nurse suggests which of the following foods to increase protein content with little increase in food expenditure?
    A) Oranges and potatoes
    B) Potatoes and rice
    C) Rice and macaroni
    D) Peas and beans

2. A client is suspected of having a fat-soluble vitamin deficiency. Which of the following is the most appropriate nursing intervention statement?
    A) "More exposure to sunlight and drinking milk could solve your nutritional problem."
    B) "Eating more pork, fish, eggs, and poultry will increase your vitamin B complex intake."
    C) "Increasing your protein intake will increase your negative nitrogen imbalance."
    D) "Decreasing your triglyceride levels by eating less saturated fats would be a good health intervention for you."

3. A new mother is breast-feeding her infant and asks the nurse about the introduction of cereals into the diet. The nurse's best response is:

A) "I'm glad you are breast-feeding, as your milk contains many antibodies that protect against viruses and bacteria."
B) "Be sure to test the temperature of the cereal if you use your microwave, as it can get too hot."
C) "You can begin feeding iron-fortified cereals between 4 and 6 months."
D) "Integrate feeding vegetables and fruit with your cereals at about 6 months of age."

4. A school nurse suspects that one of the junior-high students may have anorexia nervosa. This eating disorder is character-ized by:
    A) A lack of control over eating patterns
    B) Self-imposed starvation
    C) Binge-purge cycles
    D) Excessive exercise

5. A client is pregnant for the third time. In regard to her nutritional status, she should:
    A) Limit her weight gain to a maximum of 25 pounds
    B) Approximately double her protein intake
    C) Increase her vitamin A and milk product consumption
    D) Increase her intake of folic acid

6. After throat surgery, the client should be offered which of the following?
    A) Chicken noodle soup
    B) Ginger ale
    C) Oatmeal
    D) Hot tea with lemon

7. For a client who is HIV positive, which of the following is an appropriate consideration?
    A) The restriction of potassium, phosphate, and sodium
    B) A reduced carbohydrate intake
    C) A decreased protein and increased folic acid intake
    D) A reduced-fat diet with small frequent meals

8. When introducing a feeding to a client with an indwelling gavage tube for enteral nutrition, which of the following should the nurse do first?
   A) Irrigate the tube with normal saline solution.
   B) Check to see that the tube is properly placed.
   C) Place the client in a prone position.
   D) Introduce some water before introducing the liquid nourishment.

9. The nurse caring for a client receiving parenteral nutrition (PN) should perform which of the following interventions?
   A) Begin the infusion rates at 100–150 mL/h.
   B) Maintain a consistent infusion rate.
   C) Change the infusion tubing once a week.
   D) Monitor protein levels daily.

10. A client needs a small-bore nasogastric tube inserted for enteral nutrition (EN). Which of the following is the most appropriate nursing intervention statement?
    A) "The tube will feel uncomfortable and may make you gag at times when I am inserting it."
    B) "We will mark this tube from the end of your nose to your umbilicus to obtain the right length for insertion."
    C) "Please hold your breath when I insert this small tube through your nose down into your stomach."
    D) "Please tilt your head back after the tube passes the nasopharynx."

11. Which of the following foods is a complete protein?
    A) Eggs
    B) Oats
    C) Lentils
    D) Peanuts

12. According to *Canada's Food Guide to Healthy Eating*, the average adult's diet should include how many servings of vegetables and fruit?

A) 1–3 servings/day
B) 2–4 servings/day
C) 3–5 servings/day
D) 5–10 servings/day

13. The parent of an 8-year-old child asks the nurse if there are any special nutritional needs for this age. The nurse identifies that school-age children need to:
    A) Increase their intake of B vitamins
    B) Maintain a sufficient intake of protein, and vitamins A and C
    C) Increase carbohydrates to meet increased energy needs
    D) Significantly increase iron intake

14. A general classification of drugs that alter taste and have decreased absorption when taken with food is:
    A) Anticoagulant
    B) Antidepressant
    C) Antihistamine
    D) Antibiotic

15. A factor that interferes with nutrient absorption is:
    A) A decrease of gastric enzymes
    B) Lack of the intrinsic factor
    C) Serious depression
    D) A decrease in muscle mass

16. The nurse who is assisting a client in meal selection realizes that clients who practise Islam or Judaism share an avoidance of:
    A) Alcohol
    B) Shellfish
    C) Pork products
    D) Caffeine

17. The nurse can recommend which one of the following foods for a client on a full liquid diet?
    A) Pureed meats
    B) Scrambled eggs
    C) Soft fresh fruit
    D) Canned soup

18. The client receiving feedings through an enteral tube begins to experience abdominal cramping and nausea. The nurse should:
    A) Cool the formula
    B) Remove the tube
    C) Use a more concentrated formula
    D) Decrease the administration rate

CHAPTER 44

1. The client had a myocardial infarction that consequently decreased his overall cardiac output. Within 24 hours he developed acute renal failure. This is an example of which type of condition?
   A) Prerenal
   B) Intrarenal
   C) Postrenal
   D) Irreversible

2. The client has chronic renal failure and is contemplating dialysis. Which type of management is anticipated by the nurse?
   A) Hemodialysis
   B) Peritoneal dialysis
   C) Kidney removal
   D) Medication treatments

3. Which of the following early symptoms does the nurse expect a client with a bladder infection to exhibit?
   A) Chills
   B) Hematuria
   C) Flank pain
   D) Incontinence

4. The client has an indwelling catheter. The nurse should obtain a sterile urine specimen by:
   A) Disconnecting the catheter from the drainage tubing
   B) Withdrawing urine from a urinometer
   C) Opening the drainage bag and removing urine
   D) Using a needle to withdraw urine from the catheter port

5. The nurse should observe the client for which of the following immediately after an intravenous pyelogram (IVP)?
   A) Infection in the urinary bladder
   B) An allergic reaction to the contrast material
   C) Urinary suppression caused by injury to kidney tissues
   D) Incontinence as a result of paralysis of the urinary sphincter

6. A client with an excessive alcohol intake has a reduced amount of antidiuretic hormone (ADH). The nurse anticipates this client to exhibit:
   A) An increased blood pressure
   B) Oliguria
   C) Signs of dehydration
   D) A low serum sodium level

7. A client is going to have a cystoscopy. Which of the following reflects information that should be communicated before the procedure?
   A) "There will be no need to have a special consent form."
   B) "Are you allergic to iodine?"
   C) "You will need to have fluids restricted the evening before the cystoscopy."
   D) "You will probably be given sedatives before the procedure."

8. A postpartum client has been unable to void since the delivery of her baby this morning. Which of the following nursing measures would be beneficial for the client initially?
   A) Increase fluid intake to 2500 ml
   B) Insert indwelling Foley catheter
   C) Rinse perineum with warm water
   D) Apply firm pressure over the bladder

9. Which of the following is the least invasive alternative to urethral catheterization?
   A) Suprapubic catheterization
   B) Reinsertion of a Foley catheter
   C) Catheter irrigation
   D) Condom catheterization

10. The unit manager is evaluating the care of a new nursing staff member. Which of the following is an appropriate technique for the nurse to obtain a clean-voided urine specimen?
   A) Restrict fluids before the specimen collection
   B) Apply sterile gloves for the procedure
   C) Collect the specimen after the initial stream of urine has passed
   D) Place the specimen in a clean urinalysis container

11. Clients with chronic alterations in kidney function suffer from insufficient amounts of:
   A) Vitamin A
   B) Vitamin D
   C) Vitamin E
   D) Vitamin K

12. The assessment of a client with reflex incontinence is expected to identify:
   A) An urge to void and not enough time to reach the bathroom
   B) An uncontrollable loss of urine when coughing or sneezing
   C) A constant dribbling of urine
   D) No urge to void and an unawareness of bladder filling

13. The urinary output for an average adult should be:
   A) 800 to 1000 ml/day
   B) 1000 to 1200 ml/day
   C) 1500 to 1700 ml/day
   D) 2000 to 2300 ml/day

14. When assessing the client for possible urinary retention, the nurse should be alert for:
   A) Small amounts of urine voided 2 to 3 times/hour
   B) Large amounts of cloudy urine being voided
   C) Pain in the suprapubic region and blood-tinged urine
   D) Spasms and dysuria

15. A timed urine specimen collection is ordered. Which of the following will result in the need to restart the test?
   A) The client defecates prior to urinating and collecting the sample.
   B) The client voids in the toilet.
   C) The first voided urine is discarded.
   D) A preservative is placed in the collection container.

16. The nurse should incorporate which of the following into the teaching plan for a client with a urinary diversion?
   A) Special clothing will need to be ordered in order to fit around the diversion.
   B) A stomal bag will need to be worn only at night.
   C) Special skin care is a priority.
   D) A reduction in physical activity will be planned.

17. The nursing instructor is evaluating a student during the catheterization of a female client. Which of the following is determined to be an appropriate part of the technique?
   A) Keeping both hands sterile throughout the procedure
   B) Reinserting the catheter if it was misplaced initially in the vagina
   C) Inflating the balloon to test it prior to catheter insertion
   D) Advancing the catheter 7 to 8 inches

18. A client is receiving closed catheter irrigation. During the shift, 950 ml of normal saline irrigant are instilled, and there is a total of 1725 ml in the drainage bag. The client's urinary output is calculated by the nurse to be:
   A) 775 ml
   B) 950 ml
   C) 1725 ml
   D) 2675 ml

19. A bladder retraining program for a client in an extended care facility should include:
    A) Providing negative reinforcement when the client is incontinent
    B) Having the client wear adult diapers as a preventative measure
    C) Putting the client on a q2h toilet schedule during the day
    D) Promoting the intake of caffeine to stimulate voiding

CHAPTER 45

1. Which of the following is an expected change in elimination associated with the aging process?
    A) Absorptive processes are increased in the intestinal mucosa.
    B) Esophageal emptying time is increased.
    C) Changes in nerve innervation and sensation cause diarrhea.
    D) Mastication processes are less efficient.

2. A 6-month-old infant has severe diarrhea. The major problem associated with severe diarrhea is:
    A) Pain in the abdominal area
    B) Irritation of the perineal and rectal area
    C) Electrolyte and fluid loss
    D) Presence of excessive flatus

3. When irrigating a colostomy the nurse uses a cone that fits properly to prevent:
    A) Introducing air into the colon
    B) Leaking the solution around the stoma
    C) Administering the solution too rapidly
    D) Introducing bacteria from the stoma

4. The nurse recognizes that which of the following is true concerning ostomies?
    A) An ileostomy client will have solid, formed stool.
    B) A double-barrel ostomy refers to one created for the ileum and one for the colon.

C) Some clients will have control over when they can evacuate their colon.
    D) Family members or significant others will need to learn the care.

5. A client had a gastrectomy 5 days ago and is just beginning to drink fluids. To prevent flatulence, the nurse instructs the client to:
    A) Drink carbonated fluids
    B) Take a sitz bath
    C) Use a straw when drinking fluids
    D) Ambulate in the hall

6. A client has come to the clinic for an annual physical. An affirmative response by the client to which of the following questions should prompt the nurse to investigate further?
    A) "Do you know what caused your mother's death?"
    B) "Are you between 30 and 40 years of age?"
    C) "Do you commute to work?"
    D) "Do you eat a diet high in fiber?"

7. The client has been admitted to an acute care unit with a diagnosis of biliary disease. The nurse suspects that the feces will appear:
    A) Pus filled
    B) Black and tarry
    C) White or clay colored
    D) Bloody

8. The client asks the nurse to recommend bulk forming foods that may be included in the diet. Which of the following should be recommended?
    A) Whole grains
    B) Fruit juice
    C) Rare meats
    D) Milk products

9. A client has been experiencing abdominal pain of unknown origin. Which diagnostic test is the least invasive?
   A) An endoscopy
   B) An upper GI study
   C) A culture and sensitivity
   D) An abdominal laparotomy

10. The client is taking medications to promote defecation. Which of the following should be included in the teaching plan?
    A) Increased laxative use often causes hyperkalemia.
    B) Salt tablets should be taken to increase the solute concentration of the extracellular fluid.
    C) Emollient solutions may increase the amount of water secreted into the bowel.
    D) Bulk-forming additives may turn the urine pink.

11. While undergoing a soapsuds enema, the client complains of abdominal cramping. The nurse should:
    A) Immediately stop the infusion
    B) Lower the height of the enema container
    C) Advance the enema tubing 2 to 3 inches
    D) Clamp the tubing

12. Clients may experience which of the following 24 to 48 hours postoperatively as a result of the anesthetic?
    A) Stomatitis
    B) Paralytic ileus
    C) Gastrocolic reflex
    D) Colitis

13. For clients with hypocalcemia, the nurse should implement measures to prevent:
    A) Gastric upset
    B) Malabsorption
    C) Constipation
    D) Fluid secretion

14. The client is to receive a Kayexalate enema. The nurse knows that this is used to:
    A) Prevent further constipation
    B) Reduce bacteria in the colon before diagnostic testing
    C) Provide direct antidiarrheal medication to the intestine
    D) Remove excess potassium from the system

15. The appropriate amount of fluid to prepare for an enema to be given to an average-size school-age child is:
    A) 150 to 250 ml
    B) 250 to 350 ml
    C) 300 to 500 ml
    D) 500 to 750 ml

16. The nurse is instructing the client in stomal care for an incontinent ostomy. The nurse evaluates achievement of learning goals if the client uses:
    A) Triamcinolone acetonide (Kenalog) spray for a yeast infection
    B) Peroxide to toughen the peristomal skin
    C) A commercial deodorant around the stoma
    D) Alcohol to cleanse the stoma

17. The nurse should implement which of the following measures for a client with a nasogastric tube?
    A) Taping the tube carefully to the cheek adjacent to the nostril being used
    B) Securing the tubing to the bed by the client's head
    C) Changing the tubing daily
    D) Marking the tube where it exits the nose

CHAPTER 46

1. Which of the following is true concerning the physiological effects of immobility?
   A) Serum calcium levels decrease.
   B) Hypertension develops because of the increased cardiac workload.
   C) Caloric intake often increases.
   D) Plantar flexion occurs, which restricts ambulation.

2. A 61-year-old client recently suffered left-sided paralysis from a cerebrovascular accident (stroke). Which of the following is the best intervention for this client?
   A) Encourage an even gait when walking in place.
   B) Assess the extremities for unilateral swelling and muscle atrophy.
   C) Encourage holding the breath frequently to hyperinflate his lungs.
   D) Teach the use of a two-point crutch technique for ambulation.

3. Two nurses are standing on opposite sides of the bed to move the client up in bed with a drawsheet. Where should the nurses be standing in relation to the client's body as they prepare for the move?
   A) Even with the thorax
   B) Even with the shoulders
   C) Even with the hips
   D) Even with the knees

4. A client is leaving for surgery, and because of preoperative sedation, needs complete assistance to transfer from the bed to the stretcher. Which of the following should the nurse do first?
   A) Elevate the head of the bed.
   B) Explain the procedure to the client.
   C) Place the client in the prone position.
   D) Assess the situation for any potentially unsafe complications.

5. Which of the following is indicated when the client is to have passive range-of-motion exercises performed by the nurse?
   A) Exercise the joint beyond the point of slight resistance.
   B) Perform movements quickly.
   C) Perform each movement one time during the session.
   D) Institute exercises as soon as the client's ability to move the extremity is lost.

6. The nurse assesses that the client has torticollis and that this may adversely influence the client's mobility. This individual has a(n):
   A) Exaggeration of the lumbar spine curvature
   B) Contracture of the sternocleidomastoid muscle with a head incline
   C) Increased convexity of the thoracic spine
   D) Abnormal anteroposterior and lateral curvature of the spine

7. An immobilized client is suspected of having atelectasis. This is assessed by the nurse upon auscultation as:
   A) Harsh crackles
   B) Wheezing on inspiration
   C) Diminished breath sounds
   D) Bronchovesicular whooshing

8. The best approach for the nurse to use to assess the presence of thrombosis is to:
   A) Measure the calf and thigh diameters
   B) Attempt to elicit Homans' sign
   C) Palpate the temperature of the feet
   D) Observe for a loss of hair and skin turgor in the lower legs

9. A client is getting up for the first time after a period of bedrest. The nurse should first:
   A) Obtain a baseline blood pressure
   B) Assist the client to sit at the edge of the bed
   C) Assess the respiratory function
   D) Ask the client if he/she feels lightheaded

10. Which of the following factors may contribute to an increased risk for thrombus formation, impaired skin integrity, respiratory infection, and constipation in the immobilized client?
A) Insufficient passive range of motion
B) Emotional depression
C) Inadequate fluid intake
D) Use of hypnotic medication

11. In order to promote respiratory function in the immobilized client, the nurse should:
A) Change the client's position every 4 to 8 hours
B) Encourage deep breathing and coughing every hour
C) Use oxygen and nebulizer treatments regularly
D) Suction the client every hour

12. The nurse explains to the client that the primary purpose for the elastic stockings is to:
A) Keep the skin warm and dry
B) Prevent bleeding
C) Prevent abnormal joint flexion
D) Apply external pressure

13. To provide for the psychosocial needs of an immobilized client, the nurse should tell the client which of the following statements?
A) "The staff will limit your visitors so that you will not be bothered."
B) "A roommate can be a real bother. You'd probably rather have a private room."
C) "We can discuss the routine to see if there are any changes we can make."
D) "I think you should have your hair done and put on some make-up."

14. The use of which of the following devices will best reduce the change of external hip rotation in a client on prolonged bedrest?
A) Footboard
B) Trochanter roll
C) Trapeze bar
D) Bed board

15. For a lateral or side-lying position, the nurse should support the client with:
A) Both hips and knees flexed
B) Thick supports under the ankles
C) Both arms laying on the mattress
D) A pillow support under the upper leg

CHAPTER 47

1. The client has an alteration in skin integrity on the left heel area. The nurse decides to use the Braden Scale instead of the Gosnell Scale of Assessment. Which category of assessment will the nurse now be able to use? The degree of:
A) Mobility
B) Friction and shear
C) The effects of nutrition
D) Physical activity

2. Pressure ulcers form primarily as a result of:
A) Prolonged illness or disease
B) Restricted mobility
C) Nitrogen buildup in the underlying tissues
D) Poor nutrition

3. The nurse notes that a client's skin is reddened with a small abrasion and serous fluid present. The nurse should classify this stage of ulcer formation as:
A) Stage I
B) Stage II
C) Stage III
D) Stage IV

4. The client has rheumatoid arthritis, is prone to skin breakdown, and is also somewhat immobile because of arthritic pain. Which of the following is the best intervention for the client's skin integrity?
   A) Having the client sit up in a chair for 4-hour intervals
   B) Keeping the head of the bed in a high Fowler's position to increase circulation
   C) Keeping a written schedule of turning and positioning
   D) Encouraging the client to perform pelvic muscle training exercises several times a day

5. The physician orders a Clinitron bed for an immobilized client. The primary benefit of this bed is that it:
   A) Rotates the client every 3 minutes
   B) Allows for severely obese clients
   C) Distributes weight by temperature-controlled forced air
   D) Absorbs moisture

6. Which of the following is correct regarding wound débridement?
   A) It allows the healthy tissue to regenerate.
   B) When performed by autolytic means, the wound is irrigated.
   C) Mechanical methods involve direct surgical removal of the eschar layer of the wound.
   D) Enzymatic débridement may be implemented independently by the nurse whenever it is required.

7. The nurse prepares to irrigate the client's wound. The primary reason for performing this procedure is to:
   A) Remove debris from the wound
   B) Decrease scar formation
   C) Improve circulation from the wound
   D) Decrease irritation from wound drainage

8. When turning a client, the nurse notices a reddened area on the coccyx. What skin care interventions should the nurse use on this area?
   A) Clean the area with mild soap, dry, and add a protective moisturizer.
   B) Apply a dilute hydrogen peroxide and water mixture and direct a heat lamp to the area.
   C) Soak the area in normal saline solution.
   D) Wash the area with an astringent and paint it with povidone-iodine (Betadine).

9. A client with a large abdominal wound requires a dressing change every 4 hours. The client will be discharged to the home setting where the dressing care will be continued. Which of the following is true concerning this client's wound healing process?
   A) An antiseptic agent is best followed with a rinse of sterile saline solution.
   B) A heat lamp should be used every 2 hours to rid the wound area of contaminants.
   C) Sterile technique should be emphasized to the client and family.
   D) A dressing covering will allow the wound area to remain moist.

10. An older adult client has a large decubitus ulcer that is healing slowly at home. The client needs to be instructed regarding a "good nutritional dietary intake" because:
   A) The potential for a protein deficiency exists
   B) The client's dietary habits have probably not been adequate for a normal healthy lifestyle
   C) There may be an insufficient caloric intake, which can result in poor wound healing
   D) Practice standards require that nutritional aspects be addressed with every client

11. A client has a healing abdominal wound with minimal exudate and collagen formation. The wound is in which phase of healing?
    A) Primary intention
    B) Inflammatory phase
    C) Proliferative phase
    D) Secondary intention

12. Which of the following is the best indicator that a wound has become infected?
    A) Palpation of the wound reveals excess fluid under its edges.
    B) Wound cultures are positive.
    C) Purulent drainage is coming from the wound area.
    D) The wound has a distinct odor.

13. The nurse is concerned that the client's midsternal wound is at risk for dehiscence. Which of the following is the best intervention to prevent this complication?
    A) Administering antibiotics to prevent an infection that could cause pressure on the wound site
    B) Using appropriate sterile technique when changing the dressing covering the wound
    C) Keeping sterile towels and extra dressing supplies near the client's bed
    D) Placing a pillow over the incision site when the client is attempting to deep breathe or cough

14. Following a head injury, the client has thin, clear drainage coming from one ear. The nurse describes this drainage as:
    A) Serous
    B) Cerebrospinal fluid
    C) Serosanguineous
    D) Purulent

15. Which of the following nursing entries is the most complete in its description of a wound?
    A) Wound appears to be healing well. Dressing dry and intact.
    B) Wound well approximated with minimal drainage.
    C) Drainage size of quarter; wound pink, 4 × 4s applied.
    D) Incisional edges approximated without redness or drainage, two 4 × 4s applied.

16. A client has a large second-degree burn on her upper thorax and receives wound dressings on a frequent basis. Which of the following is the most likely type of wound dressing for this client to receive?
    A) Saline-moistened gauze pads that are not allowed to dry
    B) Pressure dressings wrapped with elastic bandages
    C) Contact dressings that are allowed to dry
    D) Self-adherent, transparent film dressing material

17. The client is scheduled for a dressing change. When removing the adhesive tape used to secure the dressing, the nurse should lift the edge and hold the tape:
    A) At a 45-degree angle to the skin surface while pulling away from the wound
    B) At a right angle to the skin surface while pulling toward the wound
    C) At a right angle to the skin surface while pulling away from the wound
    D) Parallel to the skin surface while pulling toward the wound

18. When cleaning a wound, the nurse should:
    A) Go over the wound twice and discard that swab
    B) Move from the outer region of the wound toward the center
    C) Start at the drainage site and move outward with circular motions
    D) Use an antiseptic solution followed by a normal saline rinse

19. A client has peripheral edema that causes the left leg to swell. Which of the following is the most appropriate technique in applying a bandage around the affected extremity?
    A) Increasing tension with each successive turn when applying the bandage
    B) Placing clips and tape over the area with the most swelling to prevent slippage
    C) Assessing the skin integument carefully before reapplying each new bandage
    D) Encouraging peripheral blood flow by beginning bandaging at the proximal end and working to the distal area

20. The nurse should use cold applications for a client who has which of the following conditions?
    A) Menstrual cramping
    B) An infected wound
    C) Degenerative joint disease
    D) A fractured ankle

21. Heat applications may be very therapeutic. Which of the following is a concern when considering this therapy?
    A) Blood flow is best enhanced after the first hour of application.
    B) Blood coagulation is increased at the site of injury.
    C) Local anesthesia is promoted and stiffness reduced.
    D) Capillary permeability is increased, promoting movement of waste products.

22. The nurse uses the Norton Scale in the extended care facility to determine the client's risk for pressure ulcer development. Which one of the following scores, based on this scale, places the client at the highest level of risk?
    A) 6
    B) 8
    C) 15
    D) 19

23. The nurse recognizes that which of the following is correct in regard to the use of an abdominal binder?
    A) It replaces the need for underlying dressings.
    B) It should be kept loose for client comfort.
    C) The client should be sitting or standing when it is applied.
    D) The client must have adequate ventilatory capacity.

24. In the emergency room, the nurse documents the client's knife wound as a:
    A) Contusion wound
    B) Clean wound
    C) Acute wound
    D) Intentional wound

25. The nurse is planning a program on wound healing and includes the information that smoking influences healing by:
    A) Suppressing protein synthesis
    B) Creating increased tissue fragility
    C) Depressing bone marrow function
    D) Reducing functional hemoglobin in the blood

26. To reduce pressure points that may lead to pressure ulcers, the nurse should:
    A) Position the client directly on the trochanter when side-lying
    B) Use a donut device for the client when sitting up
    C) Elevate the head of the bed as little as possible
    D) Massage over the bony prominences

27. The first step in packing a wound is to:
    A) Assess its size, shape, and depth
    B) Prepare a sterile field
    C) Select gauze packing material
    D) Irrigate the wound

CHAPTER 48

1. The nurse begins a routine sensory assessment of the client. Which of the following is an important defining characteristic for a nursing diagnosis related to the client's sensory status?
   A) Self-rating of a deficit
   B) Functional abilities
   C) Intellectual capacity
   D) Current medications taken at home

2. Which of the following normal physiological changes in sensory function occurs with advancing age?
   A) Decreased sensitivity to glare
   B) Increased number of taste buds
   C) Difficulty discriminating vowel sounds
   D) Decreased sensitivity to pain

3. The nurse teaches a client that prolonged use of the antibiotic streptomycin may result in:
   A) Damage to the auditory nerve
   B) Alteration in perception
   C) Optic irritation
   D) Loss of taste

4. Which of the following occupations poses the least risk for sensory alterations?
   A) Waiter
   B) Welder
   C) Computer programmer
   D) Construction worker

5. For a hearing-impaired client to hear a conversation, the nurse should:
   A) Use a louder tone of voice than normal
   B) Use visual aids such as the hands and eyes when speaking
   C) Approach a client quietly from behind before speaking
   D) Select a public area to have a conversation

6. The client has had slight nerve damage from an injury to the vertebral column. Which of the following is the most important nursing intervention in regard to the client's sense of touch?
   A) Reminding the client of the need to have frequent tactile contact even if it bothers the client to be touched
   B) Keeping the client covered with sheets and blankets to allow a constant tactile sensation
   C) Allowing the client to lie motionless in order to not overstimulate her sense of touch
   D) Asking the client if touch may be used as a form of therapy

7. When dealing with a client with aphasia, the nurse should remember to:
   A) Wait for the client to communicate
   B) Speak loudly to ensure that the message is received
   C) Speak to the client from the side to avoid overload
   D) Encourage writing of messages

8. When assisting a client with temporary visual loss to eat, the nurse should:
   A) Feed the client the entire meal
   B) Allow the client to experiment with foods
   C) Orient the client to the location of the foods on the plate
   D) Encourage family members to feed the client

9. The nurse is obtaining a history of the client's hearing loss. Which of the following is the most appropriate statement by the nurse during the assessment?
   A) "How long have you been deaf?"
   B) "You don't seem to be able to pay attention to me when I am speaking."
   C) "How does your hearing loss compare to a year ago?"
   D) "Do you also have vision problems?"

10. A client is legally blind in both eyes. Which of the following is the most appropriate statement for the nurse to make regarding providing the client with assistance?
    A) "I will walk in front of you, and you can hold onto my belt."
    B) "I know that you must need me to be your sighted guide to get around in this facility."
    C) "I will warn you of upcoming curbs or stairs."
    D) "I will get you a wheelchair so that I can move you around safely."

11. A 79-year-old client drives his car in the local areas near his home. Which of the following is the most appropriate driving tip to give this client?
    A) "Go very, very slow so you will have some chance of reacting."
    B) "Take your time on long road trips when you are by yourself."
    C) "Remember to keep your car maintained with regular checkups."
    D) "To avoid sun glare, you should drive at night."

12. An older adult client in a nursing home has vision and hearing losses. The nurse is alert to which of the following signs that represents the effects of sensory deprivation?
    A) Diminished anxiety
    B) Improved task completion
    C) Altered spatial perception
    D) Decreased need for physical stimulation

13. Which of the following areas in a home assessment presents the greatest risk for a client with diabetic peripheral neuropathy?
    A) Improper water heater settings
    B) Absence of smoke detectors
    C) Cluttered walkways
    D) Lack of bathroom grab bars

14. The nurse in the pediatric clinic is checking the basic visual acuity of a 4-year-old child. The nurse should have the child:
    A) Use the standard Snellen chart
    B) Read a few lines from children's book
    C) Follow the peripheral movement of an object
    D) Identify crayon colors

15. For a client with receptive aphasia, which one of the following nursing interventions is the most effective?
    A) Providing the client with a letter chart to use to answer complex questions
    B) Using a system of simple gestures and repeated behaviors to communicate
    C) Offering the client a notepad to write questions and concerns
    D) Obtaining a referral for a speech therapist

16. The nurse recommends follow-up auditory testing for a child who was exposed in utero to:
    A) Excessive oxygen
    B) Diabetes
    C) Respiratory infection
    D) Rubella

17. The family of an older client asks the nurse how the stairways and hallways in the home may be enhanced to promote safety. In addition to extra lighting, the nurse recommends the use of paint and decorations that are:
    A) Red and yellow
    B) Black and white
    C) Brown and green
    D) Blue and purple

18. To enhance the client's gustatory sense, the nurse should:
    A) Mix foods together
    B) Provide foods of similar texture and consistency
    C) Assist with oral hygiene
    D) Make sure foods are extremely spicy

19. A home safety measure specific for a client with diminished olfaction is the use of:
   A) Smoke detectors on all levels
   B) Extra lighting in hallways
   C) Amplified telephone receivers
   D) Mild water heater temperatures

CHAPTER 49

1. A 43-year-old client is scheduled to have a gastrectomy. Which of the following is a major preoperative concern?
   A) The client's brother had a tonsillectomy at age 11
   B) The client smokes a pack of cigarettes a day
   C) The presence of an IV infusion
   D) A history of employment as a computer programmer

2. An appendectomy should be classified as:
   A) Diagnostic surgery
   B) Palliative surgery
   C) Ablative surgery
   D) Reconstructive surgery

3. The client states, "I don't like the idea of 'being put to sleep'." Which area of concern should the nurse address after hearing this statement?
   A) Body image
   B) Coping resources
   C) Self-concept
   D) Feelings

4. Which of the following clients would be at greatest risk during surgery?
   A) A 78-year-old client who is taking an analgesic agent
   B) A 43-year-old client who is taking an antihypertensive agent
   C) A 27-year-old client who is taking an anticoagulant agent
   D) A 10-year-old client who is taking an antibiotic agent

5. A 92-year-old client is scheduled for a colectomy. Which normal physiological change increases this client's risk for surgery?
   A) An increased tactile sensation
   B) An increased metabolic rate
   C) Relaxation of arterial walls
   D) Reduced glomerular filtration

6. Which of the following statements concerning the laboratory tests used in the diagnostic screening of surgical clients is true?
   A) A serum creatinine level measures the potential dysfunction of the hepatic system.
   B) Complete blood counts often are used as indicators for blood transfusions.
   C) Serum electrolytes reflect the ability of the peripheral venous system to coagulate effectively.
   D) A urinalysis assists in screening the serum levels of nitrogen waste by-products seen in renal disease.

7. The nurse is evaluating the outcome: "Client describes surgical procedures and postoperative treatment" and determines that the client has not achieved this outcome. The nurse should:
   A) Obtain the consent, as this is expected with preoperative anxiety
   B) Teach the client all about the procedure
   C) Ask the unit manager to assist with a teaching plan
   D) Inform the surgeon so that information can be provided

8. Which of the following statements most accurately reflects nursing accountability in the intraoperative phase?
   A) "I would like to see the client have a regional anesthetic rather than a general anesthetic."
   B) "There seems to be a missing sponge, so a recount should be done of all the sponges that have been removed."
   C) "Did the client receive the medications and sign the consent?"
   D) "The client looks to be reactive and stable."

9. The client will have an incision in the lower left abdomen. Which of the following measures by the nurse will help decrease discomfort in the incisional area when the client coughs postoperatively?
   A) Applying a splint directly over the lower abdomen
   B) Keeping the client flat with her feet flexed
   C) Turning the client onto her right side
   D) Applying pressure above and below the incision

10. Immediate nursing action should be taken to prevent airway obstruction when the client is:
    A) Spitting out the airway
    B) Lying on his side with his face down
    C) Supine with his neck flexed
    D) Coughing after being suctioned

11. A client is in the postanesthesia care unit (PACU) recovering from a vagotomy and pyloroplasty. Which of the following is a normal function of the client in this stage of recovery?
    A) Returned normal bowel sounds on auscultation
    B) Pain that is relieved with noninvasive comfort measures
    C) Voluntary bladder control and function
    D) A subdued level of consciousness and neurological function

12. The client is scheduled for abdominal surgery and has just received the preoperative medications. The nurse should:
    A) Keep the client quiet
    B) Obtain the consent
    C) Prepare the skin at the surgical site
    D) Place the side rails up on the bed or stretcher

13. Which of the following preoperative assessment findings for an adult client indicates a need to contact the anesthesiologist?
    A) Temperature, 100° F
    B) Pulse, 90
    C) Respirations, 20
    D) Blood pressure, 138/84

14. In the postoperative period, the nurse recognizes that an early sign of malignant hyperthermia is:
    A) Fever
    B) Tachycardia
    C) Muscle relaxation
    D) Skin pallor

15. The client tells the nurse that "blowing into this tube thing (incentive spirometer) is a ridiculous waste of time." The nurse explains that the specific purpose of the therapy is to:
    A) Directly remove excess secretions from the lungs
    B) Increase pulmonary circulation
    C) Promote lung expansion
    D) Stimulate the cough reflex

16. When preparing the client for surgery, the nurse should:
    A) Provide the client with sips of water for a dry mouth
    B) Remove the client's make-up and nail polish
    C) Remove the client's hearing aid before transport to the operating room
    D) Leave all of the client's jewelry intact

17. Nurses working in the operating room and post anesthesia care units recognize that one of the greatest risks from general anesthesia is:
    A) Cardiovascular irritability
    B) Neurological damage
    C) Musculoskeletal flaccidity
    D) Respiratory infection

18. A client who is being prepped for surgery asks the nurse to explain the purpose of the medications (Demerol and Vistaril) he has been given. The nurse should inform the client that these particular medications:
    A) Reduce preoperative fear
    B) Promote gastric emptying
    C) Reduce body secretions
    D) Facilitate the induction of the anesthesia

19. A client who receives general or regional anesthesia in an ambulatory surgery center:
    A) Will remain in the phase I recovery area longer than a hospitalized client
    B) Is allowed to ambulate as soon as being admitted to the recovery area
    C) Has to meet identified criteria in order to be discharged home
    D) Is immediately given liberal amounts of fluid to promote the excretion of the anesthesia

20. Following abdominal surgery, the client is suspected of having internal bleeding. Which of the following findings is indicative of this complication?
    A) Increased blood pressure
    B) Incisional pain
    C) Abdominal distention
    D) Increased urinary output

Answer Key

Chapter 1
1. B, p. 9
2. B, p. 7
3. A, p. 16
4. B, p. 6
5. C, p. 17
6. A, p. 8
7. B, p. 10
8. A, p. 15
9. B, p. 16
10. C, p. 16

Chapter 2
1. A, p. 26
2. A, p. 22
3. B, p. 30
4. C, p. 30
5. D, p. 41
6. D, pp. 26-27
7. A, p. 43
8. B, p. 43
9. A, pp. 30-31
10. C, p. 34
11. B, p. 31
12. D, pp. 42-43

Chapter 3
1. D, p. 53
2. A, p. 55
3. D, p. 57
4. D, p. 50
5. D, p. 59
6. C, p. 54
7. B, p. 59
8. C, pp. 52, 57
9. C, p. 50
10. A, p. 50

Chapter 4
1. C, p. 68
2. D, p. 67
3. B, p. 77
4. B, pp. 68-69
5. C, p. 69
6. C, p. 69
7. B, p. 75
8. B, p. 71
9. C, p. 72
10. C, p. 81

Chapter 5
1. B, pp. 89-91
2. D, p. 87
3. A, C, D, p. 87
4. D, p. 94
5. B, p. 97
6. D, p. 92

Chapter 6
1. A, p. 106
2. D, pp. 103-104
3. D, p. 104
4. C, p. 105
5. A, p. 108
6. C, pp. 106-108
7. D, pp. 106-108

Chapter 7
1. D, p. 114
2. B, p. 114
3. C, pp. 115-116
4. C, p. 120
5. A, p. 121
6. B, p. 131
7. B, p. 128

8. A, p. 129
9. D, pp. 117-118
10. C, p. 127
11. A, p. 118
12. A, p. 119
13. C, p. 120
14. B, p. 119

Chapter 8
1. D, p. 140
2. A, p. 141
3. B, p. 145
4. C, p. 145
5. D, p. 146
6. D, p. 149
7. C, pp. 150-151
8. A, p. 143
9. B, p. 148
10. D, p. 141

Chapter 9
1. B, p. 156
2. A, pp. 158-159, 167-169
3. B, pp. 159, 163
4. D, pp. 158-160
5. B, p. 166
6. C, p. 164
7. D, p. 164
8. A, pp. 164, 165
9. C, p. 155
10. C, p. 168
11. A, p. 166

Chapter 10
1. C, p. 177
2. A, p. 182

3. A, p. 185
4. C, p. 185
5. A, p. 195
6. B, p. 196
7. C, p. 199
8. B, p. 199
9. C, p. 199
10. D, p. 188
11. A, pp. 185-186
12. A, p. 177
13. D, pp. 211-212
14. A, p. 203
15. D, p. 204
16. A, p. 206
17. A, p. 212
18. D, p. 218
19. D, pp. 216-217
20. C, p. 219
21. C, pp. 216-219

Chapter 11
1. A, pp. 232-233
2. C, p. 228
3. B, p. 236
4. B, p. 240
5. C, p. 239
6. C, p. 226
7. A, p. 227
8. B, p. 230
9. A, pp. 230-231
10. C, p. 241
11. C, p. 236

Chapter 12
1. B, p. 244
2. B, p. 246
3. D, p. 248

4. A, p. 253
5. A, p. 256
6. A, p. 256
7. D, p. 265
8. C, p. 268
9. B, p. 264
10. B, p. 265
11. C, p. 249
12. D, p. 252
13. C, p. 254
14. D, p. 261
15. A, p. 259
16. D, p. 263
17. A, p. 263

CHAPTER 13

1. D, p. 274
2. B, p. 281
3. B, p. 279
4. C, p. 283
5. D, pp. 284-285
6. B, p. 278
7. C, p. 280
8. D, p. 276
9. C, p. 277
10. C, p. 279
11. D, pp. 283-284
12. C, p. 282

CHAPTER 14

1. D, pp. 300-301
2. D, p. 306
3. A, p. 296
4. A, p. 307
5. B, pp. 295-296
6. C, p. 299
7. A, p. 306
8. A, p. 306
9. C, p. 293
10. B, p. 296
11. C, p. 297
12. A, p. 298
13. B, p. 299
14. D, p. 301

CHAPTER 15

1. D, pp. 311, 323
2. C, p. 315
3. D, p. 317
4. C, pp. 319-322
5. B, p. 318
6. B, pp. 312-313
7. C, p. 317
8. C, p. 321
9. B, p. 318
10. C, p. 314
11. C, p. 321
12. B, pp. 321-322
13. A, p. 323
14. A, p. 312
15. C, p. 320

CHAPTER 16

1. C, pp. 327-328
2. B, p. 330
3. C, pp. 331-332
4. D, p. 334
5. A, p. 342
6. C, p. 336
7. C, pp. 337, 342
8. B, pp. 343-344
9. C, pp. 327-328
10. D, p. 331
11. D, p. 333
12. A, pp. 334-335
13. C, p. 334-335
14. D, p. 332
15. A, p. 342
16. B, p. 343
17. B, p. 343

CHAPTER 17

1. A, pp. 348-349
2. A, p. 357
3. A, pp. 350, 352
4. B, pp. 352-353
5. A, p. 355
6. D, p. 356
7. B, pp. 356-357
8. C, p. 357
9. C, p. 359

10. D, pp. 355-356
11. A, p. 358

CHAPTER 18

1. C, p. 364
2. B, p. 366
3. C, pp. 363-364
4. B, p. 373
5. C, p. 372
6. C, p. 371
7. B, p. 371
8. C, pp. 365-367
9. C, p. 371
10. D, p. 366

CHAPTER 19

1. C, p. 380
2. D, p. 380
3. C, pp. 382-383
4. B, p. 385
5. D, p. 394
6. A, p. 384
7. B, pp. 384-386
8. B, p. 393
9. A, p. 381
10. B, p. 386
11. A, p. 388
12. A, p. 389
13. D, pp. 395-396
14. A, p. 391

CHAPTER 20

1. B, pp. 408-411
2. C, pp. 407-408
3. C, p. 409
4. B, pp. 408-411
5. B, p. 409
6. C, pp. 408-409
7. C, p. 408
8. B, p. 410
9. D, p. 404
10. D, p. 406
11. C, p. 406
12. C, pp. 415-416
13. C, pp. 414-415
14. C, p. 411

15. C, pp. 418-419
16. B, p. 403
17. A, p. 417
18. D, p. 404
19. D, pp. 402-403
20. C, p. 410

CHAPTER 21

1. A, p. 425
2. B, p. 426
3. A, p. 433
4. D, p. 433
5. A, p. 435
6. D, p. 435
7. B, p. 436
8. D, p. 438
9. D, p. 441
10. C, p. 426
11. A, pp. 426-427
12. A, p. 432
13. D, p. 433

CHAPTER 22

1. D, p. 448
2. B, p. 451
3. C, p. 457
4. D, p. 451
5. B, p. 461
6. A, p. 456
7. C, p. 450
8. B, p. 451
9. A, pp. 459-460
10. B, p. 464
11. B, p. 455
12. D, p. 450
13. D, p. 451
14. D, p. 447
15. A, p. 449
16. B, pp. 450-451
17. D, p. 455
18. C, pp. 459-464
19. B, p. 465
20. D, p. 465

CHAPTER 23

1. C, p. 478
2. D, p. 481
3. C, p. 482
4. D, pp. 495-496
5. C, p. 490
6. D, p. 476
7. A, p. 477
8. B, p. 477
9. A, p. 488
10. D, pp. 476-477
11. C, p. 473
12. A, p. 476
13. C, p. 488
14. B, p. 481
15. B, p. 485
16. A, p. 489
17. C, p. 493

CHAPTER 24

1. D, pp. 519-520
2. A, p. 521
3. D, pp. 504-505
4. C, p. 505
5. D, pp. 507-508
6. C, p. 514
7. A, p. 503
8. C, p. 514
9. D, p. 515
10. C, p. 520
11. C, pp. 506-507
12. A, pp. 506-507
13. B, p. 503
14. D, p. 515

CHAPTER 25

1. C, p. 529
2. B, p. 535
3. D, p. 536
4. B, p. 536
5. B, p. 531
6. D, p. 533
7. D, p. 528
8. D, p. 531
9. A, p. 534

10. D, pp. 530-531, 533-534
11. A, p. 531

CHAPTER 26

1. D, p. 543
2. A, pp. 545-546
3. C, p. 547
4. B, pp. 545, 558
5. D, p. 546
6. C, p. 546
7. B, p. 560
8. C, p. 558
9. B, p. 549
10. B, p. 543
11. C, p. 547
12. A, p. 553

CHAPTER 27

1. A, p. 568
2. D, pp. 578-585
3. B, p. 578
4. C, p. 570
5. D, p. 570
6. C, pp. 571-572
7. D, p. 578
8. C, p. 569
9. D, p. 568
10. C, pp. 575, 583
11. A, p. 573
12. B, p. 575

CHAPTER 28

1. C, pp. 595, 598, 606
2. B, p. 605
3. D, p. 595
4. A, p. 594
5. A, p. 606
6. D, pp. 592-593
7. B, p. 597
8. A, p. 599
9. D, p. 606
10. B, p. 602
11. D, p. 600

CHAPTER 29

1. B, p. 617
2. D, p. 614
3. C, p. 620
4. A, p. 631
5. C, pp. 627, 634, 636
6. B, p. 616
7. C, pp. 616-617
8. D, p. 627
9. A, p. 635
10. D, p. 623
11. C, p. 634
12. D, p. 626
13. A, pp. 631-632
14. A, p. 632
15. D, pp. 633-634

CHAPTER 30

1. A, p. 656
2. A, p. 644
3. A, p. 651
4. B, pp. 653-654
5. D, p. 653
6. B, p. 645
7. C, p. 646
8. D, p. 648
9. B, p. 650
10. C, p. 656
11. B, p. 663
12. C, p. 661

CHAPTER 31

1. D, pp. 689-690
2. A, p. 674
3. A, p. 676
4. D, p. 678
5. C, p. 697
6. B, p. 691
7. B, p. 704
8. C, p. 708
9. D, p. 717
10. A, pp. 697, 699, 708
11. C, pp. 697, 699, 708
12. B, p. 670

13. C, pp. 681-682
14. D, pp. 701, 709
15. C, p. 709
16. A, p. 716
17. D, p. 689
18. D, pp. 708-709

CHAPTER 32

1. A, p. 734
2. A, p. 745
3. B, p. 746
4. D, pp. 755-758
5. B, p. 760
6. A, p. 772
7. C, p. 778
8. B, p. 781
9. C, p. 786
10. D, p. 794
11. C, p. 802
12. D, p. 825
13. B, p. 826
14. C, p. 747
15. A, p. 767
16. D, pp. 816-817
17. C, pp. 783-784
18. C, p. 829
19. C, p. 826
20. B, p. 779
21. D, p. 813
22. D, p. 736
23. A, p. 732

CHAPTER 33

1. B, p. 840
2. B, p. 842
3. C, p. 843
4. C, p. 844
5. D, p. 845
6. B, p. 860
7. B, p. 864
8. B, p. 865
9. C, p. 839
10. A, pp. 849, 864
11. B, p. 836
12. C, p. 837
13. A, p. 838
14. A, p. 845

Answer Key 365

15. B, p. 847
16. D, pp. 850-851
17. B, p. 852
18. A, p. 859
19. C, pp. 865-868

CHAPTER 34

1. C, p. 893
2. B, p. 891
3. D, p. 893
4. B, p. 897
5. C, pp. 897-898
6. D, p. 898
7. A, p. 904
8. D, pp. 905, 909-910
9. C, pp. 932-933
10. D, p. 934
11. C, pp. 940-942
12. C, p. 944
13. D, pp. 946, 948
14. C, pp. 917, 920-921
15. C, p. 923
16. C, pp. 897, 920
17. D, p. 904
18. D, pp. 902-903
19. B, pp. 897-898
20. A, pp. 945, 947
21. B, p. 947
22. C, p. 945
23. D, pp. 939, 944

CHAPTER 35

1. B, p. 979
2. D, pp. 982-985
3. D, p. 984
4. B, pp. 968-972
5. A, p. 973
6. C, p. 974
7. C, p. 976
8. C, p. 977
9. D, p. 979
10. B, p. 981

CHAPTER 36

1. D, p. 1004
2. D, p. 998
3. D, p. 1007
4. C, p. 1008
5. A, p. 1011
6. B, p. 1011
7. C, p. 1007
8. D, p. 1006
9. A, pp. 1004-1005
10. C, p. 1003

CHAPTER 37

1. D, pp. 1019-1020
2. D, pp. 1020-1022, 1034
3. C, p. 1023
4. B, p. 1026
5. C, p. 1041
6. B, pp. 1035, 1037
7. D, p. 1044
8. A, p. 1044
9. D, p. 1046
10. D, p. 1032
11. A, p. 1033
12. D, p. 1038

CHAPTER 38

1. A, p. 1062
2. B, p. 1061
3. D, p. 1086
4. C, pp. 1076, 1078, 1091, 1100
5. B, p. 1089
6. A, p. 1088
7. A, p. 1094
8. C, p. 1098
9. A, pp. 1097, 1100
10. D, p. 1104
11. B, p. 1062
12. C, p. 1072
13. D, p. 1082

14. A, p. 1084
15. D, p. 1093
16. C, p. 1093
17. D, p. 1085
18. C, p. 1097

CHAPTER 39

1. C, pp. 1128-1129
2. B, p. 1148
3. B, p. 1135
4. B, p. 1134
5. B, p. 1138
6. C, pp. 1136-1137
7. C, p. 1139
8. C, pp. 1152-1154
9. B, p. 1164
10. C, p. 1172
11. C, pp. 1163, 1172-1176
12. A, p. 1172
13. A, p. 1177
14. C, pp. 1187-1188
15. D, p. 1140
16. C, p. 1147
17. C, p. 1149
18. A, pp. 1152-1153
19. C, p. 1157
20. D, pp. 1167-1171
21. D, pp. 1173-1174
22. B, p. 1181

CHAPTER 40

1. D, pp. 1203, 1213
2. C, p. 1198
3. A, p. 1201
4. B, p. 1204
5. D, p. 1214
6. C, pp. 1199-1200

7. C, pp. 1207-1209
8. A, pp. 1195, 1219
9. D, p. 1202
10. C, p. 1229
11. C, pp. 1220, 1224
12. B, p. 1235
13. B, p. 1244
14. B, pp. 1198, 1203, 1210-1211
15. A, pp. 1200-1201, 1210-1211
16. C, pp. 1202, 1210-1211
17. A, p. 1214
18. D, p. 1218
19. B, p. 1218
20. C, pp. 1229-1231

CHAPTER 41

1. C, pp. 1251-1252
2. D, p. 1253
3. B, pp. 1257-1258
4. C, p. 1259
5. B, p. 1259
6. A, pp. 1259, 1264
7. D, p. 1260
8. B, pp. 1255, 1261
9. D, pp. 1255-1257
10. A, pp. 1265-1266
11. D, p. 1265
12. A, p. 1271

CHAPTER 42

1. A, p. 1308
2. A, pp. 1296, 1300
3. C, p. 1297
4. C, p. 1297
5. B, p. 1292
6. A, pp. 1311-1312
7. B, pp. 1305-1306
8. C, pp. 1304-1305
9. B, pp. 1311-1312
10. B, pp. 1308-1309
11. C, p. 1315
12. D, p. 1287
13. A, p. 1290
14. B, p. 1307
15. C, p. 1315

CHAPTER 43

1. D, p. 1326
2. A, p. 1329
3. C, pp. 1337, 1340
4. B, p. 1344
5. D, p. 1341
6. B, p. 1351
7. D, p. 1379
8. B, p. 1366
9. B, p. 1374
10. A, p. 1361
11. A, p. 1349
12. D, pp. 1335, 1338
13. B, p. 1338
14. D, p. 1342
15. B, p. 1331
16. C, p. 1347
17. D, p. 1359
18. D, p. 1372

CHAPTER 44

1. A, pp. 1387-1388
2. A, pp. 1387-1388
3. B, p. 1391
4. D, p. 1398
5. B, p. 1403
6. C, pp. 1389, 1402
7. D, pp. 1404-1405
8. C, p. 1411
9. D, p. 1428
10. C, pp. 1399-1401
11. B, pp. 1385-1386
12. D, p. 1391
13. C, p. 1388
14. A, pp. 1390, 1396
15. B, p. 1398
16. C, p. 1392
17. C, pp. 1415-1419
18. A, pp. 1426-1427
19. C, p. 1431

CHAPTER 45

1. D, pp. 1440-1441
2. C, p. 1444
3. B, pp. 1472-1473
4. C, pp. 1446-1449
5. D, p. 1481
6. A, p. 1453
7. C, p. 1453
8. A, p. 1441
9. C, pp. 1452-1454
10. C, p. 1461
11. B, pp. 1463-1465

12. B, p. 1442
13. C, p. 1443
14. D, pp. 1460-1462
15. C, p. 1463
16. A, p. 1466
17. D, pp. 1477-1478

CHAPTER 46

1. D, pp. 1493-1496
2. B, pp. 1495, 1514-1516, 1539
3. B, p. 1525
4. D, p. 1536
5. D, p. 1537
6. B, p. 1491
7. C, pp. 1494, 1508
8. A, p. 1508
9. A, p. 1508
10. C, pp. 1509, 1514-1516, 1519-1520
11. B, pp. 1514-1515
12. D, p. 1516
13. C, pp. 1520-1521
14. B, pp. 1521-1522
15. D, pp. 1528-1529

CHAPTER 47

1. B, pp. 1557-1558
2. B, pp. 1545-1546
3. B, pp. 1549-1550
4. C, pp. 1578-1579
5. C, p. 1582
6. A, pp. 1584, 1593
7. A, p. 1607
8. A, pp. 1578-1579
9. D, p. 1598
10. A, p. 1565
11. C, p. 1555
12. C, p. 1556
13. D, p. 1556
14. A, p. 1556
15. D, p. 1602
16. C, pp. 1598-1599, 1603
17. D, p. 1600
18. C, p. 1606
19. C, pp. 1617-1618
20. D, p. 1619
21. D, pp. 1618-1619
22. A, pp. 1557, 1569
23. D, pp. 1613-1614
24. C, pp. 1552-1553
25. D, pp. 1564-1565
26. C, p. 1578
27. A, p. 1605

CHAPTER 48

1. A, p. 1639
2. D, pp. 1633, 1648
3. A, p. 1633
4. A, p. 1636
5. B, pp. 1651-1652
6. D, pp. 1649-1650
7. A, pp. 1651-1653
8. C, pp. 1652, 1654
9. C, p. 1639
10. C, p. 1653

Answer Key   367

11. C, p. 1650
12. C, pp. 1633-1635
13. A, pp. 1636-1637
14. D, p. 1640
15. B, p. 1642
16. D, p. 1646
17. A, p. 1649
18. C, p. 1649
19. A, p. 1651

CHAPTER 49

1. B, pp. 1667-1669
2. C, p. 1662
3. D, pp. 1669-1670
4. C, pp. 1663-1665, 1667
5. D, p. 1664
6. B, pp. 1673-1674

7. D, p. 1685
8. B, pp. 1699-1700
9. A, pp. 1682-1683
10. C, p. 1704
11. D, pp. 1700-1701
12. D, pp. 1676, 1691-1692
13. A, p. 1689

14. B, p. 1705
15. C, pp. 1679-1681
16. B, p. 1689
17. A, p. 1698
18. D, p. 1691
19. C, p. 1702
20. C, pp. 1705, 1709